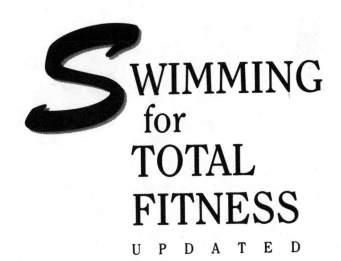

SWIMMING for TOTAL FITNESS

UPDATED

A PROGRESSIVE
AEROBIC PROGRAM

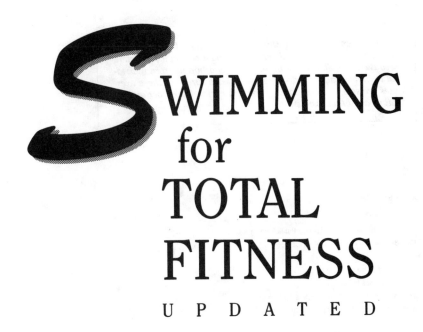

SWIMMING
for
TOTAL
FITNESS
UPDATED

BY JANE KATZ, Ed.D.

~

WITH NANCY P. BRUNING

ILLUSTRATIONS BY PHILLIP JONES

MAIN
STREET
BOOKS

DOUBLEDAY

NEW YORK LONDON TORONTO SYDNEY AUCKLAND

The advice and exercises in this book are intended to be used only in conjunction with the advice of your own personal physician. Because of the differences in physical conditioning from individual to individual, your doctor should make sure that these exercises are safe for you. Consult your physician before performing this or any other exercise program.

A MAIN STREET BOOK

PUBLISHED BY DOUBLEDAY

a division of Bantam Doubleday Dell Publishing Group, Inc.
1540 Broadway, New York, New York 10036

MAIN STREET BOOKS, DOUBLEDAY, and
the portrayal of a building with
a tree are trademarks of Doubleday, a division of
Bantam Doubleday Dell Publishing Group, Inc.

Book design by Patrice Fodero

Library of Congress Cataloging-in-Publication Data

Katz, Jane.
    Swimming for total fitness : a progressive aerobic program / by
Jane Katz with Nancy P. Bruning ; illustrations by Phillip Jones. —
Updated.
        p.   cm.
    "Main Street Books."
    Includes index.
    1. Swimming.   2. Physical fitness.   I. Bruning, Nancy P.
II. Title.
GV837.K355   1992
797.2′1—dc20   92-31877
                                                        CIP

ISBN 0-385-46821-0
Copyright © 1981, 1993 by Jane Katz and Nancy P. Bruning
ALL RIGHTS RESERVED
PRINTED IN THE UNITED STATES OF AMERICA
SECOND EDITION
10 9 8 7 6 5 4 3 2
May 1993

THIS BOOK IS DEDICATED
TO ALL SWIMMERS —
PAST, PRESENT, AND FUTURE.
MAY YOUR *JOIE DE L'EAU*
ALWAYS BE PART
OF YOUR *JOIE DE VIVRE!*

ACKNOWLEDGMENTS

Since I've been swimming all my life, acknowledging everyone who has contributed in some way to the information found between the covers of this book seems a more formidable task than writing the book itself! But here goes. I'd like to thank:

- My parents, Leon and Dorothea, who introduced me to the wonders of the water at a very early age.

- My sisters, Elaine and June, who have always been supportive of my swimming endeavors, and have shared their expertise as well.

- Particularly my brother Paul—former All-American and international swimming champion at Yale University, who, in his coaching career, has brought the La Salle College swimming team to its first conference championship since 1966—for sharing his theories and techniques with me.

- My nephews, Stephen, Jason, Justin, and Austen, who continually share their fun in water.

- Nancy P. Bruning, whose writing expertise and love of swimming have helped in large part to make this book possible; Lindy Hess; Gerry Helferich, my initial editor (a.k.a. "that swimming maniac"); to Phillip Jones, whose illustrations help prove that one picture is worth a thousand swimming lessons.

- Michele Martin, Theresa Horner, and Katharine Chang for initiating and carrying out this updated state-of-the-art version of our book, to Kacy Tebbel for copy editing, Marysarah Quinn and Patrice

Fodero for book design, Peter Kruzan for cover design, and to Liz Kurnetz.

- Lisa Harbatkin and Stuart Kampel, for their assistance in the initial stages of the book.

- Linda Ayache for her help in typing the manuscript.

- All the doctors and consultants who were generous enough to contribute their time and expertise in answering our questions.

- To Dr. Willibald Nagler, for his timely comments in the Foreword.

- To Gil Rogin and John Butterfield for their quotable quotes.

. . . and finally all my swimming and dry-land buddies who have given me their support and feedback over the years: the various staff members and officials of the U.S. Masters Swimming Committee, Inc., including June Krauser, Ted Haartz, Enid Uhrich, John Spannuth, Suzanne Rague, and Dorothy Donnelly; the past and current presidents of the International Swimming Hall of Fame—Buck Dawson, the late John B. Kelly, Jr., and Dr. Sam Freas; the members of the CCNY (my alma mater!) swim team and its staff, Jim Sinocchi, Greg Kincheloe, and particularly Elaine Fincham and coach Marcello Rodriguez; the swimmers of the Empire Swim Club and its inaugural president, Jim Forbes; fitness and competitive swimmers around the world; also Phil Moriarity, former coach at Yale University; Dr. Herbert L. Erlanger; Pat Earle; Dr. Michael Ross; Bob Fine; Louise Dembeck-Neiman; Dr. Paul Hutinger; Margaret A. Johnson; Fran Hare; Patti Robison; Roz Heitner; Elizabeth Nichol; Leslie Porte; and finally all my students and professional colleagues with whom I've had the pleasure to teach and work.

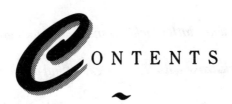

CONTENTS

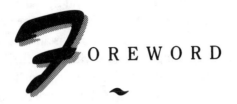

OREWORD

*T*hroughout history, water has been used to promote and restore health. *In aqua sana est* (Water is healthy) was chiseled by the Romans into the walls of their baths. And, whatever reasons the Romans had for crediting water as a source of well-being, we now know that its physical properties have a health-promoting effect. This promotion of health through swimming has been the spark behind the work of Dr. Jane Katz. In her book she sets forth a fitness program using modern training methods developed from her experience as both a teacher and a competitive swimmer. This book, which is addressed to the fledgling swimmer as much as to the experienced one, shows swimming to be a satisfying and healthy way to physical fitness.

Swimming has many advantages over other sports. Most aerobic activities (that is, those that make us out of breath), such as jogging, tennis, climbing, and aerobic dancing, place stress on the weight-bearing joints and the lumbar spine. Swimming, on the other hand, gives an aerobic effect with less stress to the joints. In addition, moving the arms and legs against the resistance of the water is the equivalent of exercising with weights, but since water doesn't allow any sudden, harmful movements, the risk of injury is lowered. Also, swimming exercises both sides of the body equally. Out of the water, only cross-country skiing even approaches this symmetrical effect.

Although swimming is ideal for people of any age, it is particularly beneficial for the older person. By the age of sixty or seventy, many people who are in otherwise excellent health are hampered in sports by minor hypertrophic arthritic changes in the spine and the weight-bearing joints, which can make it rather difficult to jog, play tennis, or take part in other sporting activities. For these people, swimming is an excellent way to reap the aerobic benefits of running or tennis without incurring any pain. In the water, the weight-bearing stress of the vertical position is eliminated, there is less stress on the joints during the contraction of the muscles, and what stress there is is distributed equally throughout the joints. For these reasons swimming is a very useful therapeutic activity for many locomotion problems. In fact, the swimmer can do much by himself to contribute to his own rehabilitation, thereby often shortening an otherwise long and expensive process.

In addition, recent reports show that often youngsters who are not able to participate in sports like track or soccer because of some respiratory illness such as asthma can become successful competitive swimmers. The air near the surface of the water is freer of dust and other pollutants, and it has been shown that exhaling against the resistance of the water can dilate the bronchi. Furthermore, everyone, not only asthmatics, can benefit from the efficient breathing techniques learned in swimming.

Whatever statistics one reads, one sees that swimmers have a much lower frequency of injury than participants in virtually any other sport. I do not know of anybody of any age who cannot learn to swim, and I do not know of anyone who has regretted doing so.

Jane Katz, Ed.D., is a professor of health and physical education at Bronx Community College and John Jay College of Criminal Justice of the City University of New York. Her academic achievements and her experience as a member of international swimming and synchronized swimming teams make her aptly suited to write an excellent, instructional book on swimming. *Swimming for Total Fitness* gives, in easily understood form, a program that will prepare the beginner for pleasurable and beneficial swimming and that will also help the experienced swimmer to sharpen his skills. Structures of the locomotion system change continuously as we mature, but swimming is one activity that can be performed with impunity at any age. Youngsters, busy executives, homemakers, and other persons who want to engage in an aerobic activity with an extremely low incidence of injury will derive much benefit from studying Dr. Jane Katz's book and following her program.

WILLIBALD NAGLER, M.D., F.A.C.P.
Physiatrist-in-chief, New York Hospital Cornell Medical Center

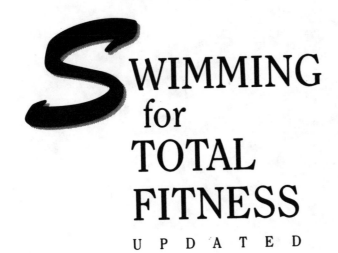

SWIMMING
for
TOTAL
FITNESS

U P D A T E D

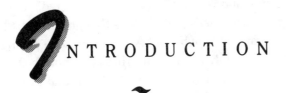

INTRODUCTION

It falls from the sky, and it comes out of the ground. Two thirds of your body is made of it. It keeps your skin from wrinkling, flowers from wilting. You wash with it, drink it, cook with it. Kids love to play in it, wars have been fought over it. Three quarters of the earth is covered with it. Some believe it cleanses the soul and purifies the mind. What is it? It's *water*— and it's also what makes swimming unique in the world of sports and physical fitness.

You know by now that exercise is good for you—physically, mentally, even emotionally. But how should you exercise? As doctors in sports medicine have focused more closely on sports-related injuries, they have learned that some sports, although in some ways good for you, can also be downright bad. How many runners do you know without shin splints, for instance, or how many tennis players do you know who don't complain of tennis elbow? And many sports seem like fun initially but soon prove boring, or expensive, or limited in scope (or all three). No wonder people hesitate to begin a program or, once they start, become disillusioned and give it up so easily. Broken arms, bad knees, hours of grueling, sweaty work, depleted bank accounts should not be the price you have to pay for physical fitness.

And it's not—if you swim! Swimming has something special: you do it in water. And that's a plus. Water is the secret ingredient that makes swimming better for you than any other sport. Did you know, for example, that every time a runner's foot hits the ground his body receives a shock of up to *three times* his or her body weight? (Multiply that by 3,000 strides for every mile run, and you're talking about an incredible pounding.) On the other hand, a swimmer's body feels as though it weighs less in water, owing to the upward force of buoyancy. And there's no jarring against any hard surface: there's only the smooth, rhythmic motion through the water. That's not to say you shouldn't run at all. But that extra wear and tear can add up over time, if dry-land exercise is the mainstay of your fitness program. More and more people are discovering that their feet, leg muscles, knees, and hip joints simply cannot stand up over the years to that kind of constant pounding. That's why swimming is the sport of the future—it lets you fulfill your fitness quota without the harmful side effects that land sports can bring.

Swimming is the closest thing on this earth to a perfect sport. It exercises all the major muscles of the body; it's the inexpensive, fun, social, graceful, sensual, safe, gentle way to achieve fitness—and it's an activity that you can enjoy for a lifetime. It can also be an athletic, artistic, intellectual, and spiritual challenge, depending upon how you want to go. So give swimming a try. But I warn you. You may never want to get out of the water. You'll find swimming one of the few things that successfully combine business (in this case, physical fitness) with pleasure.

Swimming is still among the most popular sports activities in the United States. According to the 1992 National Sporting Goods Association, over 66 million Americans went swimming at least once during the year. A 1990 Gallup poll affirms this participation: 38 percent of those polled said they participated in swimming that year: followed by fishing at 29 percent, running and jogging at 19 percent, and aerobic dance at 13 percent. So come join us . . . get in the swim!

WHAT SWIMMING WILL DO FOR YOU

~

Swimming has a lot going for it. But first I want to say a few words about what sets it apart from all the rest—water. That's because an appreciation of the water is one of the most important aspects of discovering the joys and benefits of swimming.

What's so special about water? Plenty! First of all, how long and hard will you work at something if you aren't deriving some pleasure from it? Not very long and not very hard. The fact that something is "good for you" isn't really enough in the long run. Whether it's running or swimming—or eating your vegetables—if you do it only because you "should" and not because you like it, you'll soon find excuses for stopping.

But water *feels* good and *is* good—for your body and for your soul. In water, our bodies seem to defy gravity, and we come as close as we ever will to the feeling of flying. And water is a wonderfully sensuous medium; just being in it is relaxing and exhilarating at the same time. In water every motion seems effortless, our muscles relax, and our mental walls seem to melt and float away.

Most people, no matter what their age, find water deliciously pleasurable and soothing. When you're tense or you have an ache somewhere—especially if you suffer from a back problem—don't you think about how nice it would be to soak your troubles away in a soothing whirlpool or bath?

But water's greatest advantage is its buoyancy. This buoyant quality is the swimmer's secret ally. The buoyancy is always there—holding you up while you're in the water, and keeping you feeling "up" long after you've wiped the last droplet from your skin. Water lifts your spirits as well as your body. After a swim, there's a euphoria that permeates your entire existence for hours afterward.

But enough of swimming's seemingly magical properties. What will it do for you in scientific terms?

It Helps Your Heart, Blood Vessels, and Lungs.   Swimming is an excellent *aerobic* (heart-pumping) exercise, which means that if you do it regularly and vigorously enough to raise your heartbeat to 70 percent of its Maximum Rate (see Target Rate, page 234) for a half hour or more, your cardiovascular system will gradually grow stronger and more efficient. By making your system work this way (in a sensible, progressive manner), you train your body to handle the extra demand, and it even becomes able to function better under normal conditions, when the strain is removed. This is known as the *training effect*. When you exercise aerobically, your lungs actually increase in size, capacity, and efficiency. Your heart becomes more powerful, more fit with exercise, just like any other muscle. Your blood vessels actually increase in number, and they may even become more flexible, thereby forestalling any tendency toward arteriosclerosis. Some studies also indicate that aerobic exercise reduces the cholesterol levels in the blood overall, and that it may alter the cholesterol that is found in the blood to a less dangerous type. Other aerobic benefits include lower blood pressure, improved digestion, a clearer complexion, and generally increased alertness. Aerobic exercise can also help alleviate the stress that can put a lethal strain on the heart, and, finally, if you're overweight, the weight reduction that usually goes hand in hand with vigorous exercise (more on this below) will further alleviate the strain on your heart.

Swimming has this added effect: when your body is horizontal and immersed in water, your heart is actually larger than when you're vertical on dry land and it has to pump against gravity. As a result, between 10 and 20 percent more blood is pumped with each heart contraction. This effect gives you the potential to work harder and longer than you ever could on land. And it makes swimming the ideal (and sometimes the *only*) exercise available to those who suffer from heart disease.

It Gives You Stronger, Firmer Muscles.   Swimming is the single best exercise for toning your arms, shoulders, waistline, hips, and legs all at once. And since the water cushions and supports your body, your chances of straining a muscle are greatly reduced.

It Increases Flexibility.   Swimming's long, sinuous motions, along with the increased range of movement that your body has in the water, actually elongate your muscles while strengthening them. Swimming will help loosen you up—both in the water and after you're out.

It's Easy on Your Muscles and Bones.   One of the best things about swimming is that it gives you all of the pleasures and benefits of exercising without the troublesome and often painful side effects that other sports can have on your musculoskeletal system. It's the whole-body, all-around exercise that builds endurance and balanced muscle strength, without jarring your bones and muscles. Because the resistance of the water actually helps you exercise your muscles, because the movements are relatively slow and rhythmic, and because you aren't likely to collide with other people or with equipment—the average swimmer has virtually no injuries to worry about. In fact, swimming's the one exercise that doctors—especially sports medicine specialists—unfailingly recommend to those who have sustained injuries in other sports, or in life.

The fact that swimming puts a minimum of strain on the joints of your body is especially good news for those with arthritis or chronic back problems, since it's often the only exercise these people can perform. It's also good news for those who want to avoid these problems in the future.

It Helps You Lose Weight.   In order to lose weight, your body must use more calories than it takes in. Swimming will help greatly here (see page 354). And although light or moderate exercise can stimulate the appetite, studies (and personal experience) have shown that strenuous exercise may actually diminish your desire to eat. After a vigorous swim, the last thing you'll want to do is stuff yourself. (That's why it's a good idea to schedule a swim before the biggest meal of the day.)

More importantly, exercise helps raise your metabolism—the rate at which your body burns up calories—not only during exercise, but for hours afterward. Even long after you're out of the pool, in other words, your swimming will still be helping you to lose weight. Finally, swimming is so relaxing that it may even help you control compulsive overeating brought on by tension.

It's Good for Overweight Persons. If you're on the heavy side, your adipose tissue makes you even more buoyant than your svelter counterparts. This extra support is why you're more comfortable swimming than doing any other sort of exercise. And being overweight doesn't slow you down nearly as much as it does on land; in fact, some swimmers—especially headline-making long-distance swimmers—have an extra layer of fat for warmth.

It Aids Physical Therapy. Water's buoyancy also makes swimming an excellent therapeutic exercise. It gradually and gently relaxes and rehabilitates muscles and joints that for one reason or another have atrophied or stiffened. Swimming is a sport that can be enjoyed by the injured and by the handicapped. The therapeutic benefits of immersing yourself in water are well documented, and doctors often recommend swimming to their patients who need a gentle, soothing form of activity for a temporary injury. Water is so safe, in fact, that nature uses it to protect us during the most vulnerable time of our lives—while we're still developing in our mother's womb.

It Helps You to Enjoy Other Sports and Other People. Your new-found energy and endurance will allow you to enjoy dry-land activities such as tennis or dancing till dawn. And love-making, too: the sensual swimmer knows how pleasurable it is to use one's muscles to move through the water; how it heightens physical strength, flexibility, and the awareness of one's body. And this is not simply the power of suggestion, or wishful thinking. Science has shown that swimming actually helps one feel "sexier" temporarily by affecting the body's hormonal balance. A study made of 258 swimmers (108 women and 150 men) found that 20 percent said they enjoyed a higher rate of sexual activity after they'd begun to swim regularly.

It Slows Down the Clock.   Lack of exercise is the most important factor in premature aging. Our bodies actually thrive on use. Up to a point, the more you do, the more you can do. In other words, use it or lose it.

Regular exercise can add years to your life. And if your sport exercise is swimming, it can continue to help slow the aging process for as long as you live. I've seen many persons sixty years and older who swim two miles or more every day. You should see the shape they're in. Most forty-year-olds would kill to look like that!

And did you know that some conditioned sixty-year-olds can swim 60–70 pecent as fast as conditioned twenty-year-olds? If you swim for fitness, statistics show that you'll lose only about 1 percent of your ability per year. And as the years go by you'll still be perfecting your technique, so that it's actually possible that your performance will improve over time.

It Provides Lifelong Satisfaction and Competition.   First of all, perfecting your swimming can bring you the unbeatable satisfaction of mastering a skill. You don't have to be an Olympic swimmer to enjoy pushing your abilities to the limit. You can always satisfy your urge to compete by swimming against your previous times and distances, or by racing informally with a group of friends. Or, thanks to the Masters Swimming Program, begun in 1970, you can engage in an organized competition against others in your own age group. The YMCAs and YMHAs across the country have also instituted this popular swimming program as part of their regular aquatic schedule.

The Masters Program is unique in that it provides recreational, social, and competitive programs that people can enjoy throughout their lives. Most other sports programs become too strenuous later in life, and the competition with younger and stronger athletes becomes too frustrating. But in the Masters Program, there are people in their eighties, nineties, and even a centenarian or two competing in swimming meets throughout the United States—and the world. So, not only can you be swimming through the '90s; you can swim into *your* nineties!

It's Inexpensive.   Swimming is an exercise that can fit everyone's budget, since it can cost as little as the price of a bathing suit. And swimming doesn't usually involve travel expenses, club membership, or fancy equipment. All you need is water! In fact, a recent comparison survey found that a swimmer spends *less than half* the money on equipment that he would for any other sport.

It's Varied.   So you think a swimming workout consists of jumping into a pool and swimming away, lap after endless lap, for as long as you can? Have I got news for you! Just turn to the workouts that begin on page 238, for a glimpse of how varied a swim can be.

First of all, there are four competitive strokes from which to choose (crawl or freestyle, backstroke, breaststroke, and butterfly). Then there are the recreational and resting strokes and skills (elementary backstroke, sculling, sidestroke, and treading skills), plus their variations. During a workout you can do each stroke while *pulling* (using only the arms), or *kicking* (just the legs), or *swimming* (using both arms and legs). You can vary the pace by swimming fast, slow, or in between. You can swim against the clock or at your own internal pace. You can swim long distances, short distances, or middle distances. You can try equipment such as fins, kickboards, hand paddles, and pull-buoys (see pages 327–29). And for each stroke, you have any number of dives, starts, and turns to practice each time you swim. And that's not even counting water exercises, deep-water running, etc. So you see, unlike many other aerobic or all-around exercises, swimming is anything but monotonous.

SWIMMING IS WHAT YOU MAKE IT

✌

You have your own special reasons for swimming. It can be for fitness, appearance, pleasure, or all three. Your reasons may change over the years, but no matter what your reason for exercising, fitness, as a friend of mine once pointed out, is one of the few things in life that's fair.

We're all born with different levels of ability, but within our limitations each of us has a tremendous amount of material to work with. It's a shame when we don't work up to our potential. In order to get into and remain in the best physical condition that he can be, that rich guy over there with the two Rolls-Royces and the private swimming pool has to work just as hard as that factory worker, hassled executive, housekeeper, or *you*. In other words, regardless of who you are, you'll get as much out of swimming as you put into it. What could be fairer than that?

Life has its competitive moments, no matter how much you may try to avoid them. And what you learn about yourself through swimming can help you over the roughest spots. For one thing, you'll have to assess your abilities objectively—past, present, and future. For another, the discipline involved in sticking to a swimming program increases your self-esteem. To see your distance grow, your skills improve, your body strengthen—

that's a good feeling. And your ability to set goals and to achieve them will carry over into other parts of your life. Even if you don't achieve all your goals, it's no disaster—that will help you develop a healthy acceptance of disappointment as well as fulfillment.

Swimming can be as social or solitary an endeavor as you like. You can join a team or swim club, go to meets and compete, and get your friends and family involved. Or you can compete against yourself in order to achieve strictly personal goals. You can reserve your swim as a private little pocket of time that's yours and yours alone. What's great about swimming is you don't have to spend time looking for a partner or team, but if you feel like company, you have the option.

And swimming can be your answer to this modern-day poser: Is there life without television? Here's one healthful alternative to the passive life, or what I call "spectatoritis." No more sitting around, waiting for, and accepting the prepackaged material that someone else has decided you want. When you swim, you become your own "live entertainment" and become more of a part of life—a doer, instead of an observer.

I hope by now you're eager to take the plunge. But first you have to know a few things about my program.

Whom This Book Is For
～

This book is for you if:

- You're an adult who has tried to learn to swim in the past, but without success.
- You can swim a little but want to learn swim skills better. (Haven't you said or heard, "I can swim but I can't breathe"?)
- You're an accomplished swimmer who wants to review your skills and refine your technique.
- You're a swimming instructor or coach who wants to improve the effectiveness of your classes.
- You're a person who is looking for a progressive aerobic fitness program.

If you don't swim now, this book will teach you how to swim—and swim correctly. That's a promise. Over the past thirty years, I've used these techniques with thousands of die-hard landlubbers of all shapes, sizes, ages, and abilities.

So, whether you're young or just young at heart, a total beginner or an experienced swimmer, whether you're swimming solo or with one or more partners, or even if you need a competent guide to help you teach others—this book is designed for *you*.

HOW TO USE THIS BOOK
~

This book can be used in several ways, whether you want to learn how to swim, to improve your skills at any level, to raise and to maintain your level of fitness, or to compete:

By Yourself. Everything you need to learn is here, divided into easy-to-understand progressive steps. Just follow the lessons and workouts carefully, on your own. For safety's sake, though, always be sure there is someone else around the water—preferably a lifeguard. Even the most accomplished swimmers obey this rule: never enter the water unless there is another person present who can help in case of an emergency.

Along with a Partner or Buddy. This is the best in terms of moral support, fun, and incentive. It's always nice to have someone else around, especially if he or she is at about the same level you are. A little companionship, help, and reassurance make anything go easier and faster, and swimming together can do wonders for a relationship. Instead of a night on the town, try a Saturday night at the pool!

As a Guide to Help You Teach Others. Swimming instructors, my fellow Masters fitness swimmers, and students alike have asked me to write a book for years. (Stop bothering me already.) Here it is!

This book takes a careful, step-by-step approach to swimming and fitness. Each lesson or workout builds the skills you've acquired in the previous one. I indicate which skills and what level of fitness you should bring with you to each level; you can find the place that's best for you to begin the program. Similarly, you can progress as far as you want. I do recommend, though, that no matter what level of swimming or fitness you *think* you're at you:

- at least review "The Fundamentals of Swimming"
- end your program no sooner than Level 10 of the Intermediate Phase

• consider progressing to the Advanced Phase and at least look at the chapter on Super Workouts!

Part One, "The Fundamentals of Swimming," consists of ten lessons. The first lesson goes right to the heart of the matter by teaching you how to exhale underwater comfortably. This is the mainstay of swimming well and the one thing that most people—even those who know the basics— have trouble with. The lessons in this section then go on to teach you the basic prone and supine swimming skills, as well as how to dive. So begin here, even if you were the star sprinter for your high school or college swim team. Your strokes might have become a bit sloppy, your memory of the finer points a bit shaky; your endurance might have dropped way off; or you may have been doing something incorrectly all along. Experienced swimmers can probably zip right through this section. If you can, you won't have to spend much time on it. And if you can't, it means it's a good thing you began here.

The lessons in this first section are also mini-workouts, designed to improve gradually your fitness level along with your skills. Each one becomes progressively more strenuous than the last, so that once you're through with the fundamentals you're ready to follow the workouts, which pick up where the fundamentals left off. These workout programs have four phases—Beginners, Intermediate, Advanced, and a special section of Super Workouts that has training tips and high-caliber workouts similar to the ones that competitive swimmers use to get into tiptop shape. The workouts gradually bring your distance up to 300 yards or meters (almost a quarter mile) for Beginners; 1,000 yards or meters (over a half mile) for Intermediates; 1,800 yards or meters (over a mile) for Advanced swimmers; and finally 3,000 yards or meters (almost two miles) for Super swimmers—while they expand your repertoire of swimming skills.

WATER, WATER EVERYWHERE
～

As for *where* to swim, there are facilities all over the place—if you look.

The last time the National Spa and Pool Institute took a count (in 1991) there were a total of almost three and a half million outdoor in-ground pools in the United States, and nearly three million outdoor above-ground pools. And that's not counting innumerable indoor pools and natural bodies of water—oceans, rivers, lakes, ponds, streams, bays, and in quarries—that are just begging for you to jump in and have a good time. As to *when* to swim, you can do it summer, winter, all year round.

If you prefer a pool (which I recommend for learning, practicing, and most workouts), you'll find that most facilities have low fees. Many localities maintain public pools that charge nominal fees, if any. Call the local Y, school board, community center, parks and recreation department, community colleges, universities, or continuing education programs. Or you might prefer to join one of the growing number of private health clubs and "spas" where you can enjoy steam rooms, saunas, massage, and other exercise facilities.

If you're an advanced swimmer, try to work out with a local swim club, team, or Y, with an understanding coach. If you're interested, call your local Masters swimming office. Often, they'll help you locate swim teams and coaches. In addition, articles in swim magazines are often helpful in locating this information.

FINDING THE TIME
❧

To derive the most benefit, you should exercise at least three times a week for approximately thirty minutes each time. I can hear the complaints now: "But I don't have that much time!" Take it from me, if you want to swim and reap the benefits, you'll find the time. Rearrange your priorities. I know people who get up early and join a workout before they run off to put in a whole day's work. Believe me, you'll feel better the whole day through! If you can persuade your friends or family to join you, so much the better.

As to what time of day to swim, that depends on you. I usually swim in the morning, and whether you're doing workouts or learning the fundamentals, you might like to start the day this way too. Others prefer to swim during their lunch break—what a great way to recharge your batteries for the afternoon! Still others find that the best time for them is after work, since exercise helps you unwind from daily pressures. If you don't work nine to five, you can visit the pool during the late morning or early afternoon, when it's often less crowded. You can even swim late at night as a way to relax before going to bed. Some people find late night swimming too stimulating, but others, especially after whirlpool or hot shower, are ready to drift off into a sound sleep.

It's Better to Be Safe
~

Before starting this or any exercise program, even at a beginning level, it's a good idea to check first with your doctor and, at his or her discretion, perhaps have a complete physical examination. This is especially important if you are in your middle years and have been getting no regular exercise. On the other hand, whatever your age, once your doctor gives you the go-ahead, you can look forward to a regular swimming program knowing that this is an ageless activity—one in which you can participate virtually all your life. It is a lifetime investment with increasing dividends.

Any Questions?
~

If you have any questions or problems as you go through the program, turn to "Dr. J's Q's & A's" on page 335. In that chapter, I answer those questions that swimmers ask most often. Or you can write to me in care of the publisher.

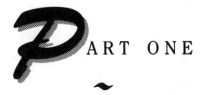

PART ONE

THE FUNDAMENTALS
OF SWIMMING

*A*ll good swimming begins with a firm grasp of the basic water skills. If you've never swum before, or have had only a smattering of experience, this section is a must. Even if you feel you know the basics, you'll benefit from reviewing them. You may or may not learn something new, but you'll definitely be able to clean up your act.

This section consists of ten lessons. Each lesson has two main parts—"Dry-Land/Prep Skills" and "Water Skills." Everything you do in the water you will first have practiced—and mastered—on land. Once the dry-land exercises have become second nature, you'll move on to the water skills. As you will see, it's not that difficult to take skills that you've acquired on land and transfer them to another medium.

WARM-UPS, COOL-DOWNS, HOMEWORK

You begin each water session with the warm-up, which includes a poolside review of the dry-land/prep skills and basic water exercises. The warm-up is an important aspect of every lesson, since it gradually prepares both your mind and your body for what's to come. It gets your blood moving and your breath going, and it makes the water feel more inviting.

Each lesson also includes a cool-down after each swim. Like a warm-up in reverse, a cool-down lets your metabolism slow back down gradually, which is the way your body prefers to do things.

15

The water-skills part of each lesson includes a section called "Homework," which lets you review your newly acquired skills at home after you've had a chance to practice them in the water. If you're using the "buddy" system, it's a good idea to do your homework together too.

TAKE IT EASY

Go slowly at first, and be sure to practice every step. If you're a beginning, this advice will be easy to follow. Not so for the experienced swimmer . . . but even if you know the basics, don't skip over and don't skip around. Review the skills in each lesson, going through them all, one by one. Even if you're sure you already know a particular skill, review it—you may be surprised to discover that you've learned it incorrectly or that you can improve upon what you already know. And, as you go through the program, you'll notice an increase in your energy and endurance, as well as your ability.

HELP

The basic "swim aid" you'll be using during this program is a kickboard (and even that's optional). Many pools don't allow devices of any kind, and besides, they're an expense, and they can be a nuisance to carry around. I also feel that beginning swimmers can become too dependent on flotation devices. However, if you like it and only rely on it temporarily to get you through a particularly stubborn phase, by all means use one. Just realize that, at some point, it'll have to go. And once you've mastered the basics, there are several pieces of equipment, such as swim fins, that I do recommend to help you master other strokes and to fine-tune your technique.

HOW LONG? HOW OFTEN?

It's up to you. Unless you're the type of person who needs to set up a real schedule, just repeat each lesson—or the most troublesome parts of it—until you've mastered each skill. Just keep practicing at your own pace until you feel confident enough to take the next step. There are no schedules to follow here, no class bells to signal that it's time to stop.

Do the dry-land/prep skills as often as possible—while watching TV, talking on the phone, as a substitute coffee break, even when you're taking a bath—any time you think of it. You're on dry land most of the time, but in this program that's no excuse for not practicing your swimming skills. The better you become at doing something *out* of the water, the better you'll do *in* the water. (And, incidentally, it also means not having to refer to this book while you're pool-side.)

As for the water skills: try to get into the water at least once a week. If possible, go three times a week; every other day is ideal for most people. The more you're in the water, the faster you'll progress. The duration of each session depends on your ambition, energy, comfort, and daily schedule. In general, though, I recommend that you go through the entire lesson the first time. This should keep you in the water about thirty minutes. After that, you needn't go through the whole lesson every time. Instead, you can practice just the particular skill or skills that you feel need the most work; and this might take only five, ten, or fifteen minutes of your time.

LET THERE BE MUSIC
➤

You might find it helpful (if it doesn't disturb others) to bring a radio or a tape player along to the pool, so that you can play your favorite music while you warm up, or maybe even during your lesson. This helps to create a relaxed, familiar atmosphere that's energizing at the same time. Swimming, when done correctly, is almost like dancing in the water, because you're moving gracefully and rhythmically. To do that, you need to be fully relaxed—that's the whole key to successful swimming. At some pools, in fact, you'll find music already piped in.

You should feel comfortable in the water. Once you've achieved that, everything else will follow easily and naturally. So do whatever you can to help you to relax. If you find yourself feeling tense, tell yourself to loosen up. Try not to fight your body's natural buoyancy. My years of teaching have taught me this over and over again: your most powerful—and sometimes troublesome—"muscle" is your brain. Once your mind is on your side, the rest will come in time.

If you can't do the strokes exactly as described, that's okay. Your body may not have the flexibility required, and this will probably improve the more you practice and loosen up. Just do the best you can, following the text and pictures as closely as possible, and remember, there's always room for individuality. Even in the world of competitive swimming, no two swimmers move exactly alike.

Above all, have a positive outlook. *TRY!* If you're hesitant about learning a new skill, just give yourself a chance. Millions of people have done it before. So can you. And you'll have fun!

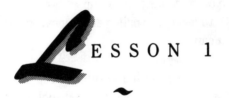

LESSON 1

*T*his is among the most important lessons in the book, because it establishes the groundwork on which all the others are based. In this lesson, you'll begin to learn how to breathe correctly, how to enter the pool safely, how to feel comfortable in the water, and how to bob and flutter kick.

DRY-LAND/PREP SKILLS

This lesson begins by teaching you how to overcome what, for many people—regardless of their swimming ability—is the biggest stumbling block of all: incorrect breathing.

Breathing

Begin by sitting up straight. Inhale, expanding your lungs fully. Then exhale.

Remember how it feels to have your lungs really full—they should feel this way every time you take a breath in the water. As you do the following exercises, try to think about nothing except your mouth and nose, isolating them from the rest of your body.

➤ HOW TO DO IT

The Mouth: Pinch your nostrils shut. Purse your lips and inhale strongly through your mouth—pretend you're drinking through a straw. Then, keeping your lips pursed, exhale just as strongly through your mouth, as though you're cooling off a cup of hot coffee. Hold a hand in front of your mouth to feel the expelled air. Repeat this ten times, breathing as deeply as you can.

The Nose: Cover your mouth and inhale deeply through your nose, as though you were smelling your favorite food cooking. Then exhale once again, expelling the air hard—as if there's too much pepper in the dish and you now need to sneeze. Repeat this ten times, each time breathing as deeply as you can.

Now inhale deeply through both your nose and your mouth. Although you may be inhaling more through your mouth, use your nasal passage as well. Exhale strongly. Begin by pretending that you're cooling off that coffee with your mouth first and then continue to sneeze from the pepper at the same time. Repeat this ten times.

All this deep breathing may make you a little lightheaded. That's because you're getting more oxygen than you really need (in other words, you're hyperventilating). Don't worry, though—you won't get that same dizziness in the water, because your body will be using the extra oxygen.

⌐ EXTRA TIPS

Make your inhale/exhale cycles as strong, even, and continuous as possible; try to get to the point where you can maintain an even stream of air for fifteen seconds. But build up to it gradually—you may find it harder than it sounds.

All new swimmers worry that the water will go into their mouths and noses. But remember this: the air flow you create when you blow out through both your nose and your mouth makes it physically impossible for the water to go up your breathing passages. As long as you're breathing air *out,* no water can get *in.*

In the water, the nose is especially important. Most people will naturally exhale through the mouth underwater, but too many people don't exhale properly out the nose at the same time, and as a result the nasal passages tend to be a perpetual problem. Therefore, be especially aware of utilizing your nose as you do these breathing exercises.

If you have trouble exhaling through both nose and mouth simultaneously, begin by exhaling through your mouth alone for a second, before joining it with the nose. If *that* isn't comfortable, try the reverse order— first the nose for a second, then nose and mouth together.

The main difference between your normal breathing and your breathing while swimming is in the volume of air that you take in and blow out.

Normally, you breathe very shallowly, using only a fraction of your total lung capacity. But when you're swimming, you'll inhale very deeply when your face is out of the water, through both your nose and your mouth. And when your head is under the water, you'll blow out hard, also through both nose and mouth, creating that protective air flow as you do so.

These exercises are also the first step in building up your cardiovascular endurance. As you take these deep breaths now, you're also strengthening and expanding your chest muscles and developing your lungs, which will help you later on in the water. Remember, even if you know how to swim, if your breathing isn't comfortable, you can't go very far—your swimming will be limited to only a few minutes.

Breathing

The next step is to get your face wet up to your hairline—and put that air flow to work.

~ HOW TO DO IT

Fill a large container with water. You can use anything—a big bowl, a large pot, your kitchen or bathroom sink, or even a bathtub.

Lean forward and just barely touch your chin to the surface of the water. Inhale, taking a deep breath, using both your nose and your mouth. Exhale through both your nose and your mouth, and watch the water. Ripples should form on the surface. If the water remains still, exhale harder next time. Repeat this ten times, making sure that the water moves each time. If you're practicing with a buddy, check each other to make sure you're breathing correctly.

Next, inhale through your nose and mouth together. Then put just your nose and mouth in the water, and exhale through both your nose and mouth, strongly, just as you did to make the ripples. Bubbles will form, indicating that you are forming the air flow mentioned earlier. You should be able to see, hear, and feel them. As soon as you run out of air to exhale, life your nose and mouth out of the water and inhale deeply. Do this ten more times without stopping.

Finally, put your whole face in the water. You can keep your eyes open or closed for now. Repeat the inhale/exhale exercise ten times, inhaling deeply and exhaling as strongly as you can.

~ EXTRA TIPS

To get rid of the excess water between dunkings, wipe your face with your hand, sweeping the water from the top of your forehead down to your chin. At this point, you might want to have a towel handy, just in case, before you start the water breathing exercises.

During your breathing cycle, especially during exhalation, try to release any tensions you may have and try to induce the feeling of total relaxation. Let your muscles relax and go limp.

This basic inhale/exhale sequence is exactly what you will be doing in the pool. That's all there is to it. As you have seen, it's fundamentally a matter of breathing the way you normally do—you're just taking more conscious control and doing it more forcefully.

Flutter Kicking

There are several other beginning exercises you can do at home. One of the most important is the flutter kick, which is the basic leg motion for both the crawl stroke and the backstroke.

～HOW TO DO IT

Sit on the edge of a chair or couch, letting your heels rest on the floor. Stretch your legs straight out in front of you, parallel to the floor, toes pointed downward, yet keeping your ankles relaxed and floppy. Lean back and support yourself with your arms on the back of the chair or couch. Now move your legs alternately up and down as though you were a wooden soldier. Keep your legs straight but your ankles loose and relaxed. The important thing is to kick with the entire leg, with the power from the hip and thigh, keeping the knees relatively straight. Repeat this twenty times, counting once for each leg change.

～EXTRA TIPS

You may find this difficult to do, especially if you have not been exercising regularly. If you experience a little muscle soreness in your abdomen and upper legs following this exercise, the important thing is to keep practicing, since this will actually help to alleviate any soreness or tightness in the water. Flutter kick while you're waiting for your hair to dry, the butter to melt, the phone to ring. Do it while watching TV—especially during the commercials, when you might be in the habit of rushing to the kitchen for another bowl of potato chips!

Gradually work up from twenty kicks, building up to a set of one hundred or more kicks, and repeat. You'll be amazed at how soon your condition will improve.

Remember: Keep your knees straight. Watch them. If they still bend, wrap a ribbon or a piece of fabric, a towel or an Ace bandage around each of them to help remind you to keep them straight.

～ BENEFITS

As with the breathing exercises, this is substantially what you'll be doing in the water. Practice on dry land familiarizes you with the kick and starts strengthening the muscles you need to do it.

Flutter Kicking and Breathing

Once you're satisfied with your progress doing the breathing and kicking exercises separately, you're ready to combine them. Of course, you were breathing before while you were kicking—now it's just a matter of combining them consciously.

～ HOW TO DO IT

Sitting on the edge of a chair, flutter kick with your legs straight, as before. Inhale and exhale strongly through your nose and mouth together, as you did with your face in the water. Try to think only about the kicking and the breathing. Don't worry about how many kicks per breath you're taking. As long as both are continuous and together, you're doing fine. Do this for thirty seconds.

～ EXTRA TIPS

When combining the breathing and kicking skills, keep the legs straight and breathe rhythmically.

～ BENEFITS

You will be combining these skills in the water, and the more you practice on land, the easier the transition will be. You are also building up your leg and abdominal muscles, as well as the breathing capacity you'll need once you start to swim.

Bobbing

The next skill is bobbing, which is similar to a knee bend.

～ HOW TO DO IT

Stand up and put both hands on a piece of furniture about waist high in front of you. Bend at the knees ten times, keeping your upper body straight. Then hold on, with your right hand only, to bob another five times. Repeat five more times while holding on with only your left hand. Finally, bob ten more times while not holding on at all.

～ EXTRA TIPS

Take care to keep your back straight and your weight distributed evenly on both feet. Increase the depth of your bobs from a half to a full knee bend (if your knees are sensitive, keep your bends shallow). Keep your back straight, with shoulder blades back.

～ BENEFITS

This helps tone the quadriceps muscles in the front of the thigh, as well as the gastronemous, or calf muscle. Later, you'll be bobbing in the pool to help acclimate your body to the water temperature, and to practice your breathing. Depending upon your physical condition, it may also begin to increase your cardiovascular efficiency.

Bobbing and Breathing

Now it's time to combine bobbing and breathing.

～ HOW TO DO IT

Hold on to the same piece of furniture with both hands, as before. Inhale deeply through both your nose and mouth as you're standing tall. Exhale strongly when you bend your knees. Repeat this ten times.

～ EXTRA TIPS

Go slowly so that you can concentrate on inhaling as you're standing and exhaling as you're bending. If you have a partner, join hands and alternate your inhaling (up) and exhaling (down), in a seesaw motion, so that you can check each other.

WATER SKILLS
～

The time has come to put your newly acquired skills to practice in the water. At this point, you may want to pick up a pair of goggles (see page 325) if your eyes are sensitive to chlorine, if you wear contact lenses, or if you just want to see better. And this is a good time to remind you never to go into the water unless there's another person around, and to stay in the shallow water until you're sure of your ability to swim in deeper water.

The Warm-up

It's a good idea to warm up the muscles in your body before you get into the water. These edge-of-the-pool or warm-up/prep skills help get your muscles ready for the "real stuff" that follows.

⌐ BREATHING

Begin by sitting on the edge of the pool or deck, at the shallow end. Let your feet dangle in the water. Start the breathing exercises you did at home, using both the nose and mouth. Repeat this breathing cycle ten times, putting a hand in front of your face to make sure you are exhaling strongly enough.

⌐ FLUTTER KICKING

Breathing normally, do the same flutter kick you did while sitting on your couch. Remember: knees straight, the power of the kick coming from the hips and thighs, ankles loose and relaxed. Move your legs alternately up and down. Kick at least twenty times, counting one for each leg.

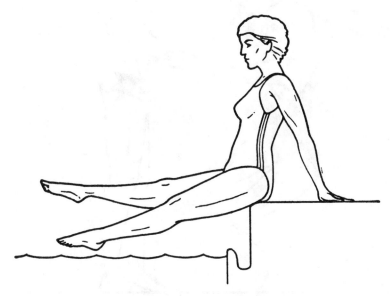

Flutter kicking on the pool deck.

⭑ FLUTTER KICKING AND BREATHING

Now combine the two, as you did at home, kicking alternately, and inhaling and exhaling forcefully. Do this for about one minute.

Bobbing

To help you adjust to the water, splash some over your arms, shoulders, face, and legs. First sit on the edge of the pool; then enter the water. Place your right hand next to you on the deck and bring your left hand around and place it next to the right, rotating your body around to the right 180 degrees. Continue this half turn to the right while letting your legs touch the pool bottom and your body slide smoothly into the water. You should find yourself facing the side of the pool, with both hands still holding on to the edge for safety. Of course, you could also turn to the left, if you find that more comfortable.

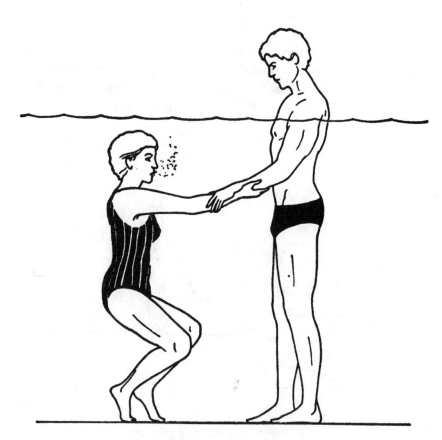

Bobbing and breathing.

➤ HOW TO DO IT

After you've entered the pool, immediately start bobbing up and down, just as you did on land. Hold on to the edge of the pool with both hands at first and bob up and down five times. Then hold on with just your left hand and bob another five times. Switch hands and bob again, gradually deepening your bends until your chin touches the water. If you're practicing these skills with a partner, face each other and join hands. Then the two of you should bob up and down alternately, like a seesaw. Do ten bobs, shaking right hands; then another ten with left hands joined.

➤ EXTRA TIPS

As you bend down, exhale deeply and be aware of how the water feels—its buoyancy will help support you later. Relax and enjoy the water. Even if you're already a swimmer, this bobbing motion will help your body adjust to the temperature change.

➤ BENEFITS

Bobbing will continue to strengthen your quadriceps (thigh) and calf muscles. As you bob, feel the slight resistance of the water; feel its buoyancy and how much lighter you seem to be than on dry land. If you noticed any feeling of discomfort doing this exercise on dry land, it will disappear when you bob in the water: the extra support will be evident in all the dry-land exercises you transfer to the water. You'll soon learn to love the delicious feeling of having water all around you.

Breathing

Let's go back to the breathing. You'll be doing the same thing you did in your sink, bowl, or bathtub—but this time in the pool.

➤ HOW TO DO IT

Return to the wall of the pool. Once more, review the breathing skills you learned on dry land; inhale very slowly and deeply as if you were yawning, then exhale forcefully, as if to cool off that cup of coffee. Try to release the air fully each time. Repeat five breathing cycles. Next, put your chin on the surface of the water, and inhale and exhale as you did at home, forming ripples on the surface of the water. Repeat five more cycles. Holding on to the edge of the pool, put your chin on the water. Inhale and, as you exhale, tip your head a little so just your nose and mouth go below the water's surface. Remember, you should be forming air bubbles just the way you did at home in your sink. Repeat five times, putting your head down a little deeper into the water each time. Take a break; then repeat five more times.

∾ EXTRA TIPS

Try to inhale fully and deeply. While exhaling, allow your body to go limp. Make sure you don't cheat: put your whole face into the water, not just the tip of your nose. If you have trouble anywhere along the way (coughing or choking), stop and go back to an earlier part of the exercise until it feels comfortable. Most people have to exhale out their noses more forcefully than out their mouths because their nasal passages are smaller. If you have a sinus condition, it may be even harder. But it's still important to exhale and create an air flow that keeps the water out.

∾ BENEFITS

Feeling comfortable exhaling underwater is the first step in a successful swimming program. Everything you've done thus far has been in preparation for this skill. Swimming, remember, is an aerobic exercise, so breathing—deeply, regularly, and comfortably—is basic. If you begin to feel dizzy, you're breathing too fast and too deeply (hyperventilating); if you feel tired, you're not breathing deeply enough (working anaerobically).

Bobbing and Breathing

You're ready to combine the two skills you've just practiced separately—bobbing and breathing.

∾ HOW TO DO IT

Hold on to the edge of the pool and, bending your knees, jump up and down very slowly, putting your whole face underwater and exhaling forcefully. Do this five times, very slowly. Next, as you bob, try opening your eyes underwater. Open one eye just slightly at first, then the other, then both. Repeat five more times.

If you're working with a partner, join hands and bob in the same see-saw motion as before. Begin bobbing with your eyes closed, then with them open.

➤ EXTRA TIPS

Don't forget to inhale above water and exhale underwater to form bubbles. Gradually open your eyes wider and wider. Try to feel, hear, and see the bubbles each time.

➤ BENEFITS

Bobbing will help you adjust to the water.

Flutter Kicking on the Wall

Now we'll move on to another skill—kicking. Let's get that water churning! Work that body!

➤ HOW TO DO IT

Supine (Face-up) Position: Stand with your back to the wall of the pool. Bend your knees until the water reaches your shoulders. Reach back with both hands over your shoulders and grasp the edge of the pool. Keeping your elbows down and next to your side for leverage, lift your legs up close to the surface of the water and do the same flutter kick you did on land. Kick thirty times, counting once for each leg motion. To return to a standing position, bend at the hips, as if you were about to sit down in a chair. When your hips touch the wall, lower your feet until they touch bottom, then let go with your hands.

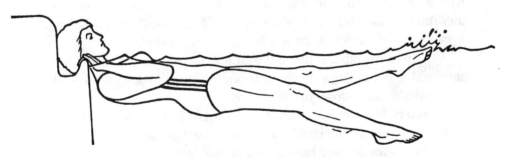

Supine flutter kick.

Prone (Face-down) Position: Turn around and face the wall of the pool. Hold on to the edge with one hand. Press the other against the wall, under the surface of the water, with your fingers facing down (this is the "bracket position"). Pull with the top arm and push with the bottom, keeping both arms straight for leverage, and lift your legs up behind you as close to the surface of the water as possible. Now do the same flutter kick you did before—legs straight, moving up and down alternately thirty times. Once that feels comfortable, add your breathing. Inhale deeply, then put your face into the water and exhale strongly. Lowering your head into the water will allow you to bring your legs up just below the water surface—this is just the beginning of good swimming form.

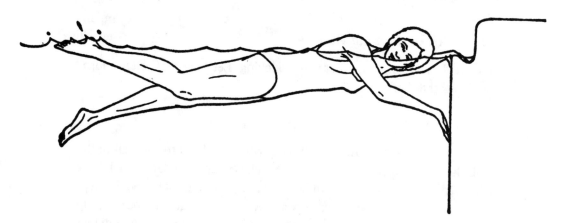

Prone flutter kick in the bracket position.

~ EXTRA TIPS

Make sure you stay relaxed and that your legs are straight but not stiff. Watch out for "bicycle riding" (i.e., bending your knees too much). Try to relax your ankles, too—it's the same flexing action as when you're walking. The trick here is to make the water bubble as though it were boiling. If your feet make a significant splash, you're overkicking.

Kick from the hip and thigh. If your legs seem to sink, you are probably "piking"—bending at the hips. Try arching your back—your legs will automatically move closer to the surface.

As you're kicking, keep Newton's third law of motion in mind: for every action, there is an equal and opposite reaction. In other words, for you to move *forward*, you have to move water *backward*. If you kick with your legs up too high, you're moving mostly air, not water. It may look impressive, but it's actually a waste of energy and won't take you very far. On the other hand, if you kick with your legs too low in the water, you're propelling your body vertically, not horizontally. As a result, you don't move efficiently through the water that way, either.

You may have to experiment a bit to find the most comfortable way of holding on to the pool edge. If may be a little rough on your arms and hands at first, until you build up their strength. Always shake them out when you're through practicing. For supine kicking, you might try stretching your arms along the wall, with your head resting on it. If possible, use the corner of the pool for this. Try as many ways as circumstances allow, until you find the one that's comfortable for you.

~ BENEFITS

This will help to increase your range of motion in the hips, to slim and tone your thighs, and to build up strength in your legs. Prone kicking will also help you become more comfortable with your face submerged. Even accomplished swimmers isolate kicking as part of their workouts to improve their form and build up that part of their bodies.

Cool-down

This part of the lesson reinforces the skills you've already learned and allows the body to make the gradual transition from strenuous activity back to lighter activity, and from being wet to being dry. Review the skills you've just learned, concentrating a bit more on those you feel unsure about. Breathe and bob, and flutter kick in both prone and supine positions. If you have a partner, practice together, watching carefully so you can correct and help each other.

To get out of the pool, use this push-up exit. Put both hands on the deck of the pool, and bob up and down three times. As you rise up on the fourth bob, straighten your arms and start flutter kicking at the same time. Lift and swirl your body up onto the edge of the pool, so that you end up in a sitting position facing the water. Besides helping to strengthen your arms and shoulders, this exit will come in handy when you're not near the pool steps or ladder.

Homework

Try to practice the dry-land exercises every day. Do the breathing exercises for five minutes, first without water, then with a sink or tub full of water. Every morning, maybe after a light breakfast, sit on a chair and practice flutter kicking. Then stand up and bob up and down in place.

If you had any problem with a particular skill, concentrate on that one, paying close attention to any extra tips that have been suggested. Try to practice with your partner—if you have one—on dry land as well as in the water. Observe each other closely so you can critique each other for further improvement. Remember, when your partner does something particularly well, tell him or her; a little deserved praise goes a long way.

If you want, start a personal homework log. It's a great way to watch how much better and stronger you're getting with every practice session.

Spend as much time as possible now learning the beginning skills. It may not look much like swimming, but it does form the basis for what you'll be learning later on. When you feel really comfortable doing everything you've learned in Lesson One, turn the page to begin Lesson Two.

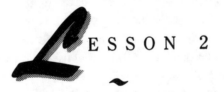

LESSON 2

*I*n this lesson you'll begin to gain even more control over your breathing, by learning to exhale very slowly. You'll also learn the prone float and recovery and you'll use the prone flutter kick to really get you moving through the water.

I've also suggested some Swimmers' Shape-up exercises to condition your body and help you warm up. These will go a long way toward improving your swimming skills and raising your fitness level, and so make learning easier and faster. I'll be adding a few more in later lessons.

DRY-LAND/PREP SKILLS

Do these general body-conditioning exercises at home, just before you begin reviewing old skills and learning new ones. Since you'll be moving around more than in Lesson One, it's advisable to wear loose and comfortable clothing during this and subsequent lessons.

Swimmers' Shape-up Exercises

Depending upon your physical condition, you may need to work your body harder than you've been doing. If you've been getting regular exercise, you're probably in fairly good shape. Even so, that's no excuse to avoid these. Since they work the parts of the body needed for swimming, you can do them as a change from, or in addition to, your regular activity. For those who have been inactive, these exercises are doubly important. Some are similar to the warm-up skills and general swimming movements; they'll also help you to release tension and so free your body for action. (See "Swimmers' Shape-ups," page 371). Feel free to incorporate as many as you like into your lessons.

These exercises will improve your overall fitness by increasing your cardiovascular capacity, your strength, and your flexibility. If done before the rest of your lesson, the exercises will relax and energize you at the same time, giving you a positive up-'n'-at-'em attitude that will make practicing and learning easier.

⌐ EXTRA TIPS

Practice these exercises any time, maybe as part of your morning routine—they're a great waker-upper! Do them all, or just a few if that's all you have time for. The more you do them, the easier they'll become. Add some of your own if you have any favorites, or if you feel that you need to work one area more than others. Exercising to music makes things more fun, as will doing them with a partner.

Review Skills

At home, review and practice the dry-land skills that you learned in Lesson One, particularly the breathing, flutter kicking, and bobbing exercises.

Controlled Breathing

Now you're just going to do a slower exhalation than you've practiced in the first lesson. For this, it's a good idea to have a watch or clock with a second hand. If one isn't available, count off the seconds by saying to yourself "one Mississippi, two Mississippi, three Mississippi," and so on.

⌐ HOW TO DO IT

Sitting up straight, inhale with both nose and mouth; then exhale. Do it at the same rhythm and with the same force you've been using to practice, but make a note of how many seconds it takes for you to exhale. Next inhale again, but this time take a full five seconds to exhale forcefully. If you can't, keep trying, adding a second or two each time. Most people will find they have some air left after five seconds. If so, lengthen your time to ten seconds, then fifteen. Now do the same thing with your face submerged in a sink or tub full of water.

～ EXTRA TIPS

If you have a partner, keep track of the time for each other. If you want to add a little competition to spur you along, both of you exhale at the same time and see who can hold out longer.

From now on, whenever you practice breathing, consciously try to lengthen your exhalation time.

～ BENEFITS

This exercise helps to increase your lung capacity and it shows you that you don't have to breathe as often as you thought and that your lungs can take in more air than you suspected. Later on, slow down your breathing. It will help you get a "second wind." It'll also help to relax you, since this type of regular, slow, deep breathing is a lot like yogic breathing.

Prone Float and Recovery to a Stand

The next step in learning the crawl stroke is really a safety measure. Before you learn how to float on your stomach, you should be able to return from the prone position to a standing one.

～ HOW TO DO IT

To practice this motion on land, stand with feet together and arms stretched out straight in front of you at shoulder level. Bend your knees as if you were doing a bob and at the same time press your arms down in front of you and to the sides. Tilt your face upward as you straighten your knees to a standing position. Repeat ten times.

～ EXTRA TIPS

As you practice this skill, repeat these key words with each motion: "Bend, press, lift, and stand." To grasp the movement better, imagine sitting down at a table and then standing up again by pressing down on the table top.

If you're practicing with a buddy, you can help your partner to recover by placing your hands, thumbs facing upward, at his or her armpits to gently support and lift the partner to a standing position.

～ BENEFITS

This is the first step toward independent swimming, since it's basic to your safety. If you're not practicing with a partner or using a wall (or lifeline or kickboard) for support, this gives you an efficient, safe way to recover to a standing position.

Prone Glide and Flutter Kicking with Assistance

This is the next step in learning the crawl stroke. Since this is the "dry run," you'll be walking instead of flutter kicking. If you don't have a partner, your "assistance" at this point will be a wall, or the edge of a table or counter top. Those with partners will assist each other now, as well as later on when you transfer this skill to the pool.

～ HOW TO DO IT

Without a Partner: Stretch your arms out straight, palms down. Stand beside a table or a wall and run one hand along it as a guide (this is your "partner"). Take five steps forward with your chin tucked to your chest and with your free arm covering your ear. As you do, exhale through both nose and mouth. Then turn around and, using your other hand to guide you, walk another five steps in the other direction so you end up where you started. Repeat.

With a Partner: Stand facing each other and grasp each other's elbows, keeping the arms straight. Have your partner place his or her hands palms up, and place your hands palms down over your partner's. Then have your partner walk backward five steps and, like an "engineer," guide you, the "train," as you take five steps forward. Next, change positions so that you support your partner's arms while he or she becomes the train. Repeat twice, remembering to let your head drop down and to exhale through your nose and mouth as you walk forward.

～ EXTRA TIPS

Make sure your arms stay absolutely straight. Get in the habit now, and you won't have to worry about your form later. Swimmers with partners can check each other. Others can check themselves periodically, with a mirror. This reminder goes for everybody: keep your chin tucked to your chest, with your arms covering your ears, when practicing this skill.

WATER SKILLS

For this lesson, you'll need a kickboard or other flotation support. Ask the swimming pool personnel what they have that you can use.

By this time, you should be noticing a definite difference while you're in the water—a new ease, new confidence, new strength. You'll find yourself feeling more relaxed and enjoying the water perhaps as you never had before.

Warm-up

As you know by now, it's important to warm up before you enter the water, which is always a lower temperature than your body. From now on, you have a choice: you may either start with the regular pool-side warm-up, which is a review of the skills you've learned so far, or treat yourself to a super warm-up and conditioning by prefacing your swimming with some of the exercises you learned as part of the dry-land/prep skills for that lesson. Or, if some form of exercise is already part of your life, why not schedule your activity for just before you practice your water skills? You'll be nicely warmed up, and nothing feels better after exercising than a refreshing swim. Do whatever you prefer, and whatever circumstances allow. Just remember pool rules, common courtesy, and safety.

Whether you add extra exercises or not, everyone should do the regular pool-side warm-up from Lesson One.

Controlled Breathing

Now you're ready to practice your breathing in the pool.

➤ HOW TO DO IT

Hold on to the edge of the pool, or join hands with your partner and take turns practicing this skill. Take three deep breaths. Then take one more deep breath through both your nose and your mouth; put your face in the water and exhale for as long as you can, again through both nose and mouth. This may take you anywhere from five seconds up to a whole minute—everyone has a different capacity. But everyone can increase whatever capacity he has, so practice this several times, each time trying to add a few more seconds to your previous exhalation, until you feel you've reached your limit for today. Partners can time each other; or you can count slowly to yourself or refer to a waterproof watch or the pool clock.

～ EXTRA TIPS

Remember, *you're not trying to hold your breath.* Your goal is to form a slow, controlled, steady stream of bubbles from your mouth and nose. Simply holding your breath is easier at first, but it doesn't form an air flow and is a guaranteed way of getting water up your nose.

～ BENEFITS

This exercise helps to increase your lung capacity while training you to utilize what you already have more fully. The more you practice, the longer you'll be able to exhale without coming up for another breath. Later on, you'll find that the less often you have to turn your face up for air, the more efficient your swimming strokes will be.

If you've been uncomfortable in the water until now, this slow, steady breathing will probably help you relax as well.

Prone Flutter Kicking with Controlled Breathing

Now that you're warmed up and have reviewed the skills you've already learned, let's go on to the next step, which combines flutter kicking with the controlled breathing technique.

～ HOW TO DO IT

Begin by holding on to the edge of the pool in your usual prone position. Start to flutter kick, then take a deep breath. Put your face down in the water, exhaling as slowly as possible, and counting (or using a watch) as you do so. Come up for air whenever you need to. Repeat as many times as you comfortably can, extending your exhalation by a few seconds each time.

～ EXTRA TIPS

Your prone flutter kicking should be pretty good by now—toes pointed, ankles relaxed and fluid, power coming from the hip and thigh, not the knee. Don't let your form fall apart because you're concentrating on your breathing. Just make the water "boil." Don't overkick or come too close to the surface, either. Partners should check and correct each other for this common mistake.

～ BENEFITS

In combining these two skills, you're coordinating what you already know. Eventually, you'll be using these skills in the crawl stroke.

Prone Float and Recovery to a Stand

～ HOW TO DO IT

Without a Partner: First practice the recovery only. Begin by standing in chest-deep water with one side facing the wall. Hold on to the wall with the nearer hand and extend the other arm forward in the water. Bend your knees, press your free arm down, lift your head up and stand. Do this

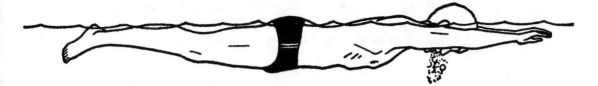

Prone float.

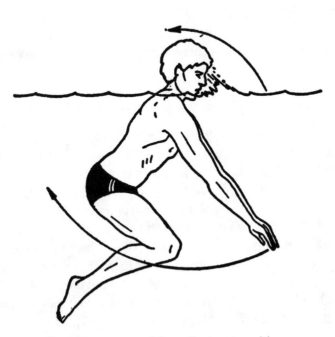

Recovery to a stand from the prone position.

five times. Next, crouch down to shoulder level. Inhale, drop your face into the water, and exhale as you push off the wall or the bottom. Let your legs come up to the surface of the water and keep your free hand straight in front of you. As you glide through the water, slide your other hand along the wall of the pool. When you need to come up for air, recover to a stand. Practice this ten times (five times on each side), until you are comfortable doing it.

Then move a step or two away from the wall and repeat the procedure: practice the recovery first with both arms; then crouch down, head in the water, and push off. Make sure your arms are straight out in front of you in a streamlined position. When you run out of air, recover to a stand. Practice this ten times.

With a Partner: Assist each other while practicing the recovery to a stand. Stand facing each other, an arm's length apart. One partner (the floater) places his or her face in the water, sets one foot in front of the other and pushes off the bottom of the pool, allowing the feet to rise toward the surface. The legs should be straight, the back arched slightly, and the arms extended straight forward. The helper places his or her hands, thumbs facing upward, under the armpits of the floater. As the floater bends and then straightens the knees to stand, the helper supports and lifts the partner. Then assume the train-and-engineer position with just the hands touching. As one partner does the float, let go with your hands during the recovery, but be prepared to assist if your buddy needs it. Practice the rest of the procedure according to "Without a Partner," above.

～ EXTRA TIPS

You'll see how the water's resistance helps you to make a smooth transition from a horizontal floating position to a vertical standing position. Remember, to coordinate the movements, repeat to yourself: "Bend, press, lift, and stand." If you feel that you're ready, add a slight flutter kick to the float to help you move along. Then let go with one hand and recover to a stand. Keep practicing, alternating hands, and letting go for a gradually longer length of time before you recover. You can also practice the recovery with your back against the wall: push your hands back flat against the wall as your knees bend and your head lifts.

Partners should try this without assistance at first, but with the other watching, and being there to help, if necessary, during the recovery. This method is better than grasping each other by the arms or hands, which immobilizes the floater and prevents him from helping himself.

～ BENEFITS

This is the first step on the road to "swimmer's lib"—once you know how to resume a vertical position safely, you can throw away your kickboard and swim on your own with more confidence. By working on the recovery to a stand, you're also improving your coordination—getting your arms, legs, and head to do what you want them to do, when you want them to do it.

Prone Glide and Flutter Kicking with Assistance

You've *practiced* flutter kicking enough. Now it's time to *use* that power to propel your body through the water.

～ HOW TO DO IT

Without a Partner: Stand in the corner of the pool, with one wall at your back and the other to your side. Bend your leg and place your foot flat against the wall in back of you; bend down so the water is shoulder level. This is the *push-off* position. Place the hand that's nearer the side wall on the edge of the deck or gutter—that's what you'll be using as a guide and support instead of the table edge or wall that you used at home. Place the other hand straight out in front of you, palm down, on the surface of the water. Now straighten your leg and push off so your body *glides* into the prone position. Immediately begin to flutter kick, letting your hand slide along the top of the wall. When you get to the other side of the shallow end, turn around and repeat in the opposite direction. Flutter kick across the pool at least five times.

With a Partner: Assume the train-and-engineer position you practiced on dry land. The "engineer" will hold his or her arms straight, with palms up, at water level, and the "train" will hold his or her arms straight, palms down, on top of the engineer's. Whoever is the train begins in the push-off position described above, but away from the corner, since you won't be needing the support of the side wall. As you push off, start to flutter kick. Your engineer walks backward, guiding you, as he did on land. Each time you repeat this skill, let your grip inch closer to each other's hands until only your fingertips are touching. Then switch positions and

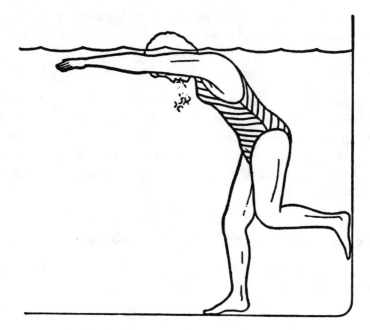

Push-off into a prone float without a partner.

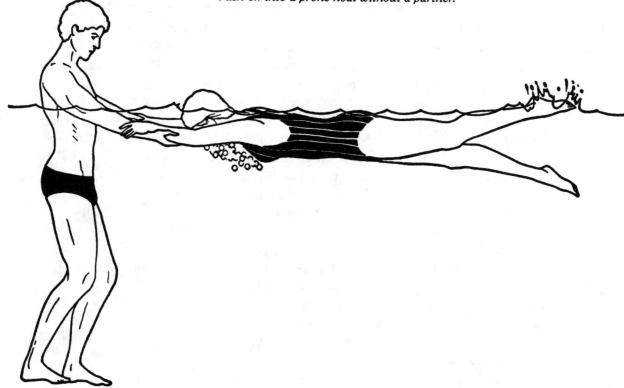

Train-and-engineer support position.

repeat, until each swimmer has flutter kicked across the width of the pool at least five times.

This is the same skill you practiced on land, except now you're flutter kicking instead of walking. Remember, it's actually easier in water, since your body feels as though it weighs less than it does on land.

After the first five times, try putting your head in the water and exhaling as you kick. Don't try to control the length of your exhalation for now unless you feel ready. Just exhale as usual, and recover to a stand whenever you need to come up for air. Then exhale again as you resume kicking.

Remember your form. Just because you're adding something new to a skill you've already learned doesn't mean you should get sloppy. Keep your legs just as straight, your feet just as pointed, your ankles just as relaxed as when you're holding on to the edge of the pool. And keep your arms straight—don't collapse at the elbow.

⌐ BENEFITS

You may not realize it, but once you've mastered this step, you're combining three skills needed for swimming the crawl stroke—flutter kicking, exhaling underwater, and keeping your arms straight. This is the correct, streamlined body position that makes kicking so much easier and more efficient. The push-off will also give you a glimpse of how exciting moving your whole body through the water can be.

Prone Glide and Flutter Kick with Kickboard (Optional)

It's time you got around to using a kickboard to help support yourself. (This step is optional, since some pools don't allow flotation devices, or just might not have a board available.)

⌐ HOW TO DO IT

Without a Partner: Stand near a wall, in the push-off position. Hold the kickboard with both hands, halfway up its sides, with the rounded end facing away from you. Make sure your arms are perfectly straight ahead of you, then crouch down so that the water is at shoulder level. Inhale, and push off as you lower your head into the water and flutter kick your way across the width of the pool. Remember, make those bubbles underwater, and come up for air (by turning or lifting your head or by recovering to a stand) only when you have to. Now you'll appreciate how important it is to keep your eyes open underwater so you can see where you're headed. As you kick, stay close to the side of the wall along the shallow end.

When you get to the other side, turn around and flutter kick back the other way. Repeat at least five times.

With a Partner: If you want, you can take this intermediate step to make the transition to using the kickboard more gradual. Flutter kick using the kickboard as I describe above, but have your partner hold on to the sides near the rounded tip of the board to give you additional support. Flutter kick across the width of the pool, five times each. Then each partner should repeat the exercise alone, using only the kickboard for support.

~ EXTRA TIPS

Keep thinking about stretching your arms and legs to keep them straight and streamlined. Make sure you keep the good form you've learned, and kick from the hip. Be certain your arms cover your ears; partners should check each other on this.

~ BENEFITS

This exercise will further improve your form by helping you to keep your body straight and moving smoothly through the water. It will also help to give you confidence in the water's buoyancy, and in your increasing ability to swim.

Cool-down

Review all the skills you've learned, especially the new ones: controlled breathing and flutter kicking across the pool. End with a few bobs and maybe some of the gentler conditioning exercises you've been doing on dry land. Everything is easier and more relaxing when you do it in water. And remember to use your push-up exit from the pool.

Homework

Continue to practice your controlled breathing, gradually extending the exhalation. When you practice in a tub of water, get used to opening your eyes and taking a good look at those bubbles that are keeping the water out of your nasal passages. Also, practice flutter kicking to continue to build your strength and technique. Every once in a while, stand in front of a mirror, raise your arms straight above your head, with thumbs locked, and carefully check your form and get accustomed to how it feels to be in this position—it's so easy to forget and bend at the elbows when you're in the water, without even realizing it. Continue to update your homework log, particularly concerning your controlled breathing. Do the conditioning exercises as often as possible, or substitute some of your own. For instance, you might prefer bike riding or a good brisk walk. Add to your dry-land activity whenever you can. Walk, bicycle, or roller skate instead of driving or taking a bus. Jog when you walk the dog. Do a few exercises on your lunch break—they're great tension relievers as well as conditioners. And don't forget to work on your water skills whenever you can, even if your partner isn't available. You'll find that a few minutes here, a few minutes there, will really add up and speed you on your way to fun, fitness, and health.

LESSON 3

This is the lesson where the pieces of the puzzle really come together—controlled rhythmic breathing, flutter kicking, and the crawl arm motion. At the end of this lesson you'll be doing the crawl stroke—some for the first time, some for the first time correctly, and everyone with a real understanding of the components and mechanics of the stroke.

If at any time you feel you are having too much trouble mastering the crawl stroke, or if you just feel more comfortable on your back, skip to Lesson Six, where you'll find the beginning of the backstroke. (I know I said not to skip around, but there are exceptions to every rule.) The important thing is not to let some hang-up about putting your face in the water, or a problem with your rhythmic breathing, stop your progress. Meanwhile, keep practicing the beginning skills you learned earlier until you feel comfortable enough in the prone position, then go back to the crawl stroke.

Since you're going to begin really moving through the water in this lesson, you might want to put on a bathing cap (if you haven't done so already) to keep your hair protected and out of your eyes. You may also want to get goggles (see page 325), if you've been experiencing some discomfort from swimming-pool chemicals.

DRY-LAND/PREP SKILLS

If you have the time, the energy, and the inclination (and I hope you do), begin this lesson with the conditioning exercises you learned in Lesson Two.

Review Skills

First review these dry-land/prep skills from Lessons One and Two: breathing, flutter kicking, bobbing, and prone flutter kicking with assistance.

Crawl Stroke (Hand-over-hand Arm Motion)

This is the familiar hand-over-hand motion that is the basis of the crawl stroke. It's simple, really, but many people have learned it incorrectly, or have simply gotten a bit sloppy over the years.

Actually there are two stages in learning the crawl stroke. The first isn't considered the most efficient by today's standards, but it's easier for novice swimmers because it's a simpler, more direct motion. After you've mastered this first stage, we'll move on to the second, which makes for a more efficient and powerful stroke.

➤ HOW TO DO IT

To begin, put your left hand on your left hip for now so that you can concentrate on your right arm. Extend your right arm straight out in front of you, fingers together and pointed downward. Then *pull* your right arm straight down, until your thumb brushes the outside of your right thigh. With your arm still straight, bring it back as far as it will go. Then bring it back even further. When you've really reached your limit, bend your elbow, *recovering* it up as high as it will go—as if you were a puppet and someone were pulling on your elbow with a string. Keep lifting the elbow as high as it will go as you bring the arm forward, then straighten it when it comes back to the starting, or *catch*, position. Repeat with the right arm five more times; then shake out your arms and practice the motion with your left arm, keeping your right hand resting on your right hip so that you can isolate the movement.

When you've got that, it's time to try the *catch-up stroke*, where you move both arms alternately, making sure that your thumb touches (or "catches up" to) the other before you begin the next downward movement. Begin in the prone position, arms straight out, thumbs touching. Do the crawl stroke with your right arm: press your hand straight down and back (the *pull*), bend the elbow high up toward the ceiling and bring the arm forward (the *recovery*), then touch thumbs with the left hand (the *catch*), and immediately repeat with the left arm to complete the stroke cycle. A *cycle* is when the right and left arm each pull once. Repeat the cycle ten times.

Next, repeat this procedure, but walk forward simultaneously to sim-

Practicing the crawl-stroke arm motion (catch-up position).

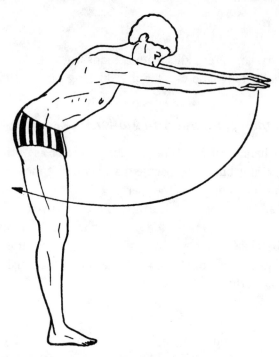

The pull.

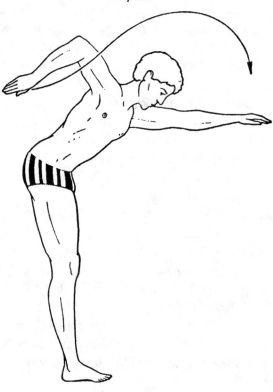

The recovery.

48

ulate the flutter kicking you'll be adding later. Make sure, as you're walk-ing, that you lower your head and look in front of you.

❧ EXTRA TIPS

This will be much easier in the water, I guarantee you. On land, your arms may feel heavy and get tired; but in the pool you'll feel lighter and more graceful because of the water's buoyancy. You'll definitely feel your shoulders and arms working—that's why those conditioning exercises are so important. Make sure you consciously relax your neck and shoulders. To get the flow of the movement, go very slowly, as if you were in a slow-motion film, and repeat the key words as you practice: "Pull, bend, re-cover, and catch."

❧ BENEFITS

The crawl stroke takes a lot of coordination; by practicing the motion on land, you'll find it that much easier in the water. Also, by actually moving your arms and stretching your shoulders on land, you're increasing your range of motion.

WATER SKILLS
❧

Warm-up

As usual, the warm-up consists of conditioning exercises, plus a review of the skills you've learned thus far.

Review Skills

Practice your controlled breathing, flutter kicking, bobbing, prone glide and flutter kicking with assistance, and/or with a kickboard.

Prone Glide to Wall with Flutter Kicking (Unassisted)

Now that you've seen how easy it is to flutter kick your way through the water and to recover to a standing position, it's time to let go of the kickboard.

～ HOW TO DO IT

Step back about ten feet from the wall of the pool. To begin the prone glide, walk toward the wall with your arms stretched out in front of you. Then lower your face into the water, and continue walking forward, exhaling those bubbles. Return to your starting position and take a step forward—one leg in front of the other, knees bent, ready for push-off. Then push off the bottom, letting your legs slowly float up to the surface and continuing to move toward the wall without kicking. This results in a beautiful, peaceful glide as the push-off propels your body smoothly through the water.

Try this a few times without kicking, then give in to the natural tendency to kick. Stop, and recover to a stand if you need to come up for air; but try to reach the pool wall before you need air.

Keep practicing, moving a little farther back from the wall each time so that you glide more.

～ EXTRA TIPS

Aim for a graceful, continuous movement. Give an energetic push-off, starting with knees bent and shoulders at water level. Glide until you begin to lose momentum, then begin to flutter kick. Remember your form (partners check each other): arms stretched out straight, covering your ears, body fully extended and streamlined. If your legs are sinking, it's probably because you're piking (bending at the waist) in the water. Push your hips forward, arch your back slightly, and stretch your legs. Think of yourself as a torpedo gliding through the water.

Crawl-stroke Arm Motion (Assisted)

～ HOW TO DO IT

Crouch down in chest-deep water and bend forward slightly, with your arms straight out in front of you, thumbs touching. Just as you did on dry land, get the feel of the stroke by working one arm at a time at first and resting the nonworking hand on your hip. Bring the arm straight down, brush your outer thigh, and continue to stretch the arm straight back as far as it will go. Then bend the elbow and carry it high as you bring the arm forward. Straighten the arm and return to the starting position. Next, work each arm alternately, repeating to yourself, "Pull, recover, catch." Repeat each complete stroke cycle at least ten times.

Now, still crouching, begin walking as you stroke, so that you get the feel of your body moving through the water. Inhale, put your face into the water as you exhale, and begin the arm stroke. Feel how pushing the water back with your arms moves your body forward. (This is Newton's third law of motion in action.) Begin walking at just the speed that you push the water. Repeat the crawl-stroke arm motion ten times, trying to travel further each time before you run out of air. Now you're ready to take your feet off the ground.

Without a Partner: Crouch down so that the surface of the water is at shoulder level. Inhale, place your face into the water to hairline level, exhale, and push off with one arm straight in front of you. Begin the crawl-stroke arm motion with that arm, letting your other hand slide along the pool wall as you move through the water. Turn around and practice in the other direction, working the opposite arm. Practice at least ten times on each side. As the arm motion becomes more comfortable, alternately release and grip the wall, gradually increasing the length of each release.

With a Partner: Assume the train-and-engineer position. One partner does the prone glide, adding the crawl-stroke arm motion. As the swimmer begins the stroke, he or she lets go of the "engineer's" hand with that hand, but still holds on with the nonworking hand. As the swimmer completes the stroke, he or she replaces the hand on the partner's arm, and slips off the opposite hand to continue the stroke. Important: one hand must be in contact with the "engineer" at all times—stay with your partner. The partners alternate until both have done at least ten cycles.

➤ EXTRA TIPS

Now that you've practiced it in the water, you're ready to learn some of the finer points of the stroker's mechanics. Your hands should enter the water at a 30- to 45-degree downward angle, and pull down and back through the water in a 90-degree arc before you begin the recovery. If you find it natural to add the flutter kick at this point, go ahead. If you find that too much to do for right now, hold off. A lot depends on your buoyancy: if you find that your legs are sinking, a smaller flutter kick can help make the difference. So can your form—remember, stretch out straight and press your hips forward in the prone position.

～ BENEFITS

You're isolating the crawl-stroke arm motion without adding the flutter kick right now so that you can concentrate on your form. That's also the reason that you're doing the catch-up stroke. It may feel a little awkward now, and you may complain that it slows you down in the water. Exactly! That's what you want to do right now—the slower you move, the more time you have to think about and to *feel* what you're doing.

Crawl Stroke (Unassisted)

～ HOW TO DO IT

Step back about three body lengths from the wall. You will begin exactly as for a prone glide, but instead of keeping your arms outstretched in front of you at shoulder level, you'll do the crawl stroke. Crouch down so that the water is at shoulder level, inhale, put your face in the water, exhale, and push off toward the wall. Immediately begin doing the crawl stroke, alternating arms and remembering to pull down and back, bend the elbow and lift it high, bring the arm forward, straighten it and touch your other hand as your arm enters the water at a 30- to 45-degree angle. Practice just the arm stroke a few times until you're sure you have it, then combine it with a little flutter kicking.

～ EXTRA TIPS

Don't forget about your form, which will make swimming much easier and more enjoyable. If you find yourself tensing up and crumpling into an ineffective, splashing fetal position, try to relax. Straighten out. Streamlining is the key; think about natural swimmers—fish, eels, and so on—and elongate your body.

Cool-down

Review all your water skills, especially the new ones you've learned in this lesson: the prone float and recovery (assisted and unassisted), the crawl stroke (walking with assistance, and without it if you're up to it).

End with some flutter kicking, using the kickboard or holding on to the wall of the pool, and a few bobs with controlled breathing. Don't forget the push-up exit.

Homework

You have a lot to practice this time. Review the recovery to a stand in front of the mirror or have your partner check your position. Work on your crawl stroke standing in front of a mirror every day. Continue to practice your bobbing and flutter kicking on land to develop your strength, and do some shape-ups or your favorite activity as often as possible to improve your overall fitness. Practice controlled breathing whenever you think of it—at home watching TV, washing your face, or even in an elevator. Add this and your new skills to your Homework Log.

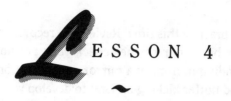

L ESSON 4

*T*his is the breakthrough lesson for new swimmers. You're now ready to take the final step in learning the crawl stroke: coordinating your controlled breathing with your arm and leg motions. First you'll learn a new skill: how to make your breathing regular and rhythmic. Then you'll combine the various components of the crawl stroke first in pairs: the arm motion with the flutter kick; then the arm motion and rhythmic breathing; then the flutter kick with rhythmic breathing. Finally, you'll put it all together, and you'll have the total picture: the arm motion with flutter kicking and rhythmic breathing.

When you're through with this lesson, you'll be a real swimmer who does the crawl stroke *correctly*. That's something to be proud of. How about buying yourself a new bathing suit as a reward? You deserve it.

DRY-LAND/PREP SKILLS

First do some conditioning exercises. As you do them, notice how your endurance has improved since you first started. Since you'll be needing more and more strength and flexibility in the arms and shoulders as you do the crawl, concentrate on exercises that work those areas. (See "Swimmers' Shape-ups." page 371.)

Review Skills

Run through the skills you've learned so far, paying particular attention to the crawl arm motion.

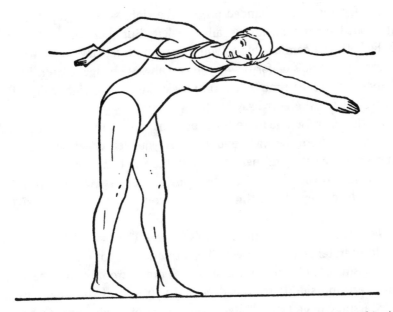

The Law of Opposites (Crawl-stroke arm motion and rhythmic breathing).

Crawl-stroke Arm Motion and Rhythmic Breathing

At long last, here's the ultimate piece to the crawl-stroke puzzle—a method of coordinating your rhythmic breathing with your arm movements. To illustrate this coordination, I've coined "The Law of Opposites," which I'll explain below.

ᳱ HOW TO DO IT

Begin by sitting up straight. Turn your head to the right, then return it to forward; turn your head to the left, then forward again. Keep your head level as you move it; don't tilt it up or down, but only from side to side. Imagine that you're watching a tennis match, and your gaze is following the ball back and forth. Repeat ten times for each side.

Next, add your rhythmic breathing: inhale deeply as you turn your head to the side, then exhale forcefully as you face forward. Repeat another ten times for each side. Exhale continuously as you rotate your head back to the face-front position.

Now do this exercise, turning your head to only *one* side, then forward again. Then repeat on the other side a few times. Remember, inhale as you turn, exhale as you return. One side will probably feel more natural to you. For most right-handed people, the right side will feel better; for left-handed swimmers, it's usually the left. But there are exceptions—maybe both feel comfortable to you; maybe both feel awkward. Whatever the case, pick one side for now—you can always change it later. For simplicity's sake, I'll assume that you're breathing on the right side—if not, just read "left" wherever I say "right."

Do this exercise one more time, but imagine that you're in the water. Lean forward from the waist and visualize your left cheek resting on the water's surface with your head turned to the right. It may help if you rest your hands on your hips or thighs. Inhale, then, as you turn your head down, exhale. Repeat ten times, turning your head only to the right to inhale.

Next, add the arm motion. Here's where "The Law of Opposites" begins to operate: as you turn your head to one side to inhale, the arm on the opposite side of your body is stretched out in front of you; the arm on your breathing side is stretched behind you, out of the way. This way, you're assured of getting a "bite" of air—and not of your arm. Once that's clear in your mind, try to put it into practice. Sit or stand, leaning forward, arms straight ahead, thumbs touching. Put your face down as if it were in the water, and exhale. As your right arm pulls down and back, turn your head to the right and inhale. As you bring your arm back to the starting position, touch thumbs, and exhale as your left arm pulls down and back.

Return your left arm to the starting position, and begin the cycle all over again. Repeat ten times; rest, then repeat another ten times.

If you have a buddy, the next step is to go back to your train-and-engineer position and practice the crawl-stroke arm motion with the rythmic breathing you've just learned.

～ EXTRA TIPS

Make sure that you're *pivoting* your head; don't lift it at all to come up for air. And turn your head to only one side. Whether it's the right or left doesn't matter as long as you're comfortable, and you stick to the same side each time you inhale. Remember, it's "Turn and inhale, return and exhale." If your neck feels a little stiff, don't worry. It will loosen up in time. Also remember to inhale and exhale continuously; try not to hold your breath even for a moment.

WATER SKILLS

～

Warm-up

Do the conditioning exercises you've been doing, concentrating particularly on stretching and strengthening the arms and shoulders in preparation for doing the crawl stroke, and head circles to loosen up your neck for rhythmic breathing. Then go right into a review of the skills you've learned so far.

Review Skills

Practice your bobbing, controlled breathing, flutter kicking, prone float and recovery to a stand, prone glide to wall with flutter kick, and crawl-stroke arm motion.

Crawl-stroke Arm Motion and Flutter Kicking

Some of you may be doing this naturally already: for others, it will be a new exciting step, even though it's only combining the last two skills.

～ HOW TO DO IT

To begin, bend down so that the surface of the water is at your shoulder level. Place your arms out straight in front of you, thumbs touching. Inhale deeply and begin to walk forward, putting your face in the water as you exhale. Start the crawl-stroke arm motion as you push off and begin to flutter kick. Recover to a stand when you need more air; then immediately repeat until you've done this drill at least ten times. When you're comfortable, and you're sure your form is good, you can progress beyond the catch-up stroke and begin the natural alternating stroke, where you pull one arm back while the other is still coming forward.

～ EXTRA TIPS

You may at first find yourself concentrating on either the kick or the arm stroke, to the detriment of the other. Don't worry. The easier and more habitual one becomes, the easier it'll be to transfer your attention to the other. But that doesn't mean that you should avoid practicing your weak area in the meantime. If putting it all together is still a problem, try this intermediate step: practice your arm motion in chest-deep water, walking forward to simulate the flutter kick. Remember your form: arms straight during the pull, elbows high during the recovery. If you still need a little assistance, whether it's your partner, a kickboard, or placing one hand on the wall of the pool, rely on it for support as long as you need to. But *only* for as long as you need to. Gradually wean yourself away from all assistance, by letting go with your supporting hand for gradually longer periods of time.

Or you may find it easier to begin with the flutter kick after the push-off, then add the arm motion, instead of the other way around.

～ BENEFITS

Once you've combined these two skills, you've reached a milestone in your swimming career. There's only one more skill to learn before you're a real swimmer.

Flutter Kicking and Rhythmic Breathing

If you can combine your kicking with your breathing, you're well on your way to putting together all the components of the crawl stroke.

～ HOW TO DO IT

Begin by crouching down so that the surface of the water is at shoulder level. Turn your head to your breathing side and rest your cheek on the water. Inhale; then exhale and pivot your face down into the water. When you run out of air, pivot your head back up to the side and inhale. Exhale as you pivot your face into the water again. Your head should be parallel to the bottom of the pool, and you should be looking straight down toward your feet. Repeat this at least ten times. Rest, and repeat another ten times.

Now let's add the kicking. Hold on to the wall in the prone flutter kick position—one hand grasping the top of the wall and pulling, the other placed flat, fingers facing downward, against the wall below the surface and pushing. So breathing will be easier, make the lower arm the one on your breathing side, and place it a little farther below the water's surface than usual.

Begin rhythmic breathing as you did before, but let your legs come up to the surface, and begin flutter kicking. Continue flutter kicking and breathing rhythmically for ten cycles; rest, and repeat.

Practice flutter kicking and rhythmic breathing, using the same progression as for regular flutter kicking—first with assistance (a partner, a kickboard, or the wall), then unassisted—until the coordination is comfortable.

～ EXTRA TIPS

If you find that your body begins to bend, make sure that both arms are perfectly straight. If you're not getting enough air, you may not be turning your head enough. So straighten out—stretch those arms and legs, and push those hips down. Streamline your body, and try to turn your head fully to get a good bite of air. If you're having trouble, try going back to just kicking or just breathing for a while. Then come back and combine them.

～ BENEFITS

By combining your breathing skills with one other skill at a time, you are coordinating in gradual steps this most important component for comfortable swimming. The breathing is the key—once you know you can get enough air whenever you want to, you'll have the confidence to add other skills to your swimming repertoire.

Crawl-stroke Arm Motion and Rhythmic Breathing

Now to combine the last two skills you've learned, the crawl-stroke arm motion and rhythmic breathing, just as you practiced on land.

～ HOW TO DO IT

Remember the "Law of Opposites"—when you inhale to the right, your left arm is forward and your right arm is back out of the way. To put the law to use, stand in chest-deep water, bending forward so that the water is at shoulder level. If you breathe to the right, drop your right arm down and back, stretch your left arm straight ahead, and rest your left cheek on the water. Inhale; then exhale underwater as you complete the stroke cycle. Rest, then repeat the arm motion, combining the exhaling and inhaling with each stroke just as you did on land. Practice this skill until it's comfortable.

When you're ready, do the same progression that you did for the crawl-stroke arm motion without the breathing—first walking through the water, then in the prone position with assistance from a partner, kickboard, or the pool wall, then without assistance.

～ EXTRA TIPS

Be sure to get the opposition that the "Law of Opposites" demands. If you have trouble coordinating the breathing and the arm motion, go back to the catch-up stroke to slow the whole process down. And remember the 30- to 45-degree downward angle of the hands on entry, along with the 90-degree downward and backward pulling arc.

Crawl Stroke, Flutter Kicking, and Rhythmic Breathing

This is it, the last and most exhilarating step in doing the crawl stroke.

～ HOW TO DO IT

Review just the arm motion and the kicking for a minute. Then take a deep breath and swim as far as you can before coming up for air. Repeat about five times. The next time, when you need to come up for air, try to take a rhythmic breath by inhaling on your breathing side *once;* then continue until you have to come up for air again. Stop, rest, and continue, trying to improve your form and to increase steadily the number of consecutive rhythmic breaths you take each time.

～ EXTRA TIPS

Remember, your elbow is the last thing to enter the water during the catch, and the first thing to break the surface after the pull.

～ BENEFITS

The combination of these three skills is the basis of the crawl stroke, or freestyle. If you've swum before, I hope that this will break forever your habit of doing what I call the "Coney Island crawl"—head above water, flopping awkwardly from side to side with every stroke. That's an inefficient and tiring way to swim. With rhythmic breathing, you'll find that you can do the crawl for much longer than you ever thought possible.

Cool-down

Time to relax with some gentle swimming movements. Practice the crawl-stroke arm motion, first standing in place, then walking forward. Remember your technique: put your thumbs together, stretch your arms straight out in front of you, pull your arm straight down and back as far as it'll go, then bend the elbow high as you return to the starting position.

The crawl stroke.

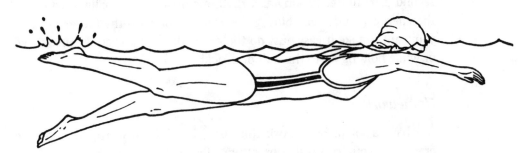

The catch.

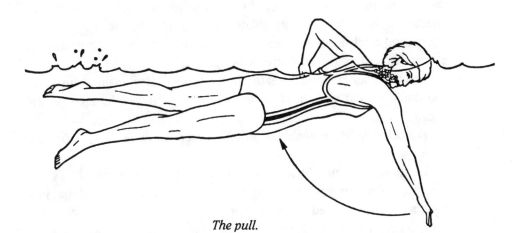

The pull.

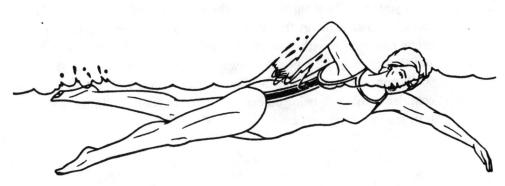

The recovery.

Next, practice the pairs of skills you learned today—rhythmic breathing and the crawl stroke, first standing in place, then walking forward as the pull of the stroke propels you through the water. Next move on to the second pair: flutter kicking and rhythmic breathing. Finally, if you have the energy, practice combining the arm motion with the flutter kick. (If you want to take it easy, just do the prone flutter kick, either unassisted or while holding on to the wall or a kickboard.)

Homework

You have a lot of homework this time, but it'll be worth it. Continue practicing your controlled breathing, flutter kicking, bobbing, and the crawl-stroke arm motion. It's tough to combine the arm motion with the flutter kick on dry land, so try to get yourself to the water as often as you can. In the meantime, practice the arm motion in front of a mirror to check your form. If you want, isolate each arm at first, then go on to the alternating catch-up stroke. Add rhythmic breathing to your arm motion practice as well as to your flutter kicking.

Practice your rhythmic breathing in a tub of water, making sure that you don't just lift your head up for air—you should really pivot at the neck.

For best results, do some conditioning exercises *at least* three times a week.

It might take you a little longer to feel that you've mastered this lesson. But really, this final step is simply one of coordination—and that just takes some getting used to. To do that, you must practice, practice, practice. You can do it—just keep at it, slowly but surely, to ensure that your form stays as good as it is when you practice the skill separately.

If you're really struggling with the coordination, don't worry. Go on to learn other skills in the next lessons if you're uncomfortable in the prone position, or with your head in the water. Don't ignore your prone skills completely; keep plugging away at what you *can* do, and gradually you'll notice improvement. Besides, mastering other skills will give you confidence that will help you eventually to conquer the things that are a little stubborn right now.

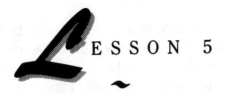

LESSON 5

Today you're going to learn a simple safety skill that will enable you to stay afloat in deep water for a long time while using very little energy.

As before, you'll first familiarize yourself with the motions on dry land. Each part—sculling with the arms and bicycling with the legs—is explained separately first; then you'll learn how to combine them.

DRY-LAND/PREP SKILLS

I hope you've been doing your conditioning exercises regularly. Do them again today as part of your prep skills.

Review Skills

Practice your controlled breathing, flutter kicking, bobbing, and prone skills.

Sculling for Treading

This is the first step in learning how to move on your back. It's also similar to what the top half of you is doing when you're treading water, which you'll be introduced to in this lesson.

～ HOW TO DO IT

Sit with your arms extended in front of you, parallel to the floor, with thumbs up and palms facing each other. Now create a figure 8 motion with each arm like this: holding your hands at about waist level, fingers held loosely together, turn your thumbs down and press your arms out away from each other until they're about shoulder width apart; then turn your thumbs up again and press your arms toward each other until the palms touch. You're now back to starting position.

Continue forming the figure 8 until you're sure of this skill.

～ EXTRA TIPS

On the outward press, make sure that your hands extend out to the sides and back beyond your shoulders.

～ BENEFITS

This is a smooth, effective stroke that plays an important role in treading. Even if you already know how to tread, your technique can probably stand improvement. Wait till you try this in the water—you'll see what a difference an efficient sculling motion can make.

Bicycle Leg Motion for Treading

Now for the other half of this skill. Relax a moment, and take this one sitting down.

～ HOW TO DO IT

Sit up straight on the edge of a chair. Then simply imagine that you're pedaling a bicycle. Bring alternate legs up, knees bent toward your chest. As one leg comes down, flex that foot (which means ankle is bent upward, with the toes now pointing up) and raise the other. Continue alternating the legs, letting each foot rest only a moment on the ground before you raise it up again.

～ EXTRA TIPS

If you need to, hold on to the edge of the seat for leverage. No need to hurry when you kick this way, either now or when you get into the water.

⌁ BENEFITS

This exercise works the quadriceps or thigh muscles.

Treading (Sculling and Bicycle Leg Motion Combined)

On land this looks like an egg beater gone wild, but it really works well in the water, so practice the coordination before you get into the pool.

⌁ HOW TO DO IT

From a sitting position, begin the sculling motion with your arms. This time, add the bicycle leg motion, really bringing those knees up.

⌁ EXTRA TIPS

Make sure you don't forget the proper form for each individual skill when you combine them. Keep your hands relatively flat and sweep your hands way out to the sides and back beyond your shoulders. Keep your arm motions large and relaxed.

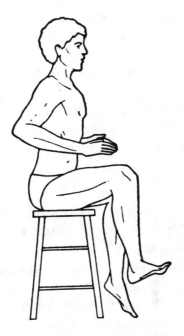

Dry-land practice for treading.

WATER SKILLS

～

Warm-up and Review Skills

After your conditioning exercises, review your breathing, flutter kicking, bobbing, and prone skills while sitting on the edge of the pool.

Buoyancy Check

And now for something completely different. This is an interesting little test to prove what I've been telling you all along: the water makes you so buoyant that it's actually difficult for a person to sink!

～ HOW TO DO IT

That depends on what's available. Ask the lifeguard whether the pool has an extension pole, which is usually used as a lifesaving device. If not, improvise with a broom handle or reasonable facsimile. For this you also need someone to hold the pole for you. Go to water about as deep as you are tall. Have your helper hold the pole vertically near the wall, with the tip touching bottom. Wrap your feet around the pole, crossing them at the ankles; this will prevent your legs from floating up. Grasp the pole with both hands, one under the other. Take a deep breath, and begin to exhale slowly with controlled breathing as you work your way down the pole, hand under hand, as if sliding down a rope. Go down as far as is comfortable, stay there for a few seconds; then loosen your grip a bit (don't let go completely) and you'll pop right back up.

Notice how much effort it took to get your body underwater—and to stay there. Did you feel how easily you rose to the surface? That's because the buoyancy of the water naturally pushed you up.

～ EXTRA TIPS

If you can't find a suitable pole, and if you're practicing on your own, you can use the pool ladder. Slide down, hand under hand along the railing; or use the ladder's steps as handholds and climb down that way. (You'll have to hook your feet under each step to keep the lower part of your body from floating up.)

Make sure that you take a deep enough breath before you slide down, and that you release it underwater as slowly as you can. This is where your controlled breathing comes in handy. While you're down there, take a look around, try to absorb the feeling of being underwater, and relax!

～ BENEFITS

This will add to your confidence and should help you to stop fighting the water and let it start working *for* you. Many people make the mistake of struggling in the water; they try to stay *on top* of it instead of *in and through it*. They don't realize that the water will support the body weight of an average human being. That's a fact—whether you're male, female, skinny as a rail, or big as a whale. You don't even have to move to float; the water will *hold* you up, if you let it.

Deep-water Tour

Next, do a little traveling—to the deep end of the pool. You'll discover that everything you've learned works in deep water too.

～ HOW TO DO IT

Since we're moving into deep water, make positively sure that someone capable of helping you is around. My method for getting you there and back is absolutely safe, but regardless of your level of ability, you should never swim alone.

To get there, begin by grasping the edge of the pool with both hands. Then slide one hand toward the deep end and bring the other hand to meet it. Continue "side-stepping" with your hands along the edge of the pool wall until the water is at least over your head. Now you're going to try some of your warm-up skills.

Bobbing: Holding on to the edge of the pool with both hands, bob down as far as your arms will let you. Make sure you extend them as straight as possible. Repeat at least ten times. Now let go with one arm and bob another ten times; switch hands and bob ten times again.

Buoyancy Check: Interrupt your warm-up here to see how the buoyancy test works in deeper water. Again, have someone hold the pole for you (or improvise with the steps of a ladder). Cross your ankles around the pole and, in a hand-over-hand motion, slide down the pole. Slide up—you'll pop up out of the water.

Flutter Kicking: Holding on to the wall, do some supine kicking first. Then do some flutter kicking in a prone position, adding your rhythmic breathing. Remember, to give your head enough room, you may need to slide the hand on your breathing side farther down along the pool wall.

Think about your controlled breathing, slowing it down, just as you do in shallow water.

Prone Skills: Just go as far as you comfortably can this time. Start by holding on to the pool edge with one hand, your side to the wall. Begin bobbing up and down, sliding your hand along the wall and moving forward, still holding on to the edge. Then go into the prone float position and begin to do the crawl stroke with your free arm. When you're comfortable with that, add rhythmic breathing and flutter kicking in whatever sequence feels best for you. Then turn around and try this on your other side. If you can, let go of the wall completely and swim the crawl stroke across the width of the pool, staying close to the end wall, and with a partner or lifeguard nearby.

～ EXTRA TIPS

Try to keep just as relaxed in deep water as you are in shallow water. As I've said before, you will naturally float in water. Here's why: Archimedes' Law states that a body submerged in liquid is buoyed up by a force equal to the weight of the liquid it displaces. The specific gravity of water is 1.0; yours is less than that. So the water your body displaces weighs more than you do, and therefore holds you up. Just how buoyant you are depends upon your body type. Bones and muscle are denser than adipose tissue (fat), so thin, big-boned, or muscular people are less buoyant than those with a layer of fat.

～ BENEFITS

This "tour" may be to a totally foreign country for some of you; for others, deep water is a welcome old friend. For everybody, it's a reminder that, no matter how deep the water is, it's only water—there's just more of it under you, helping to buoy you up. Relax and let that buoyancy work for you.

Treading (Chin-deep Water)

Back to familiar ground. It's time to learn how to tread in the water.

～ HOW TO DO IT

To begin, stand in chest-deep water and review the sculling motion. Make a figure 8 with each arm, keeping your arms at approximately chest level.

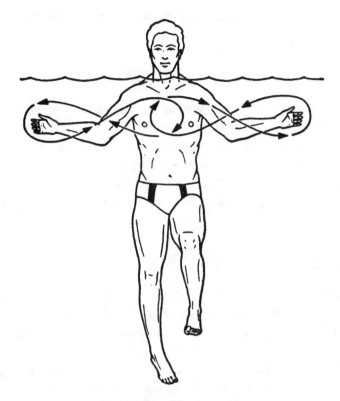

Treading in chin-deep water.

Then bend your knees and add the bicycle motion, keeping your knees up high, as if you were bicycling. Try not to let your feet touch bottom.

When you have the feel for this sculling and bicycling, walk your way to chin-deep water. You should still be able to touch ground when your legs are straight, but not when they're bent in the bicycling position. As your feet come off the pool bottom, bend forward at the waist in addition to at the knees, so that you have more room to kick.

～ EXTRA TIPS

Remember to use a wide, figure 8 motion with your hands—the more water you push down, the more easily you'll stay up. If your feet touch bottom now and then, just push off again and continue.

～ BENEFITS

Treading is a skill that may save your life someday, so, although it's not a swimming stroke per se, it's important for you to know. It can also become a part of your fitness program, as a relaxing skill between more strenuous swims.

Cool-down

Practice your prone skills—individually if any are still proving less than perfect, then together in whatever combination you like. Next, put it all together—crawl-stroke arm motion, flutter kicking, and rhythmic breathing—and try to swim across the entire width of the pool. If you can't do it, that's okay, but it's not too early to begin to push yourself, to ask yourself to do a little more than you're used to. After all, that's how you progress.

Homework

Practice everything you can on land. Do the crawl-stroke and sculling arm motions, either sitting down or standing. Add rhythmic breathing to the crawl stroke, and the pistonlike bicycle motion to the sculling. Practice your controlled breathing in a basin of water until it feels more comfortable and natural. Whenever you can, get to the water and do what parts of the lesson that you can, or that you feel need work. When you're ready, go on to the next lesson.

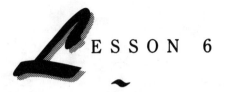

L ESSON 6

In this lesson you'll learn how to float and flutter kick in the supine (face-up) position. You may prefer this position to the prone position, because here your face remains above the water line, and you don't have to coordinate your breathing with each stroke. In this lesson you'll also move your treading to deep water.

Dry-Land/Prep Skills

First prepare yourself with some Swimmers' Shape-ups.

Review Skills

Practice your breathing, flutter kicking, bobbing, prone skills, and treading.

Now you're ready to begin something new—the first step toward swimming the backstroke.

Supine Float and Recovery

~ HOW TO DO IT

Begin this skill by lying in bed or on the floor. Stretch out on your back, arms to your sides with palms facing down. Notice how your chest is

71

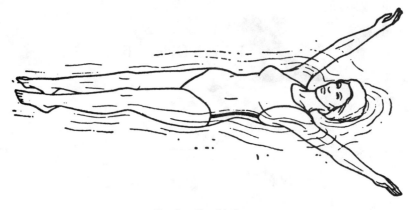

Supine (back) float.

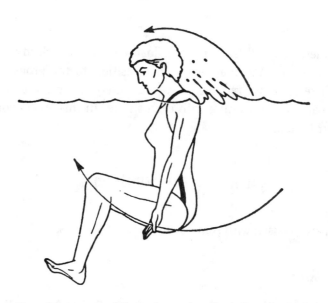

Recovery to a stand from the supine (back float) position.

slightly raised and your abdomen completely flat. Everything is level and you're relaxed because your mattress or floor is supporting you. That's the position you'll take and the feeling you'll get when you try this in the water.

So much for the "float." To practice the *recovery,* stand up with feet together, arms straight out to your sides at shoulder level and parallel to the floor. To initiate the recovery, imagine that someone has punched you—hard—in the stomach. In addition to uttering a few choice words, this would cause you to bend over at the waist with the hips back, in what's known as a *pike* position. Assume this position. Then bend your knees and drop your chin. Reach behind you with straight arms in a forward scooping motion. As your arms continue to brush the back of your knees, begin to straighten your legs. Continue to move your arms forward until they're in front of you, straightening and extending your legs completely as you do so, until you're standing up straight. Practice this movement five times. Each time, repeat to yourself the key words, "Pike, bend, scoop, and stand."

If you're working with a partner, practice supporting each other during the recovery. The helper stands directly behind the floater and places his palms, fingers down, at the small of the floater's back to support him as he recovers.

➤ EXTRA TIPS

To help you get a better feel for the recovery, pretend that the punch was so hard that you need to sit down. Grab in back of you for an imaginary chair; then sit down as you bend your knees. Finally, change your mind and stand up instead, raising your arms in front of you, as if you were carrying a tray of hot soup, until they're parallel to the floor.

➤ BENEFITS

This exercise will help you to remember to stretch out and relax during the supine float. The recovery, conversely, will let you return to a standing position smoothly and safely.

WATER SKILLS
➤

Warm-up

Get your body ready for the water by doing some Swimmers' Shape-up exercises and by reviewing all of your dry-land/prep skills.

Then continue your warm-up in the water by practicing your bobbing and prone skills.

Supine Float and Recovery

➤ HOW TO DO IT

First practice just the recovery to see how the water's natural resistance will help you return to a standing position. Stand in chest-deep water with your arms extended straight out to your sides, parallel to the bottom of the pool. Pike from that punch, reach back and down, bending your knees and dropping your head to look at them; finish the upward arm movement and straighten your legs. When that feels comfortable, try it for real from a floating position as follows.

Without a Partner: Go to the corner of the pool—once again, it's the best seat in the house—and support yourself by grasping the sides as you did for the supine flutter kick (page 29). Squat down so that your shoulders are at water level, with one foot slightly in front of the other. Put your head back (rest it on the gutter if you can), arch your back, and push up with the back foot; let both legs float up to the surface of the water. Stay there for a few seconds; then recover as you did before, by bending your hips and body forward. Release your hands from the wall and scoop forward as your legs touch bottom.

When you're ready, practice this using only one arm as a support. Stand with one shoulder against the side of the pool and grab the edge of the wall with the nearer hand. Then bend down so that the water is up to your shoulders, tilt your head back, and let your chest and legs rise into the floating position; your free arm is relaxed and floating palm up. Then recover, using one arm to scoop. Repeat five times; then practice holding on with your other arm. Finally, when you feel ready, let go of the wall altogether and use both your arms to recover.

With a Partner: The floater stands with his arms out to his sides, palms up. With his partner supporting him at the small of the back, fingers pointed downward, the floater begins the supine float as described above. Float for at least five seconds; then recover to a standing position. Repeat, adding a few seconds each time, until you can float for fifteen seconds. Then switch with your partner. When this position feels comfortable, try using gradually less support until you are floating unassisted.

⌁ EXTRA TIPS

In the recovery, the more you pike, the easier it will be to go from a horizontal to a vertical position. If your partner is having trouble piking enough, put your hands around his or her waist, fingers forward, as you did during the dry-land practice. During the recovery, pull back gently to help the piking action.

Another way to practice this skill is to hold a kickboard over your abdomen as you float. Hold it lightly, with your fingertips just resting on the side edges. Then bring the board to one side of you and hold it there with one hand while you scoop with the other hand to perform the recovery. As your feet approach the bottom, let go of the kickboard.

Check to see that you aren't doing the Irish jig (or any other dance) during the recovery. Keep your legs primly together the whole time: while you're floating, while they're bending, and while they're straightening out. And make sure that both feet touch bottom together. Remember, form counts.

～ BENEFITS

The supine float is the basis for swimming on your back. This is also another step in establishing your water confidence. And since you've learned the recovery to a stand, you know that you can safely right yourself at any time.

Supine Float with Flutter Kicking

～ HOW TO DO IT

To begin the supine float, walk backward, lean back, and lift your feet from the floor of the pool. Once you're floating, begin to flutter kick. As before, use a partner or the wall to assist you if you need to at first; then gradually use less and less help until you can float and flutter kick unassisted. Practice until comfortable.

～ EXTRA TIPS

Try to get a relaxed, stretched, and streamlined feeling along your body and all across your abdomen, chest, shoulders, and upper arms. Tuck your hips in and under. Avoid "sitting" in the water; don't bend at the waist until you're ready to recover to a stand. Keep your chest high and your head back. Arch your back slightly—especially if your hips tend to sink.

Remember your kicking form—legs straight, ankles relaxed, just making the water "boil." You can sneak a peek at your legs in the supine position, so use the opportunity to acquire a feel for how a perfect flutter kick is done.

～ BENEFITS

Adding the flutter kick to the supine float helps you maintain a better body position: chest high, legs close to the surface. It also prepares you for the next step in learning how to swim on your back—the sculling arm motion.

Deep-water Treading

HOW TO DO IT

～ *Without a Partner:* Standing in chest-deep water, with one side toward the pool wall, hold on to the edge with the hand. Begin the bicycle leg motion, and start sculling with your free arm. Tread water for approximately one minute; then grasp the wall with both hands, turn around, and tread for another minute, sculling with your other arm. Next, with your hand still on the wall, relax into the prone float (or supine float, if you prefer). Go completely limp, and hold your body absolutely motionless while you exhale during the prone float. When you need to come up for air, recover, using your free arm to pull you back up to a vertical position; immediately resume treading water. Repeat the treading on the other side. Keep alternating sides, lifting your arm and letting go of the wall—for a second or two at first, then for gradually longer periods until you feel comfortable sculling with both arms.

With a Partner: Take this intermediate step. Both partners face the same direction, holding on to the wall with the nearer hand. The person in front is the treader; the one in back is the supporter. The supporter grips the treader's bathing suit by the strap or by the waist and pulls upward. The treader begins to bicycle with his or her legs and to scull with the free arm. Then, when the treader feels the upward tug on the suit, he or she lets go of the wall and starts to scull with both arms at the same time. Alternate positions five times; then gradually lighten the support and let your partner tread water more and more on his or her own.

When you feel comfortable doing this exercise in shallow water, move into deep water (as you did for the buoyancy check) and practice this skill there.

～ EXTRA TIPS

Remember, this is the same thing you've done in shallow water. The buoyancy check showed you how difficult it is to sink even if you do absolutely nothing. By treading, you should stay up easily. So relax. Use a slow, sweeping motion, crossing your hands in front—and reaching your back in order to get the most vertical thrust.

～ BENEFITS

Your ability to tread in deep water enables you to remain calm and afloat whenever your other strokes are interrupted—say, by another swimmer. Any time any disturbance changes your position in the water, just tread until you can resume normal swimming. When you're treading, your arms and legs stay completely underwater—that's a very efficient use of energy, which is why you can tread water for so long, especially when you combine it with the prone or supine float.

Cool-down

Review all your skills, both the new and the old—prone float, kicking, recovery, crawl stroke with rhythmic breathing (separately, then together), treading in chin-deep water, supine float, and supine kicking on the wall.

Homework

In front of a mirror, practice your form for the crawl stroke, prone and supine recovery, and sculling. Do your flutter kicking and bicycling in spare moments. Review your rhythmic breathing in a basin of water. Concentrate on stretching out your arms, shoulders, and sides when you exercise—you'll need those muscles even more for the next lesson.

LESSON 7

*N*ext you'll learn a variation of the sculling motion that you can do while on your back. And you'll get ready for a new kind of plunge into the water—a head-first entry.

DRY-LAND/PREP SKILLS

Begin as you usually do, with Swimmers' Shape-ups, to prepare you mentally and physically for water action.

Review Skills

Practice your breathing, flutter kicking, bobbing, prone skills, treading, and supine skills.

Supine Sculling

This is one of the intermediate steps in learning the backstroke and is a variation of the sculling motion that you have already used for treading.

~ HOW TO DO IT

Stand up straight and begin to do the sculling motion—figure 8s with both arms—that you learned for treading. Now modify it a bit: begin to make smaller movements, about shoulder width apart. Then gradually

78

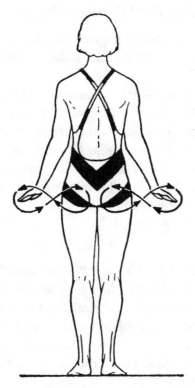

Practicing sculling.

drop your hands to hip level, and finally bring your hands behind your hips, still forming figure 8s.

⌣ EXTRA TIPS

This is a variation of the treading arm motion, so it shouldn't present a problem. And supine sculling will feel more natural underwater, where you will use it to propel you backward while your feet flutter kick. For more power and leverage, remember to keep your hands sculling as close under your hips as possible.

⌣ BENEFITS

This arm motion will help you to feel more balanced and more comfortable on your back.

Sculling is also a great and relaxing way to really tone up your arms. So don't give it short shrift. It's simple but effective, and it has a part to play in your personal fitness program.

Introduction to Head-First Entries (Diving)

Until now, you've been entering the water feet first. Head-first entries are a more efficient way to initiate prone skills, are more exciting, and are fun!

The progression of head-first entries is called the diving sequence. For shallow surface and sitting entries, your feet begin in the water rather than on the pool deck. For safety considerations, these entries should take place in water at least five feet deep. All other dives should be done in water not less than nine feet deep, as recommended by the American National Red Cross. These dives include kneeling, tip-in, standing, and racing, and will be highlighted in Part Three.

❧ HOW TO DO IT

Begin by sitting up straight in a chair. With feet shoulder-width apart and knees bent, rise up on your toes, hips back, and heels resting against the legs of the chair. Extend your arms straight in front of you and put your head down, as you would for the prone glide. Make sure that your arms cover your ears, and that your chin is tucked to your chest. Then just straighten your knees and stand up into the prone glide. Finally, practice your recovery to a stand.

❧ EXTRA TIPS

A head-first entry is really only an extension of the push-off into the prone float, which you already know. To help you to keep your chin tucked firmly into your chest, imagine that you're holding a gold pencil there, or something else that you wouldn't want to drop.

WATER SKILLS
❧

Warm-up

Do some Swimmers' Shape-ups on dry land or in shallow water followed by a review of these skills while pool-side: breathing, flutter kicking, bobbing, prone skills, treading, and supine skills.

Then continue the warming-up process in the water.

Review Skills

Practice your bobbing, prone skills, treading, and supine skills.

Supine Sculling with Flutter Kicking

Now to add some arm and leg action to the back float.

❧ HOW TO DO IT

Standing in chest-deep water, review the sculling arm motion that you learned as part of treading. Make figure 8s with each arm, weaving them first away, then toward each other. Gradually bring the motion down around your hips, making the loops smaller and smaller, then move your hands behind your hips. Next, begin to walk backward (this is the direction you'll be moving while on your back), as you push water forward.

Next, stand with one foot slightly in front of the other and push off into the supine float, still sculling; after a few sculls, add a flutter kick to help your legs stay up and to help propel you through the water. When you're ready, recover to a standing position.

❧ EXTRA TIPS

This is a matter of getting your coordination together. You will probably find it easier than the crawl stroke, where you have to coordinate rhythmic breathing, and where your arms are moving alternately. Here, your head stays above water, and both arms are doing the same thing at the same time, so this should be an easy stroke, and a welcome change.

If you need it, have your partner support you, or support yourself on the pool wall as you did when you learned the supine float. Do whatever is comfortable. If you find it easier to begin kicking first, then add the sculling, go ahead and do it that way. But when you combine the two skills, don't concentrate on one to the exclusion of the other. Make sure you're doing them both simultaneously, in a continuous motion.

Try to keep splashing to a minimum; it's a waste of time and energy. Remember, in order to move forward, you have to push water, not air.

❧ BENEFITS

This is the final step before learning the elementary backstroke. Your coordination should be superb by now.

Introduction to Shallow Surface Entry

~ HOW TO DO IT

Begin by practicing the prone glide and recovery. As you do, be particularly conscious of the push-off from the wall and of your streamlined body position.

Then sit on the edge of the pool or on the top step of the ladder or the steps at the shallow end. Push off from the side of the pool, as you did before to start the prone glide, but this time tuck your chin tightly to your chest and angle your arms down about 30 degrees to propel your body just beneath the surface. As you start to lose momentum, arch your back slightly and lift your chin a little to the surface in a prone glide. Recover to a stand. Repeat this shallow surface dive at least five times, or until you're comfortable with it.

~ EXTRA TIPS

If you have trouble with this part, relax and go on to something else, then come back to the shallow surface dive in a little while. If you've never dove before, getting over this first hurdle is the most challenging part, so don't push yourself too fast.

If you get water up your nose, check to see that you're beginning to exhale, expecially through your nostrils, just before your head enters the water.

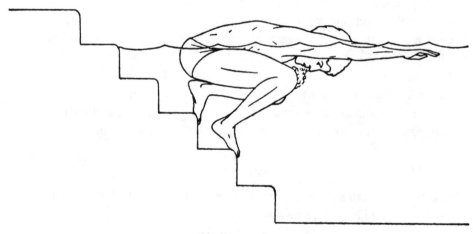

Shallow surface entry.

Speaking of heads, make sure to keep yours tucked down. Remember that gold pencil you're holding. Raising the head is the single most common fault divers make, and it's the cause of all those belly whops. The body follows the head through space, so if the head pops up, so does the body—and, in a dive, you want to enter the water in a smooth, downward arc. Get into the habit of really tensing your abdominal and leg muscles when diving, for an extended, clean body line.

Whenever you're making a head-first entry, be sure that your arms cover your ears, and that your hands are stretched out straight in front of you to protect your head. If your hands tend to separate on entry, hook your thumbs or grasp one wrist with your other hand.

Cool-down

Practice all your skills—supine, prone, and treading—for a few minutes, paying particular attention to your form. Remember to be conscious of the *whole skill* and not just the individual parts—think about your kicking and arm motion together. If you need to, go back and practice the parts individually until you're sure of them. Add rhythmic breathing when you practice prone flutter kicking on the wall; add controlled breathing during the prone float. Do some push-offs and practice a few head-first entries, using the pull-up exercise instead of the stairs to get you out of the water.

Homework

Keep practicing your rhythmic breathing in a basin of water, and when you review your crawl stroke on land. This is the part most people have trouble with, no matter how long they've been swimming. Remember the "Law of Opposites." Practice your other skills, too—sculling, treading, bobbing, and flutter kicking—while watching TV or in front of the mirror. Not only will this improve your form, it'll help tone and strengthen your muscles.

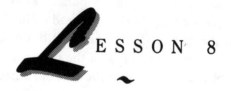

$\mathcal{L}$ ESSON 8

~

$\mathcal{I}$n this lesson you'll learn the elementary backstroke. This is primarily a resting or survival stroke and is quite easy and pleasant to do. Since both arms do the same thing at the same time, it's simpler than the alternating ("windmill") backstroke that you'll learn next. Eventually, the elementary-backstroke arm motion will be combined with a new kick, which is explained in the next lesson.

This lesson will also teach you how to dive from a sitting position, which is the next step in learning this other new skill.

Of course, you'll also continue to practice and improve the prone and supine skills you already know, as well as your treading.

DRY-LAND/PREP SKILLS

~

Do your favorite Swimmers' Shape-ups, paying particular attention to arm circles to help prepare you for the elementary backstroke. Then add other arm and shoulder stretchers.

Review Skills

Practice your breathing, flutter kicking, prone skills, treading, and supine skills.

Elementary Backstroke Arm Motion

You'll like this one—even on dry land it gives you a nice stretch, but wait until you try it in water and you feel the restful glide from this stroke.

～ HOW TO DO IT

Stand up straight, with your back arched slightly and your hands at your sides. This will be your resting, or *glide,* position. For the *recovery* of this stroke, imagine that you have an itch all along the sides of your torso. Slide your fingertips along your sides, keeping your elbows back and close to your body as they bend. When your fingertips are near your armpits and you just can't go any higher, straighten your arms, still keeping them as far back as they'll go, and raise them in a V shape, out behind your

The elementary backstroke.

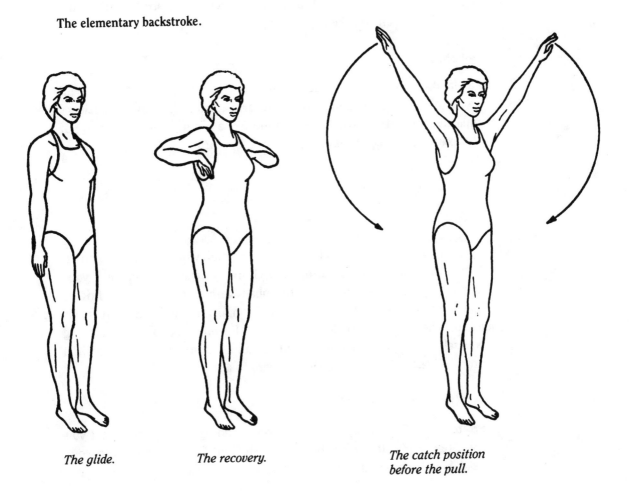

The glide.   *The recovery.*   *The catch position
                                                        before the pull.*

head, palms facing downward and out. Pause a second (this is the *catch* of the stroke) and try to reach back another inch.

For the power part of the stroke, or the *pull,* keep your arms straight and snap them down quickly so that they slap your outer thighs. Hold them in this position for a second (the glide) before you begin the cycle all over again. Repeat five to ten times while standing in place; then walk backward as you do the arm stroke, to simulate the flutter kicking that you'll be doing in the water.

～ EXTRA TIPS

Make sure that you slide your hands *along* your sides and that you keep your chest forward. If you're wearing clothing with a side seam, run your fingers along the seam as you raise your arms in the recovery. To help you remember the motion, repeat the key words "up (recovery), out (catch), together (pull), and glide." You can also practice this stroke while lying on the floor or on your bed.

～ BENEFITS

On land, the elementary backstroke gives you an excellent stretch all along the upper chest and through the arms, and it develops your triceps muscles. (This stroke will have even more of a toning effect when you put the extra resistance of the water to work for you.)

Sitting Dive Entry

～ HOW TO DO IT

Again, review the prone float and diving position while sitting on a chair. Extend your arms forward, drop your chin to your chest, and cover your ears with your arms. Hook your thumbs together and point your fingers downward at a 30- to 45-degree angle. Lean forward and press your heels against the chair legs. (Later, you'll push off from the pool trough, lifting yourself into a piked-standing position, and ending up in the water in a prone glide.) Then simulate the recovery to a stand. Repeat five times.

～ EXTRA TIPS

Stretch and straighten your body as you stand up to make sure that you don't tend to "collapse" in the water later on. Remember to keep your head down—chin tucked to chest, body streamlined in a perfect stretch.

WATER SKILLS

～

Warm-up

Again, do some arm and shoulder stretches during the Swimmers' Shape-ups. Then practice these skills pool-side: breathing, flutter kicking, bobbing, prone skills, treading, and supine skills.

Review Skills

Once you're in the water, keep moving, and practice your bobbing, prone skills, treading, and supine skills.

Elementary Backstroke with Flutter Kick

Let's see how great this stroke feels in the water.

～ HOW TO DO IT

Review this stroke while standing in chest-deep water. Begin in the glide position with your arms down at your sides, palms against your thighs. Start the *recovery:* bring both your arms up, bending the elbows, until your fingertips are as close to your armpits as you can get them. Then begin to straighten your arms and extend them up, out, and back (think of the statue *Winged Victory*). Try to move them back a little more for the *catch.* Then, for the *pull,* snap your arms straight down until they slap your thighs. Repeat five times.

Next, bend your knees so that the water is just below your chin. Arch your back slightly and practice the elementary backstroke while walking backward. Begin to think about coordinating your breathing with the stroke: inhale as your arms reach up and your chest expands, and exhale as your arms snap down. Practice this five times.

The next step is to add the supine flutter kick to the float. First, review the recovery to a stand a few times. Then, as you begin the float, start to flutter kick. Next, add the elementary-backstroke arm motion. Remember, reach up and back in the water, hold a second, then snap your arms down to your sides, keeping them under the water the entire time. If you need to, hold on to the wall with one hand at first and practice a few strokes with one arm at a time, alternately. Or practice with your partner, using the train-and-engineer position you used to learn the prone skills.

Either way, use gradually less assistance until you're eventually doing the stroke on your own.

Remember, if you find it easier, you can begin the stroke with either the arm motion or the flutter kick.

~ EXTRA TIPS

After you snap your arms down, hold them by your side a moment so you can really feel the glide that this stroke gives you. You'll see how powerful the stroke can be and what a restful, fluid motion you can get in the water.

~ BENEFITS

This smooth, flowing stroke gets you accustomed to swimming on your back and so leads right up to the familiar windmill backstroke. In the water, the resistance will make your arm, chest, and shoulder muscles work even harder than on land, thus helping to fight flabby arms and droopy chest.

Sitting Dive Entry

When first practicing this head-first entry, you may want to remove your goggles, if you're used to wearing them, since they can sometimes shift annoyingly from the impact of entering the water. Or, if you want to keep your goggles, just wear them a bit tighter than usual. For safety's sake, always make sure that you're diving into water that's at least five feet deep.

Sitting dive entry.

Initial position and entry.

➤ HOW TO DO IT

Practice a few shallow surface entries; then push up and exit the pool. Sit on the edge of the pool, resting your heels on the back wall of the gutter, with toes curled around the gutter's edge, or trough. (If your pool has no gutter, find a ladder rung or other suitable way to brace yourself.) Extend your arms, locking thumbs and covering your ears with your arms. Point your hands down at a 30- to 45-degree angle, tuck your chin to your chest, and look at the water's surface three to five feet in front of you. Begin to exhale as you bend forward from the waist and roll into the water, pushing against the gutter with your heels and toes and straightening your legs and body as you do so.

Enter in a streamlined position, making a downward arc in the water and keeping your arms together and extended in front of you, head still down. Then point your fingers upward to help your ascent to the surface. When you approach the surface, you'll be in the prone glide position. Recover to a stand, or do a few crawl strokes and then stand. Rest, and repeat at least five times, using the push-up exit from the pool.

➤ EXTRA TIPS

Practice, practice, practice! Other than that, the most important thing to remember is to keep your body as taut and streamlined as possible so that you enter the water cleanly like a knife, fingers first. Tighten your abdominal and leg muscles and point your toes hard. The head leads the body, so keep your head tucked down until you're ready to surface.

Make sure you keep your eyes open at all times so that you know exactly where you are during the entire dive. Keep your body extended during the dive, especially during the push-off. Put as much spring and energy into it as possible, as if you were sprinting for a bus.

Recovery to the surface to prone float position.

~ BENEFITS

Perhaps learning to dive has been your particular stumbling block. This can be the case even for good swimmers. But thinking of it as an extension of the push-off and prone glide you know so well will help you to overcome any hesitation you've felt up to now. Remember, your mental outlook is an important as your physical performance.

Entering the water head first puts your body in the correct, streamlined position for beginning the crawl stroke (and the other prone skills). And the momentum from the dive drives your body forward, giving you a boost to begin the crawl stroke.

Cool-down

Review all the prone and supine skills you've learned thus far, plus treading. Run through each component separately if you need to concentrate on some aspect of your form; then combine them to work on your coordination. Finish with a few practice surface dives or push-offs, always surfacing into a streamlined prone glide, and perhaps adding a few crawl strokes. Remember your rhythmic breathing while swimming the crawl. If you feel particularly energetic, try a sitting dive from the pool deck to finish off your lesson.

Homework

Go over all your skills, preferably in front of a mirror if there's no partner around to check your form. Stretch your body as long as it will go during the elementary backstroke. And think about your streamlined position while you do the crawl-stroke arm motion, first by itself, then with rhythmic breathing.

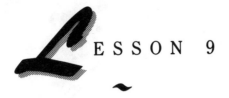

L ESSON 9

In this lesson the elementary-backstroke arm motion combines with another leg motion—the whip kick. This is a new, more efficient version of the old frog kick that you may have seen or learned. First you'll learn this kick alone; then you'll see how to coordinate it with the elementary-backstroke arm motion, with and without assistance.

DRY-LAND/PREP SKILLS

Do a few Swimmers' Shape-ups to begin.

Review Skills

Practice your breathing, flutter kicking, bobbing, prone skills, treading, and supine skills.

Whip Kick (Supine Position)

Different from any kick that you've learned so far, this is the leg motion that you'll be using along with the elementary-backstroke arm motion that you learned in the last lesson. The good news is that both legs do the same thing at the same time, so you've only one set of movements to think about.

91

The whip kick.

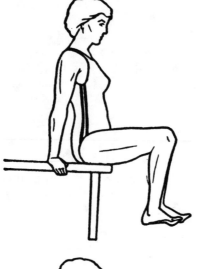

*Knees bent, legs together,
heels dropped toward floor.*

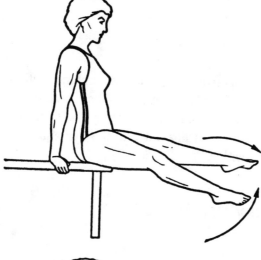

Legs snap together.

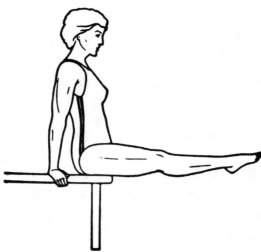

*Finish with legs together,
fully extended, toes pointed.*

～ HOW TO DO IT

Sit up straight in a chair, grasping either the edge of the seat or the arms for leverage. Press your legs together and lift them straight up off the floor, toes pointed, similar to when you begin flutter kicking. Keep your knees and thighs close and parallel to each other; then, bending your knees, drop your heels toward the floor. Keeping your knees close, flex your feet and rotate them outward, separating them by about hip width. For the propulsion part of the kick, move your lower legs in an outward semicircle, snapping them toward each other as they straighten at the knees. End with your legs together, in a fully extended position with toes pointed and streamlined; glide for a second. Repeat this five times; rest; then repeat another five times.

～ EXTRA TIPS

Try to keep your knees as parallel as possible. Let them come apart slightly when you rotate your feet outward, but they should still be closer together than your feet. Your feet and calves should do most of the moving; the thighs do move, but not as much. To help you remember the action, repeat the key words: "Bend, extend, snap together, and glide."

～ BENEFITS

Since this is so different from flutter kicking, getting the coordination correct on land is especially important. The whip kick is useful for trimming and toning the abdominal muscles and the legs, especially the inner and outer thighs—areas hard to reach with other forms of exercise. It also gets your knee and hip joints moving in a new plane, which will help keep them from stiffening up.

NOTE: The whip kick is a relatively new, more effective version of the old frog kick. If you prefer to use the frog kick for any reason (you already know it, or you have a knee problem) turn to page 150, where it is described as an alternate kick to use with the breaststroke.

Elementary Backstroke with Whip Kick

～ HOW TO DO IT

Review the arm motion again: bend, extend, snap down, and glide. Then review the leg motion: bend, extend, snap together, and glide. Notice that the key words are almost exactly the same, because both arms and legs move together.

First practice while balancing yourself on the edge of a chair. Do both motions at once—as you bend your knees, bend your arms; as you extend and straighten your legs, extend and straighten your arms; as you bring your legs together, bring your arms down; and as you hold your legs together, hold your arms at your sides for the glide.

Next, try the coordination standing up. Begin with your arms down at your sides, legs straight and together. Then bend, extend, and straighten arms and legs simultaneously—jump with legs apart for the extension, then jump and bring your legs back together for the snap.

～ EXTRA TIPS

Both the arms and the legs move in a simultaneous, similar motion. For the legs, repeat the key words to yourself: "Bend, extend, snap, and glide." This corresponds to "recover, catch, pull, and glide" for the arms. Begin to coordinate your breathing with your arm and leg movements for a steadier, more regular stroke: inhale as you bend your legs and stretch your arms up, and exhale as you snap down with both arms and legs.

～ BENEFITS

This particular set of movements stretches your shoulders, sides, arms, and entire rib cage. And the jumping-jack action will help strengthen your thighs.

WATER SKILLS

～

Warm-up

Concentrate on stretching out your arms and sides during the Swimmers' Shape-ups.

Review the swimming skills you've learned so far, beginning on dry land: breathing, flutter kicking, bobbing, prone skills, treading, and supine skills.

Continue the warm-up in the water with bobbing, prone skills, treading, and supine skills.

Whip Kick (Supine Position)

⌣ HOW TO DO IT

Begin by standing with your back against the pool wall, your arms extended out away from your sides, and your hands grasping the pool edge as you do when practicing the supine flutter kick. Pull your legs up and, keeping them together, extend them just below the surface of the water, with your toes pointed. Keeping your knees and thighs underwater, flex your feet and drop your heels down toward the bottom of the pool. Next, rotate and flex your feet away from each other so that your toes face outward. Then snap your legs together in a semicircular motion, being careful not to break the surface of the water. Hold the extended position for a moment before you begin the next kick. Do ten kicks; rest, then do ten more.

⌣ EXTRA TIPS

If you already know the frog kick, remember that this new version is narrower. The power comes not so much from the snap of your legs together as from the pressure exerted when your feet form the semicircles.

Make sure that your legs come completely together; try to feel your ankles touch.

As you do the whip kick, keep these key words in mind: "Up (bend knees), out (extend legs), together (snap legs together), and glide."

The "egg-beater" variation (see page 378) is an excellent way to improve your whip kick and to strengthen your inner thigh muscles. (It can also be used during treading as an alternate to the bicycling motion.) To do it, go to the deep end and, extending your arm straight out to your side, hold on to the pool wall with one hand. Holding yourself in a nearly vertical position, do the whip kick with the leg nearer the wall. Try to touch the wall with your foot while keeping your knee directly under your chest, then straighten your leg and extend it under your body. Switch hands and repeat on the other side. Then, while facing the pool wall and holding on to the edge with both hands, move both legs in "egg-beater" fashion so that, instead of bending and extending together, they rotate alternately: as one leg bends, the other is straight.

⌣ BENEFITS

Now you'll see how this kick works against the resistance of the water, giving your legs and abdominal muscles even more of a workout.

Supine Float and Whip Kick

～ HOW TO DO IT

First practice the supine float and recovery to refresh your memory. Then lean backward and give a good push-off from the pool bottom, so that you assume a supine glide. Your feet should be close together and close to the surface, and your toes should be pointed. Begin the whip kick and continue for a minute or so. As before, use some assistance at first if you need to, then gradually come to perform the skill alone.

～ EXTRA TIPS

If you're not using any assistance, you can add some easy sculling to help keep your upper body afloat and moving. Listen and look carefully for any splashing—remember, in this kick your feet and legs should stay underwater at all times. Aim for a smooth, continuous motion, with a slight pause at the end for the glide.

～ BENEFITS

This exercise is an intermediate step in learning the elementary backstroke. And, as you practice, you're toning your leg muscles, particularly the inner thigh.

Elementary Backstroke with Whip Kick

You're now ready to put two and two together (two arms and two legs) to swim the elementary backstroke. You've done all the parts separately in the water, and you've put them all together on land, so this part should be a snap.

～ HOW TO DO IT

Floating on your back, review the elementary-backstroke arm motion with the flutter kick. Practice the recovery to a stand, too. Then, standing in shallow water, review the arm motion with the whip kick, doing a "jumping jack" in the water as you did on land. Remember, "up, out, together, and glide," with both arms and legs moving together.

Next, push off into the supine float. Your arms should begin the stroke down at your sides; your legs should be together and straight, with toes pointed. Begin moving your arms and your legs simultaneously. "Up, out, together, and glide." Stop whenever you need to by recovering to a stand.

The elementary backstroke.

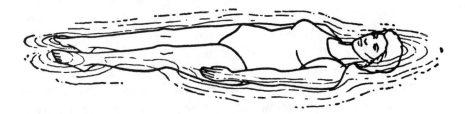

The glide.

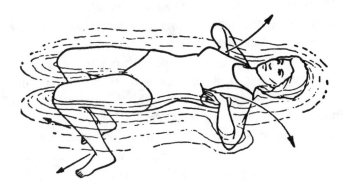

The recovery.

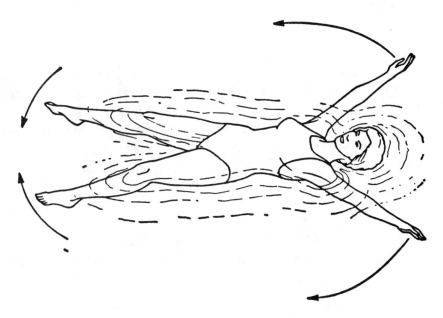

The catch, ready for pull.

ᕁ EXTRA TIPS

Remember, in this stroke the arms and legs "bend, extend, snap, and glide" together. During the glide, rest a moment. Relax and do nothing—just feel yourself being propelled through the water from the momentum of the stroke. When you start to lose that momentum, it's time to stroke again, so use this moment to think about beginning the next stroke. Try to make each complete arm and leg motion carry you as far as possible (stretching out in a streamlined position helps, so do good form and muscle strength).

If your body tends to sink, you may be piking at the waist. Be sure to arch your back, lifting your chest, hips, and abdomen high in the water. If your face should dip below the surface at any time, remember to exhale out your nose and mouth until they resurface.

Make sure your arms and legs stay underwater throughout the whole stroke. There should be no splash. Really flex your feet for propulsion. Squeeze your legs together quickly and smoothly, and use all of your muscles to streamline your body during the glide.

When you're doing this stroke, make sure that you pay attention to the approaching wall. Sneak a peak in back of you every now and then, and recover to a stand when you get to the wall. (You could also count the number of strokes needed to get you across the pool, or make note of some nearby landmark such as the stairs, a ladder, or an object lying on the edge of the deck.)

ᕁ BENEFITS

This is by no stretch of the imagination a racing stroke (although the early competitive backstroke did resemble it closely), but the elementary backstroke is a nice, easy, restful skill that also tones and stretches your arms, thighs, and abdomen. Later on, it will play a part in your fitness program by allowing you to vary your swims and your pace. Until then, stretch, relax, and enjoy the stroke.

Cool-down

Swim through all your new and old prone and supine skills. Finish this lesson with a few shallow surface dives, then a sitting dive, and a push-up exit.

Homework

Practice the crawl and backstroke arm motions in front of a mirror. Check your form. Remember, the better your technique, the easier and more pleasurable swimming will be. Continue to practice your rhythmic breathing in a vessel filled with water.

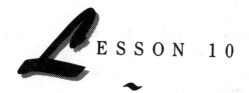

L ESSON 10

Only two more things to learn and practice—the windmill-backstroke arm motion, and how to turn your body over (to go from a prone position to a supine position, or vice versa) and change direction in the water. Once you know how to do that, you'll have mastered the fundamentals of swimming and you'll know all you need to have a safe and pleasurable time in the water. Moreover, you'll be in a position to improve your fitness and your skills even further by following the Workout Program that begins on page 221.

DRY-LAND/PREP SKILLS

Begin with some Swimmers' Shape-ups, including arm circles, to prepare you for the windmill backstroke. Then review your skills (even though some may seem old hat by now, you can always improve on them).

Review Skills

Practice your breathing, flutter kicking, bobbing, prone skills, treading, and supine skills.

Windmill-backstroke Arm Motion

This alternating arm stroke is the final step in the progression of supine skills. Later on, you may wish to refine your technique by learning the bent-arm pull (see page 119), but to understand the basics of this stroke, begin with the simpler straight-arm pull described here.

〜 HOW TO DO IT

Begin by doing the stroke as a catch-up drill, employing the same principle used to introduce the crawl stroke a few lessons ago. Standing up, extend both arms straight out in front of you at shoulder level, with the backs of your hands touching and your palms facing out. Your thumbs will be down and your pinkies up, fingers held loosely together. To begin the *recovery* of the stroke, lift one arm straight up and overhead, just approaching the midline of your body. Then move your hand back, pinky

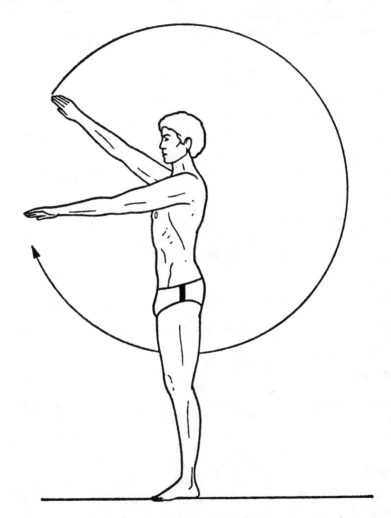

Windmill-backstroke arm motion (catch-up position).

downward, another six inches for the *catch* of the stroke, still keeping your arm straight. For the *pull,* simply swing your arm in back of you in a semicircle. As your thumb brushes past your thigh, rotate your hand so that your little finger once again leads the action. Then continue the circular motion until your hand meets your other hand extended in front of you. Touch the backs of your hands and hold a moment for the "catch-up." Then begin the stroke with the other arm.

When you have the hang of that, begin to alternate arms, so that, as one is pulling, the other is recovering, and you have a 180-degree angle of opposition. Do this while walking backward to simulate the propulsion of the flutter kick. As you walk, move your arms alternately in a constant motion, rather than one at a time. As a result, they will never actually touch (or "catch up" with) each other, but will always rotate directly opposite each other, like the blades of a propeller or windmill.

～ EXTRA TIPS

This stroke is very much like the arm circles that you've been doing for quite a while now. Really stretch up and back as you rotate your arms from the shoulders. Remember to keep your elbows straight but not rigidly locked throughout the motion.

～ BENEFITS

This stroke will be faster than sculling or the elementary backstroke when you try it in the water. In the meantime, practicing it on land will help firm and stretch your chest, shoulders, back, and arms.

WATER SKILLS

～

Warm-up

Concentrate on arm and shoulder exercises. Then begin your dry-land review.

Review Skills

Practice your breathing, flutter kicking, bobbing, prone skills, treading, and supine skills.

Enter the pool with a sitting dive, swim to the deep end, and continue your warm-up in the water. Practice some bobbing, prone skills, treading, and supine skills.

Windmill-backstroke Arm Motion

It's time to transfer your dry-land skills to the water, and once again to see how well Newton's Third Law of Motion Works.

～ HOW TO DO IT

Begin with a review of the catch-up backstroke in shallow water. Bend your knees so that the water is at shoulder level. Brace yourself by placing one foot in front of the other. Extend both arms in front of you at shoulder level, palms facing outward. Begin the *recovery* with one arm by bringing it out of the water (little finger up), lifting it straight overhead at shoulder width. Press your arm back another six inches for the *catch;* then sweep it behind you and down under the water for the *pull.* As you brush your thigh with your thumb, rotate your arm so that the little finger faces up again, and continue the circular motion until your active hand meets the extended one. Hold a moment, and then begin the stroke with your other arm.

Then proceed to the alternating arm motion. As you did on land, alternate your stroke so that your arms move continuously and in opposition to each other. Begin to walk backward in the water. If you can, lean back slightly in the water to get a body position that more closely approximates the supine float.

～ EXTRA TIPS

Remember the three parts of the arm motion—the catch, the pull, and the recovery. Check to see that your arm position is correct during the recovery—little finger up, arm straight and directly above your shoulder. As your hand passes overhead, make sure it stays at shoulder width, with your little finger first so there's no splash later on. During the *pull,* try to keep your arm straight, and remember to rotate your arm prior to the *recovery,* so that pinky lifts first (no splash here either).

Windmill Backstroke with Flutter Kick

This is the last step in learning the basic windmill backstroke. As with all the other skills, begin with assistance if you need it; then gradually come to do it unassisted.

The windmill backstroke.

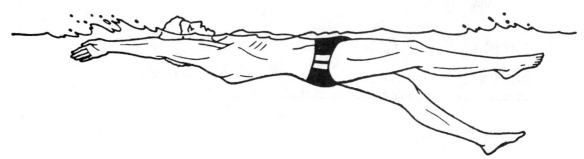

The catch.

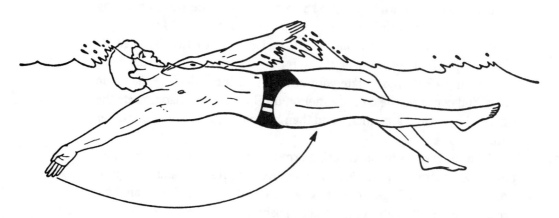

The pull.

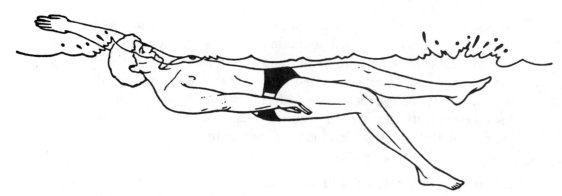

The right arm is about to begin the recovery, as the left arm is about to begin the catch.

～ HOW TO DO IT

Begin in a supine float. Then coordinate the arm motion with the kick by starting with either motion first, then adding the other. If you need assistance and you have a partner, have him or her stand in back of you and support you in the train-and-engineer position (engineers, beware of flying arms), alternately supporting and releasing the hands as they stroke. If you need some assistance but have no partner, support yourself by sliding one hand along the pool edge as you flutter kick and do the backstroke with your free arm. Then turn around and reverse directions, using the other arm to do the stroke. Use gradually less assistance until eventually you can do the arm and leg motions together on your own. When you get tired, recover to a stand.

～ EXTRA TIPS

Keep your chin near your chest and look toward your feet, so the water line is just at ear level. If you begin to pike, or "sit," in the water, try to keep your chest and shoulders up by pressing your shoulder blades back and together. If just your legs tend to sink, your head may be too high. To get a clean, knifelike entry into the water, make sure that your hand enters with the little finger first. Then to further minimize splash, turn your little finger up again before you lift your arm from the water for the recovery. The arm motion accounts for most of the power behind the stroke, so concentrate on the form and power of your arms, and keep your kicking relaxed. The kick should be rhythmic and constant, with about six beats per arm cycle, or three kicks per arm pull. Remember, kick from the hip, not the knee. Inhale and exhale regularly and continually, approximately one breathing cycle per arm cycle. If your face should become submerged for a moment, exhale through both nose and mouth until it resurfaces.

～ BENEFITS

In the windmill backstroke, the head, shoulders, and chest ride slightly higher than your legs. This is called *hydroplaning,* and, as you'll see, it's an important concept in improving your technique in all the strokes. (In the backstroke, it has the added benefit of also keeping your head higher in the water, which makes breathing easier and visibility better.)

Changing Direction and Turning Over

These are two handy safety skills that may come naturally to some, but may be a mystery to others. If you want to change the direction in which you are swimming, or change from a prone to a supine position (or vice versa), here's how.

～ HOW TO DO IT

To *change direction,* reach with your forward arm in the direction you wish to go, and move your body in a wide semicircle through the water. Turn your head in the same direction simultaneously, and keep kicking to maintain a high enough body position.

To *turn your body over* from one position to another, simply press your head and one shoulder down into the water, so that your entire body rotates along the longitudinal axis, like a log.

～ EXTRA TIPS

If you have trouble mastering the change of direction, you may want to try going through the vertical treading position as a transitional stage; scull with one arm to turn your body to face the opposite direction, with your legs bending, tucking, and then bicycling as they help you make the change.

Once the head turns in the direction you wish to roll, the shoulders and hips will follow.

Cool-down

Rest a few minutes before you put all the skills you've learned together into a mini-workout.

Exit the pool, push-up style. Then reenter the water with a sitting dive, and surface into a prone glide. When the glide slows down, begin the crawl stroke with rhythmic breathing; swim toward the deep end, and rest whenever you need to by recovering to a vertical position and treading water. Then resume swimming until you reach the other end. Tread water for one minute at the deep end; then return to the shallow end, using your supine skills: the elementary or windmill backstroke or sculling, or any combination of the three. When you've finished, do one minute of bobbing before exiting the pool. As you repeat this lesson, keep trying to swim farther and farther before you have to tread to rest. Also practice changing direction and rolling over from the crawl position to the back-stroke position (and vice versa).

Homework

Practice, as they say, makes perfect. That's especially true for you now. All you need to do now is perfect your skills so that you're efficient, and graceful, too. You can stay at this level the rest of your life and call yourself a swimmer. Or you can keep going (and I hope you will), by learning new strokes and further refining the ones you already know. You can also continue to improve your level of fitness by following the progressive program that begins on page 221. Whatever you decide, there's a whole new world open for you to enjoy.

Now that you've achieved your first major goal, why not treat yourself to a new bathing suit, a bathing cap, a new pair of goggles, or a membership in a health club or other pool facility?

And by the way, welcome to the world of swimming!

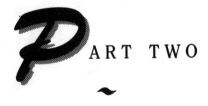

PART TWO

THE TECHNIQUES
OF SWIMMING

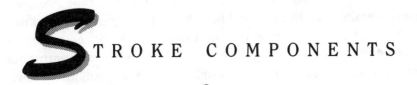

STROKE COMPONENTS

Considering how many centuries man has been splashing around, the swimming techniques used today are relatively recent innovations. These refinements are largely the result of the needs of competitive swimmers, for whom every little advantage counts in their endless quest to swim faster. The old styles were largely a product of simple trial and error. But recently, swimming techniques have been elevated to a science, making today's competitive styles remarkably different from those of even a decade or two ago. As a result, swimmers' times have plummeted to the point where an Olympic champion of ten years ago would have trouble even qualifying for today's games.

THE ART OF SWIMMING

What does this have to do with your average fitness swimmer? Well, swimming faster comes from a more efficient technique, which is more natural and graceful, and therefore ultimately easier. So, even if you don't choose to pit yourself against another swimmer or against the clock, sharpening your technique will make swimming more pleasurable. Even if you think you know these strokes, browse through the following pages. You will almost certainly find tips that will help you improve your form. You may not be doing the S pattern in the crawl stroke, for instance. Or perhaps you're doing the old frog kick instead of the whip kick with your breaststroke. Take a look at your breathing, your body position, the angle of your hand as it enters the water. And wouldn't you like to know how to make a smooth, fast transitional turn when you reach the wall of a pool? Or how to enter the water in a clean, graceful dive?

Swimming is a sport, but it's also an art. And if it's to become a part of your life, wouldn't you like to do it as well as possible? No matter how well you swim, you will always be able to do it a little bit (maybe a lot) better. There's always a new challenge. I'm still reviewing and perfecting things I thought I learned years ago.

THE BASICS AND BEYOND

❧

This section picks up where the ten lessons in Part One left off. To get the most out of it, you should be acquainted with "The Fundamentals of Swimming": you should be comfortable floating on your back and on your stomach (supine and prone positions), you should be able to do the crawl stroke (also called freestyle) with rhythmic breathing, the elementary and windmill backstrokes, sculling, deep-water treading, and, ideally, a sitting dive. If any of these elements are a mystery to you, go back and review them; they are the foundation on which all strokes, starts, dives, and turns are built.

Once you've learned a skill, always aim for a constant, smooth, rhythmic motion, with no wasted effort. As you learn and practice, try to develop your kinesthetic sense—your ability to perceive the relative position of each part of your body in space (or water). Only when you have an idea of your body position will you be able to tell when you're doing something correctly, or, if you're performing a skill incorrectly, how to go about correcting it. Some people have a keener kinesthetic sense than others, but everyone can improve upon what he has.

So work in front of a mirror first to practice a movement. Then, during your regular workout at the pool, concentrate on learning or improving a specific skill. (You'll see that the workouts in this book do this for you already.) Practice with a steady buddy or swimming partner as often as possible. As you progress, watch, ask, and listen to other swimmers.

Regardless of your level, you can still help and correct each other.

SUCCESS WILL COME

◆

You may feel a little stiff and awkward at first, depending on your physical condition, your age, and your past swimming experience. You may not be able to do a movement exactly as pictured or described. Your legs may not snap together briskly, your elbow may not come up quite high enough, you may have a tough time getting some of the coordination. If you're relearning a stroke the right way, you may find it tough to eradicate years of habit.

Just hang in there and do the best you can. As long as you have the basic idea, you will approach the ideal more and more every day. If you have a bad back, stiff shoulder, or trick knee, you may need to individualize a stroke or two. So, although these techniques work best for most swimmers, if a particular technique doesn't work for you after you've given it a good chance, give in to your idiosyncrasies and modify the technique so that it comes closer to being correct for you.

PRINCIPLES OF GOOD STROKE MECHANICS

◆

As I've mentioned earlier, swimming is an art, a sport, and a science. No matter what the stroke, start, dive, or turn, there are certain basic principles that apply. Here's a crash course in fluid mechanics that will help explain why strokes are done the way they are.

Buoyancy, or Archimedes' Law: The specific gravity of water is 1.0; yours is less, which means that you will float. There is a simple, unchanging principle that explains this phenomenon. Basically, when any weight is submerged, the water presses in on it from all sides. In the case of a buoyant object, such as your body, more pressure is exerted upward than in any other direction. This difference in pressure causes an upward force, called buoyancy. Since people are naturally buoyant (big-boned and heavy-muscled types are less buoyant; fat floats better) very little effort is required to keep afloat. So when you swim, don't try to swim *on top* of the water; swim *through it*. Devote your energy to propelling yourself forward, not to staying up. However, the faster you go, the higher in the water you'll ride; this is a natural by-product of greater speed.

Newton's Third Law of Motion: This one says that, for every action, there's an equal and opposite reaction. Swimmers move *forward* by pushing *back* against the water (instead of pushing *up* and *out* as many do). The greater the resistance of the water, the greater the forward thrust. And since still water provides greater resistance than water that's already moving backward, the old straight-arm pull isn't the most efficient way to swim. The most effective stroke, instead, is one that's curved so that you're always pushing against a column of "new" or still water. We'll discuss this concept in more detail later on.

Bernoulli's Principle of Streamlining: In order to move through water most efficiently, your body must pose as little resistance (drag) as possible. This streamlining effect with Bernoulli's Principle or Lift Law allows you to swim faster the higher your upper body rides in the water. To streamline your body, keep it generally horizontal along the central axis (your spine) so that all your energy is used for propelling your body *directly forward,* and none is wasted by moving it vertically, to the side, or even backward.

Next, you have to keep in mind how to generate the most power to propel you forward without destroying the streamlining effect. If you were an eel or a submarine, this would pose very little problem. But we land creatures have to move our arms and legs up, down, and around in order to move, and this interferes with streamlining by increasing our surface area. The greater the area exposed to the water, the greater the drag. This is the dilemma that faces every swimmer: how to obtain the greatest power (using your arms and legs to make the most of the water's resistance) while sacrificing the least streamlining (creating as little resistance as possible on the other parts).

Resistance Check: An Experiment

To help you get a feel for the three principles of stroke mechanics discussed here—Newton's Third Law of Motion, streamlining, and resistance—try this exercise the next time you're in the water. Although the experiment deals with only hand position, the principles apply to the rest of a swimmer's body as well.

Stand in shoulder-deep water, with one arm extended straight out in front of you at water level. Pull your arm downward and backward in an arc, holding your hand in each of the following positions consecutively:

1. Flex your wrist and extend your fingers upward toward the ceiling (water slides off your hand).

2. Make a fist (feel pressure on your arm, but there is no "paddle" or "lever" effect of hand).

3. Flex your hand at the wrist, at a 90-degree angle ("overdigging"—pushing water out and back too soon).

4. Spread your fingers apart, pulling with arm straight downward (arm slips through water without much power).

Now try this: Slide your hand into the water at a 30- to 45-degree angle downward, thumb side down. Keep your elbow higher than your hand, and pull straight through, describing the same arc as you did before. You will feel a big difference—this is the most efficient way to press against the water, and you will now feel your body start to move forward. That's Newton's Third Law of Motion using the water's resistance to propel you forward.

This experiment also gives you a good "feel" of the water. With every stroke you should try to hold as much water as possible. Try to get a good "grip" on it. (However, you should also keep your hand somewhat relaxed, with fingers straight but slightly apart.)

THE STROKES
➤

In this section, you'll study the four competitive strokes (the crawl or freestyle, the backstroke, the breaststroke, and the butterfly) plus a fifth (the sidestroke).

Which Is the Hardest Stroke? The Fastest?

Of course, it depends on how hard you're swimming and how efficient your technique is, but in general terms, here are the strokes ranked from most strenuous to least strenuous:

  Butterfly
  Crawl (freestyle)
  Backstroke
  Breaststroke
  Sidestroke

And here are the strokes ranked from fastest to slowest:

Crawl (freestyle)
Butterfly
Backstroke
Breaststroke
Sidestroke

Everyone has a favorite stroke and a least favorite stroke, with the others falling somewhere in between. But it's a good idea to learn and practice as many strokes as you can, because it makes for more interesting workouts, and because each stroke works your muscles differently.

Stroke Basics

Body Position: In general, the higher your body rides in the water, with the shoulders slightly higher than the legs, the easier it will be to swim. But don't get carried away—remember, we humans move *through* water, not on top of it. The water should come to about your hairline.

Arm Motion: No matter how different they seem, all the arm strokes in this section have these three components in common:

1. They begin with the *catch*—the angled entry of your hand so that air bubbles don't get trapped and your hand doesn't slip through the water. This is the ready position during which you should get a good hold on the water.

2. Next comes the two-phase underwater *pull*—always some variation of an elongated S-shaped path that makes the most use of the water's resistance. Phase 1 is a diagonal, outward, and downward movement; you pull water in a semicircle from about shoulder width back inward to about the mid-line of the body. Phase 2 is a shorter, accelerated press backward. Ideally, the second phase supplies most of the power of the arm stroke.

3. Finally, there's the *recovery,* which occurs either over or under the water, depending on the stroke. This component, which brings the arm back to the starting position and gives it a short rest, should be done with as little resistance as possible.

When learning and doing each stroke, review the basic S-shaped path that your hand and arm follow; this allows you continually to press "still" water backward.

Leg Motion: The main power from any kind of kick comes from the large muscles in the hips and thighs. The aim of all strokes is to push water backward, not to splash water into the air. So make sure your feet and legs barely break the surface.

Breathing: There should be a continuous exchange of air, whether your head is above the water or below. Inhale fully and exhale slowly and fully through both nose and mouth. Exhaling through the nose is especially important when your face is underwater, since that's what keeps the water from getting in.

Another factor to bear in mind is the ratio of arm power to leg power. Most people will be surprised by this comparison:

COMPARISON OF LEG AND ARM POWER

	Percentage of Stroke's Power from Kick	*Percentage of Stroke's Power from Pull*
Freestyle or crawl	20	80
Backstroke	25	75
Butterfly	30	70
Breaststroke	50	50
Sidestroke	50	50

These percentages are meant to give you an idea of what to strive toward. Think of them as a goal that you're constantly trying to achieve; whether you do depends on your own relative strengths and weaknesses. If you have an especially good kick, for instance, that will naturally supply more power. And in competition the percentage varies, too: sprinters use more leg power, and distance swimmers rely more on their arms.

If you find these general ratios hard to believe, try this: just pull for one lap; then just kick; finally, swim (use both arms and legs) for one lap. Time yourself for each lap—then compare.

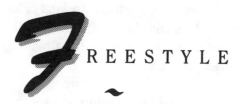

FREESTYLE

The crawl stroke is just about everyone's favorite, whether they are recreational or fitness swimmers, or competitive swimmers, who often call it the freestyle. The words "crawl stroke" and "freestyle" are used interchangeably. The crawl stroke is the easiest to learn for most people. As your crawl stroke improves, you will be developing your "freestyle" stroke techniques for faster and more efficient swimming.

The present-day crawl had its origins in Australia, around 1893. The stroke supposedly got its name when a swimming coach, amazed at the unusual stroke used by twelve-year-old Alick Wickham (and at the boy's resulting speed), exclaimed: "Look at that kid crawling!" Although this original "Australian crawl" has been greatly refined over the past century, the basic idea of combining a hand-over-hand arm motion with a vertical kick and a prone body position was a remarkable improvement over the strokes then in common use.

Word began to spread of the crawl's speed and efficiency, and gradually more and more competitive swimmers adopted the stroke for speed swimming. It became supreme among all others for long-distance swimming as well when Gertrude Ederle used it in her English Channel swim in 1926. ("Doc" Counsilman used the freestyle in his 1979 Channel swim, too–at the age of fifty-eight!) Since then, many swimmers have contributed to the popularity and refinement of this all-purpose stroke, including Esther Williams, Johnny Weissmuller, and Buster Crabbe, who literally swam their way to fame and fortune. More recently Mark Spitz, winner of seven Olympic gold medals in Munich in 1972, set four Olympic records in freestyle sprint events. Since then, such swimmers as Matt Biondi,

118

Tracy Caulkins, Ambrose ("Rowdy") Gaines, Janet Evans, and Tom Jager have continued to shatter freestyle records.

LEARNING THE FREESTYLE

The basics of this stroke have already been taught in Part One, "The Fundamentals of Swimming." Here you'll learn a few refinements to your technique, including the more efficient S-pattern arm pull. This technique is more powerful than the traditional straight-arm pull because your hand moves a column of still water, instead of water that you've already set in motion. This gives you a better "hold" on the water and increases the resistance against your hand, enabling you to push yourself forward with more force. The backstroke, breaststroke, and butterfly also utilize an S-pattern pull, so once you understand the principle you can transfer this technique to the other strokes as well.

Remember, the arms account for about four fifths of the forward propulsion in the crawl stroke/freestyle. Actually, long-distance swimmers

The freestyle.

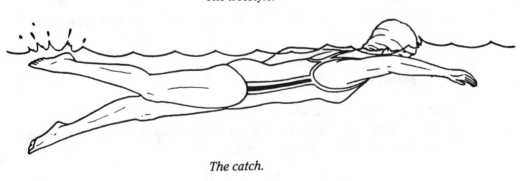

The catch.

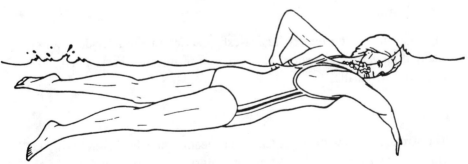

The pull (phase 1).

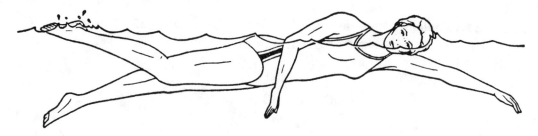

The pull (phase 2).

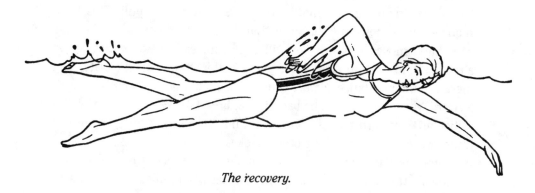

The recovery.

use their legs even less, while competitive sprinters may get more of their power from the kick.

Body Position

Your body should have a long, stretched-out feeling. It should be streamlined along its central axis (your spine), and the water level should come between your eyebrows and your hairline.

Arm Motion

Practice the motion on dry land. Next, practice in shoulder-deep water, walking forward at the speed at which you push water back. Then move on to the arm drills.

THE CATCH

The stroke begins with the *catch*. Slice cleanly into the water, with your elbow up and your hand and forearm entering the water at a 30- to 45-degree angle. Keep your hand relaxed, thumb down, and palm facing slightly diagonally outward. Then extend your arm into the water fully, four to eight inches below the surface, before beginning the first phase of the underwater pull. Throughout the stroke, keep your elbows higher than your hands.

THE PULL

This part of the stroke makes an S shape for your left arm, a backward S for your right arm. As the illustration shows, the S should be done so that it is "bottom heavy." For the best leverage, keep your elbow bent slightly during the entire pull.

PHASE 1: With your arm slightly bent, your hand pulls back, down, and out. When it reaches just past shoulder width, pull in toward your stomach. During this first part, feel as if you are gathering up an armload of water and then pressing it back. This first phase should also give you a feeling of leverage or lift.

PHASE 2: From this position, press diagonally back toward your thigh. Straighten and extend your arm as you accelerate the movement at the end of the stroke; imagine that you're throwing a ball behind you. The speed of the pull is actually greatest here, at the end.

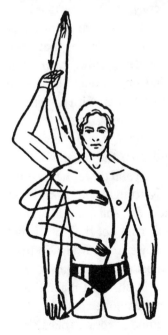

The S-shaped bent-arm pull for the crawl/freestyle.

THE RECOVERY

For the *recovery*, bend your elbow as you lift the arm out of the water. Keep the elbow higher than the hand, and initially lead the swing forward with the elbow. The fingers point back and trail behind for half of the recovery. Midway, the fingers take over the lead, and the hand enters the water at a 30- to 45-degree angle, thumb downward, for the catch.

Body Roll

As one arm recovers, there's a natural tendency for the body to roll 45 degrees or more toward the arm that's pulling.

As the right arm pulls, the right shoulder rotates deeper into the water, contributing further to the body roll. This body roll gives more leverage to the pulling arm. It increases lift and streamlining on the recovery side, because the shoulder, more above the water, encounters less resistance.

As a result of body roll, you can think of your fingertips tracing a path close to the center line of your body during phase 1 of the pull.

Leg Motion

The leg motion of the crawl stroke/freestyle is called the flutter kick. Although this kick is technically known as the six-beat kick (i.e., three kicks per arm motion), it's more important that the kicks are rhythmic and continuous than that you get exactly six per complete arm cycle.

Practice while sitting on the edge of the pool, then practice while holding on to the pool wall, then with a kickboard. Try some of the kick drills described below.

To flutter kick, move your legs up and down alternately. Keep your legs close together, and keep the up-and-down span to about twelve to eighteen inches. The action and power here come from the hip and thigh, so keep your knees fairly straight, but not locked. Your ankles should be loose and floppy; let them flex and point in an undulating or almost whip-like movement as an extension of the flutter motion of your legs. When used correctly, feet add power to your kick in the same way that swim fins do. Your toes should almost point as your leg begins the downward movement of the kick. Don't splash—just make the water "boil" for the most efficient kick. Kicking, when done correctly, helps you to maintain your body position and the tempo of your stroke. Most of the propulsion of the kick comes on the "downbeat." In the freestyle, the kick serves mainly to stabilize the stroke and to help keep your legs from sinking too far below the surface. An inefficient kick, however, can slow you down by creating resistance drag and making your arm pulls less effective.

Many swimmers find that the legs naturally cross over slightly at the ankle; there's no harm in this. Another variation of this kick is called the *trudgeon,* which is a scissors kick that occurs when the swimmer inhales. If one of these kicks happens naturally and feels comfortable, by all means go ahead and use it.

Breathing

Rhythmic breathing, the correct way to breathe while doing the freestyle, consists of pivoting your face out of the water to inhale, then pivoting it back down into the water to exhale. Remember, pivot your head; don't lift it.

Coordinating Arms and Breathing

Learn to breathe rhythmically and to coordinate the head action with the arm motion. Follow the "Law of Opposites" as described in "The Fundamentals of Swimming, " page 56: as your head turns to inhale, the arm on the opposite side extends and enters the water; at the same time, the arm on your breathing side has completed the last part of the S pattern. If you breathe on the right, for example, begin to turn your head just as the fingers of your left hand enter the water. Inhale as your face breaks the surface; exhale completely as it pivots back into the water. You'll probably prefer one side more than the other, but practice breathing on both sides; eventually, you should try alternate breathing, where you breathe first on one side, then, three arm strokes later, on the opposite side. Ideally, you should be swimming efficiently enough for your head to create a "wake," or air pocket, that will allow you actually to breathe with your mouth below the surface of the water. Finally, remember to inhale and exhale continuously throughout rhythmic breathing; don't hold your breath at any time. The entire cycle should take about three to five seconds.

Coordinating Arms and Legs

Many swimmers are comfortable doing a six-beat kick. This means coordinating three downward kicks, or beats, per one arm pull, with the downward kick of one leg coordinating with the catch of the opposite arm.

Other swimmers develop a two-beat kick—one downward beat per arm pull—because it's less tiring when you ease up on the legs. Sometimes they add a cross-over, too.

There are several variations, but you should work out whichever coordination works best for you—just remember, your goal is to move smoothly and constantly through the water.

CHECKLIST FOR A BETTER FREESTYLE
~

Once you've gotten the basics, keep these pointers in mind to help you swim more efficiently:

- Keep your body position as stretched and streamlined as possible, with your shoulders riding higher than your legs. (Feet should be approximately one foot below the surface of the water at the lowest point of the kick.)

- Aim for a full arm extension (straight but not locked) at the beginning and the end of each stroke.

- Accelerate your stroke during phase 2 of the pull.

- Keep your elbows higher than your hands at all times during the stroke. Turning the thumb downward helps keep the elbow up, in addition to cutting down on the amount of air entrapped into the catch (remember, you want to push water, not air).

- At the highest point of the recovery, your elbow is bent at a 90-degree angle, with the wrist flexed slightly back. Initially the elbow leads during the recovery, until the hand extends for the catch.

- Make sure that you take time for the catch of the stroke.

- When inhaling, rotate your head just enough so that your mouth clears the water. The less you turn, the better, so that you get a clean, quick "bite" of air. Some swimmers actually twist their mouths up toward their breathing side to minimize head movement even further. When you breathe, you should be looking diagonally toward the far end of the pool (not at the bottom or at the ceiling, or behind you).

- Don't overkick; this will tire you out, and may even decrease your speed. Just make the water "boil." And try to keep your ankles loose and supple to get a whipping action.

FREESTYLE STROKE DRILLS: ARMS

❧

These drills may be done with or without a *pull-buoy* for support. Advanced fitness and competitive swimmers may also use additional *resistance devices* such as an inner tube and/or hand paddles.

NOTE: Even though these are arm drills, some may require kicking to maintain body position and smooth motion during the drill.

1. Catch-up Freestyle: To slow down the stroke and feel the S-pattern pull.

As you do the arm motion, touch one thumb to the other before beginning the next pull. Maintain a steady kick throughout the drill.

- Practice this drill standing on land, then standing in shallow water, then walking forward in shoulder-deep water.
- Do one lap of catch-up; then swim normally for one lap.
- Do half a lap of catch-up; then complete the lap by swimming.
- Pull for four catch-up strokes; then complete the lap by swimming.

(If you have a problem with the catch-up drills, do them while holding on to the end of a kickboard with the nonpulling hand.)

2. One-arm Pulls: To even out the stroke, so both arms pull with the same power. This drill may be done with or without kicking.

Pull with one arm at a time, keeping the nonpulling arm stretched out in front of you.

- Pull with the same arm for an entire lap, or alternate the number of strokes done with each arm (i.e., eight right, eight left). May be alternated in a descending/ascending progression (8R, 8L; 4R, 4L; 2R, 2L; 1R, 1L; 2R, 2L; 4R, 4L; 8R, 8L).

3. Glide Freestyle: To get a better "feel" for the water with a deeper, more efficient pull, and to allow for body roll. This drill may be done with or without kicking.

Hold your hand in the catch position for as long as possible, and glide in the water with the body roll; try to minimize kicking.

- Pull for one lap doing the glide freestyle; then swim for one lap.
- Pull for half a lap doing the glide freestyle; then complete the lap by swimming.
- Pull for four glide freestyle strokes, then complete the lap by swimming.

4. DPS (Distance Per Stroke): To maximize the efficiency of each stroke.

Count the strokes needed to complete a lap while pulling; on the next lap, try to decrease the number of strokes needed. Try to do this for a number of consecutive laps.

The glide freestyle drill works wonders for your DPS. Incorporate the S-pattern pull to maximize your efficiency. As a goal, maintain the same speed (watch the clock!) as you decrease the number of strokes on each lap.

5. Fist Closed Pulling: To develop pulling power from the whole arm, not just relying on the hands for propulsion.

- Curl your fingers into a fist, placing the thumb over the middle fingers. Keep elbows high through each armstroke.

6. Dig Freestyle: To practice lifting elbows high on the recovery.

- Begin swimming one length of the pool with very short strokes; where hands enter the water at your ears, elbows are high on the recovery. Then gradually stretch out each successive stroke so that the final strokes to the wall are "normal."

7. Head-up Freestyle: To develop a high body position and proper hand entries. Swim with your eyes above water; hold head in position looking forward. The water line is at the bridge of your nose.

FREESTYLE DRILLS: LEGS

~

These drills may be done with or without fins or a kickboard. When kick drills are done without a board, you will develop a "feel" for the water with your hands. Because kick drills are done without using the arms—

which in the freestyle account for four fifths of the stroke's power—they give you a good chance to work your leg muscles more than you would ordinarily.

1. Sit and Kick: To get the "feel" of the water with your feet.
Sit on the edge of the pool, feet dangling in the water, and practice the flutter kick. Keep your ankles flexible and moving as you kick.

2. Wall Kick: To practice good kicking form and leg position.
Assume the bracket position (see page 29), holding on to the edge of the pool, with one hand grasping the edge and pulling outward, the other dropped below the water surface and pushing against the wall for leverage. Flutter kick in the prone position, with the power coming from the hip, just making the water "boil."

3. Free Kick: To strengthen the leg muscles; to practice good kicking form with the body in proper swimming position. A kickboard is optional.
With arms extended straight in front of you, flutter kick for several laps. If you use a kickboard, you can either keep your head above water and breathe normally, or you can practice your rhythmic breathing. If no kickboard is used, take a rhythmic breath, when needed, by lowering the arm on your breathing side and sculling during the inhalation.

4. Kick and Roll: To get a different feel for the water during kicking; to practice the body roll. This drill should be done without a board.
Do the free-kick drill, and after every ten kicks rotate your body a quarter turn, so that you first kick in a prone position. (Use your topmost arm to scull whenever you need to inhale, and use the S-pattern underwater pull to change positions.)
A variation of this drill is kicking on your side for a specified distance (i.e., half a lap), then rotating onto the other side.

FREESTYLE DRILLS: BREATHING

～

Breathing, the hardest part of the freestyle for many people, requires both coordination and good breath control. The arm and leg drills can be adapted to include breathing practice, as you will see.

1. Catch-up Freestyle: To prolong the stroke, giving you time to think of the breathing and to coordinate it with the arm movement.

Practice the catch-up drill as described on page 125, adding rhythmic breathing.

2. Wall and Free Kick: To coordinate rhythmic breathing with flutter kicking.

Do the wall and free-kick drills (page 127), incorporating rhythmic breathing. During the wall kick, inhale on the side of the underwater arm. During the free kicking, hold the kickboard far enough away from you to allow your head to rotate into and out of the water as you practice your rhythmic breathing. Try adding the crawl-stroke arm motion during both drills by alternately grasping and releasing the pool wall or the kickboard between strokes.

3. Bilateral Breathing: To help balance the stroke; to streamline your technique; to improve your breathing capacity.

Breathe every third stroke instead of every second stroke, so that you turn your head to your accustomed breathing side for only every other inhalation.

- Practice this standing on land, then walking in shoulder-deep water as you stroke.
- Swim one lap breathing bilaterally; then swim normally for one lap.

(This drill also gives you greater visibility as you swim—important in a crowded pool, or in a race where you want to check out the competition on both sides of you. Over long distances, alternate breathing also gives your sternocleidomastoids an even break—these neck muscles can become overworked if you continually turn your neck to the same side. It gives your arm muscles on your nonbreathing side a rest, too, since that arm tends to pull a bit harder during the inhalation.)

4. Controlled Breathing: To develop endurance and breathing capacity; to enhance your ability to get a "second wind."

- Inhale on every other stroke cycle (every four strokes—alternate breathing); then increase your breath control by inhaling on every third cycle (six strokes).

- Do bilateral breathing, increasing and decreasing the number of strokes between breaths (i.e., inhale every third, fifth, seventh, fifth, then third strokes).

COMMON FREESTYLE ERRORS AND WHAT TO DO ABOUT THEM
〜

Body Position

Error	Correction
Body not streamlined and/or too low in water	Stretch and straighten body—*think* streamlined. Body level depends upon individual buoyancy, head position, and arm and leg motions. The faster you go, the higher your body rides in the water.
Head too low in water during exhalation	Keep water at hairline or cap level. Do head-up freestyle drill.
Rear end sticks up (body too piked)	Arch lower back slightly; press hips toward bottom and tuck in the buttocks.
Irregular or bouncy stroke	Check rhythm of all parts of stroke; practice skills in pairs (arms and legs; legs and breathing; arms and breathing).
No body roll	Do glide-freestyle drill.
Low body sways, but upper body is still	Do glide-freestyle drill, letting upper body roll from shoulder and legs follow through.
Uneven stroke because of too much body roll on breathing side	Do bilateral-breathing drill; rotate head past midpoint during exhalation to even out roll; practice late breathing.
Body is off balance to one side	Contract muscles slightly along sides of torso to shift balance and to place hips in horizontal and lateral alignment with rest of body; do glide-freestyle drill. Pull with small kickboard between your legs.

Arms: S-Pattern Pull

Error	Correction
Fast and/or sloppy stroke	Do catch-up freestyle drill.
Hands enter too close to head and cross beyond midpoint of body during underwater pull, causing body to zigzag	Practice S-pattern pull, making sure hands enter water shoulder width apart; practice in front of mirror, in shallow water, swimming.
Hand enters at wrong angle to miss catch of stroke; hands pointed upward, or flat (causes splash), or catch air upon entry	Slide arm downward at 30- to 45-degree angle, four to eight inches under surface. Slice water smoothly like a knife with fingertips; thumb slightly downward to begin pull.
Fingers tight and stiff, cupped, or spread apart	Relax fingers, keeping them close together but not clamped tightly.
Pulling straight-armed and/or "slipping" through water	Keep elbows bent and higher than hands; pull with an exaggerated S pattern and press a still column of water back to get most leverage and power; be certain to brush thumb past thigh before recovery.
Elbows are lower than hands, slipping through water	Do catch-up and fist-closed drills.
Unbalanced stroke (one side stronger than the other)	Do one-arm pull drill; apply S pattern evenly. Do dig freestyle drill.
Straight, high, or wide arm recovery	Lift elbows out of water first, with elbow bent at a 90-degree angle. Let fingertips skim the surface of the water and then reach forward for the catch.
Tremendous effort required for arm recovery; arm drags through water during recovery	Recover arm with elbow leading and high above surface, so that forearm and hand clear water.

Error	Correction
Hesitation during stroke; arms remain in catch position too long	Catch-up is a drill only; when swimming, move arms in opposition.

Legs: Prone Flutter Kick

Error	Correction
Bicycle riding (bent knees and rubbery legs)	Do kick drills—begin thrust of kick from hip and thigh.
Breaking surface and splashing (kicking too high)	Do kick drills—make water just "boil"; lower legs and lift shoulders; check to see if head is too low.
Flexed feet and/or stiff ankles; inefficient kick; little forward movement; foot cramps	Do sit-and-kick drill; use fins for swimming and other drills to get a better feel for water, increased flexibility and greater strength.
Uneven kick, or forced, uncomfortable kick	Pick most comfortable kick (two-beat flutter, six-beat flutter, with or without crossover or trudgeon) and stick to it; keep rhythm constant during kick drills.
Shallow kick (less than twelve inches)	Use fins during kick drills for greater range of motion, greater strength, and better feel for the water.

Rhythmic Breathing

Error	Correction
"Coney Island" breathing (head turns to both sides above water)	Practice rhythmic breathing during drills.
Getting a mouthful of water instead of air; arm blocks inhalation	Remember "Law of Opposites" when doing rhythmic breathing; inhale in air pocket created by "bow wave."

Error	Correction
Running out of breath too quickly	Inhale and exhale fully and continuously; practice controlled breathing drill.
Breathing irregularly; holding your breath	Practice continuous rhythmic breathing.
Neck discomfort during rhythmic breathing	Do bilateral-breathing drill to determine most comfortable side.
Head goes too far underwater during exhalation	Lift head up to hairline or cap level, and look slightly forward to approaching wall during exhalation.
Head turns too far and/or too long to side during exhalation	Turn head just so lower edge of mouth is at water level to get "bite" of air in pocket created by "bow wave."
Looking backward over shoulder during inhalation	Look diagonally forward during inhalation.
Chin lifts during inhalation	Pivot head from side to side as if it were a doorknob.
Stroke hesitation during inhalation	Practice rhythmic breathing on other side.
Mouth and nose stay underwater during rhythmic breathing	Lift head slightly forward and maintain steady, strong pull and kick during head rotation to keep body position as high as possible.
Mouth stays closed during exhalation; no sign of air bubbles	Begin steady exhalation through both nose and mouth as soon as face reenters water; continue exhaling until next inhalation.
Water enters nose	Exhale out nose when face is underwater.

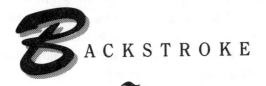

BACKSTROKE

The backstroke is popular, largely because breathing poses no problem—since you swim on your back, your nose and mouth stay above the surface and you can breathe normally during the entire stroke cycle. Many swimmers find that the supine position also allows for efficient leg action, which helps compensate for the relative inefficiency of the angle of the arm stroke. Of course, the disadvantage of the backstroke is that when you're on your back you can't see where you're going, only where you've been.

The earliest backstrokers did a variation of the inverted breaststroke. The elementary backstroke (taught in Part One), which uses the whip kick, is similar to this old style. Since many people find this variation relatively easy to master, it's often used to introduce the more familiar windmill backstroke.

The big hero of backstroke history is Harry Hebner, who introduced the alternating arm pull during the 1912 Olympics. Since that time the backstroke has undergone many subtler changes, too, including the powerful and efficient bent-arm pull you'll find here, which is similar to the S-pattern pull in the freestyle. John Naber won his Olympic medals in 1976 using these same techniques.

LEARNING THE BACKSTROKE

The backstroke is often called the back crawl—and that's the easiest way to visualize it: you lie on your back, your arms moving alternately and

133

rotating from the shoulder like a windmill, while your legs do an inverted flutter kick. The backstroke used today incorporates a bent-arm underwater pull, which is a refinement of the traditional but less efficient straight-arm pull. In this stroke, the arms should supply about three fourths of the forward propulsion, the legs one fourth.

"Where am I?" To keep from bumping your head on the pool wall, count the number of strokes you need per lap the first time you swim it, and for each lap thereafter. Or, to save counting, spot a landmark, such as a ceiling mark, a ladder, or a depth indicator, and fix the number of strokes to carry you from that point to the wall. (Most pools have flags strung across them five yards from each end for just this purpose.) If you're not sure how close you are to the wall, leave one hand overhead and "kick in" rather than overpull and risk bumping your head.

Body Position

Your body is in a supine position, with your legs stretched out straight. Your head should be facing straight up, your chin should be tipped slightly

The bent-arm backstroke.

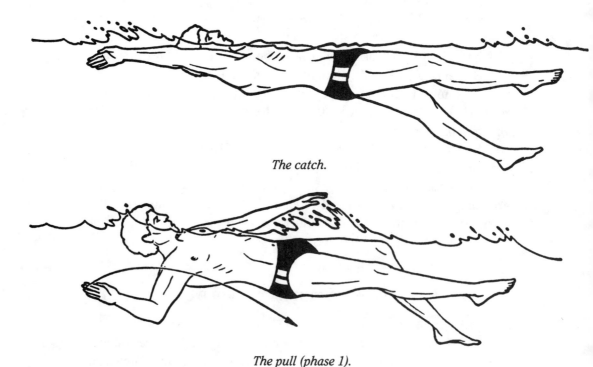

The catch.

The pull (phase 1).

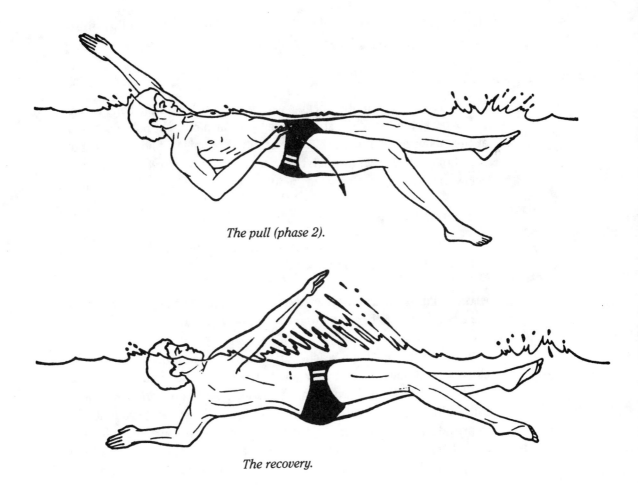

The pull (phase 2).

The recovery.

toward the chest, and your eyes should be looking diagonally toward your feet. The water level should be at the middle of your head, with your ears just submerged. Keep your back straight but not rigid. Your hips should be as close to the water's surface as possible, but lower than your shoulders.

Arm Motion

As with the freestyle, each arm rotates alternately from the shoulder, with one pulling underwater while the other returns to the starting position by recovering upward out of the water. In the bent-arm pull the arm bends in and down toward the legs at the beginning of the second phase.

Practice the arm movement standing on land first, then standing in shoulder-deep water, leaning backward to feel the stroke in the water;

then begin walking backward as the arm stroke propels you in that direction.

THE CATCH

The backstroke arm motion begins with the *catch,* where the hand enters the water at the top of the stroke. Keep your arm straight but not locked at the elbow, and your hand in line with the shoulder. Slide your hand, little finger first, down through the water like a knife, four to eight inches below the surface, to get a good "hold" on the water.

THE PULL

Once you've gotten a hold on the water, begin the two-phase bent-arm pull from the catch position.

PHASE 1: Pull your arm backward and downward. As the pull continues, the elbow begins to bend and to move in toward the waist.

PHASE 2: When your hand reaches shoulder level, continue to bend your elbow in and down toward your waist. Then pivot the forearm, pressing "still" water straight down toward your feet, as if you were throwing a ball behind you. During this last phase of the pull, accelerate your stroke to provide as much power as possible, and end with your hand fully extended below your leg. (This is similar to phase 2 of the freestyle, where you pull under your stomach in order to push still water back toward your feet.)

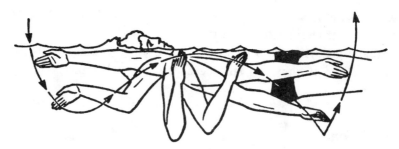

The bent-arm pull for the backstroke.

THE RECOVERY

Lift your arm (thumbs up) and brush your hand past your outer thigh to begin the *recovery.* Continue the upward motion with the arm extended but relaxed, and swing it straight up and overhead in a semicircle. At this point, your thumb position should be whatever is most comfortable for you; the recovery should give your hand, arms, and shoulder muscles a chance to relax. Enter with the pinky down for the catch, to begin the stroke again.

Body Roll

As your arms move, your body will tend to roll through the water. This rotation should occur smoothly and naturally around a central axis—your spinal column. As your right arm enters the water, your right shoulder follows and dips down at an angle of about 45 degrees to the water line; your left shoulder simultaneously rotates up 45 degrees from the water line. As your right arm pulls, your shoulders return to the normal horizontal position; then you roll to the left as your left arms enters the water. The roll originates in the shoulders and chest and travels down the body to the hips. (The head stays straight during the roll.) Body roll helps your stroke efficiency by allowing the pulling arm to pull deeper (and so to press continuously against new water), and by cutting down on the resistance meeting your recovery arm (since that shoulder is now out of the water).

Leg Motion

The backstroke uses the flutter kick, with legs close together and moving up and down alternately, similar to the action in the crawl. The kick is more important in the backstroke than in the crawl, however, because of the supine body position—much of your below-the-waist weight is beneath the water line. The flutter kick also serves to stabilize the body position during the shoulder roll. Practice flutter kicking while sitting on a chair, sofa, or pool deck. Make sure that the kick originates in the hip and thigh. Then practice while holding on to the pool wall or steps, and finally progress to free kicking (see the drills that follow).

To do the flutter kick, move your legs up and down alternately, as if you were walking. Keep your legs close together and kick twelve to eighteen inches deep. The action emanates from your hip and thigh; your knees should stay loose and flexible. The knee actually bends slightly on the upbeat of the kick, supplying more of its energy there, then straightens on the downbeat. The feet should flex and bend easily at the ankle in a whipping action to add to the propulsion. Keep your feet just below the surface of the water when you kick and just make the water foam or boil.

Breathing

Since your face stays above the water throughout, breathing during the backstroke is simply a matter of keeping a steady rhythm for both inhalation and exhalation, usually with one breath cycle per arm cycle. Be certain not to breathe too fast or too shallowly.

Coordinating Arms and Legs

The usual is a six-beat kick: six kicks per arm cycle, or three kicks per arm stroke. Variations on the six-beat kick, such as the four-beat or two-beat kick, are very rare in the backstroke. Again, though, you should just aim for a consistent rhythm and not worry too much about actually counting your beats.

CHECKLIST FOR A BETTER BACKSTROKE

～

After you have the basics of the backstroke, keep these pointers in mind as you practice.

- Keep your back straight and your head still throughout the stroke. If you tend to "sit" in the water, arch your back upward slightly and look at the ceiling.
- Tighten the buttocks but relax the waist.
- Keep your arms working continuously and in opposition to each other. There's no glide in this stroke—as one hand enters the water above your head, the other is emerging at your hip.
- Slice your hand cleanly into the water, pinky first, for the catch.
- Let the body roll naturally during phase 1 of the pull.
- As you bring your elbow close to the waist and complete phase 2 (the "ball-throwing" phase) of the pull, come close to the surface of the water, but be careful not to break it. Remember, you don't get anywhere by pushing air.
- During the recovery, keep your arm fully extended but not tense, with the wrist relaxed; imagine that your shoulder is leading the action.
- Accentuate the upbeat on the kick.

- Keep your legs underwater throughout the kick, which is a rapid but relaxed action. Although the knees bend slightly, make sure that the power comes from the hip and drives whiplike down through the leg and toward the feet. The idea is to propel a column of water backward.

- The kick accounts for one quarter of the power of this stroke, but don't overkick—just make the water "boil."

BACKSTROKE DRILLS: ARMS

These drills may be done with or without a pull-buoy for support. You might also like to try the new smaller hand paddles made especially for the backstroke, in order to provide additional resistance and a better "feel" for the water; inner tubes supply extra resistance for the more advanced swimmer, too (see page 330).

NOTE: Even though these are arm drills, some may require kicking to maintain body position and smooth motion.

1. Catch-up Backstroke: To slow down the stroke in order to articulate the bent-arm pull.

Begin by flutter kicking in the supine position with your arms extended overhead. Do the bent-arm S pull with each arm alternately, touching one to the other at the catch position before beginning the next stroke.

- Practice while standing on land, then while standing in shallow water, then while walking backward in shoulder-deep water.
- Pull for one lap doing the catch-up; then swim for one lap.
- Do half a lap catch-up; then complete the lap by swimming.
- Pull for four catch-up strokes; then complete the lap by swimming.

(If you have trouble keeping your lower body up during this drill, kick slightly, or use a pull-buoy to support you, or alter the drill by extending your arms along your sides during the catch-up (so that your arms don't touch, and you begin the stroke with the recovery instead of the catch).

2. One-arm Pulls: To even out the stroke; to develop shoulder roll; to isolate the bent-arm S pull with each arm. This drill may be done with or without kicking.

Pull with one arm at a time, keeping the nonpulling arm stretched out in the catch position.

- Pull with one arm per lap, or alternate the number of strokes done with each arm (for instance, pull eight times on the right, then eight times on the left). Or alternate in a descending/ascending progression: 8R, 8L; 4R, 4L; 2R, 2L; 1R, 1L; then 2R, 2L; 4R, 4L; 8R, 8L.

A practice variation is to swim close enough to hug the side wall of the pool in order to develop your sense of proper hand position during the bent-arm pull. Another variation is to do this drill with the nonpulling arm held at your side.

3. Glide Backstroke: To get a better "feel" for the water; to slow down the stroke in order to concentrate on stroke details; to practice body roll, and to accentuate phase 2 of the pull. This drill may be done with or without kicking.

Move both arms alternately but, at each extension of the pull, hold the hand in the overhead catch position for as long as possible, and glide in the water, feeling the body roll.

- Pull or swim for one lap doing the glide backstroke; then swim the regular backstroke for one lap.
- Pull or swim for half a lap doing the glide backstroke; then complete the lap by swimming.
- Pull for four glide backstrokes; then complete the lap by swimming.

NOTE: This is a *drill* only; when doing the backstroke, a glide is undesirable—aim for a constant motion with your arms.)

4. DPS (Distance Per Stroke): To increase the efficiency of each stroke.

Count the strokes needed to complete one lap while pulling only. On successive laps, try to lower the number of strokes needed.

Incorporate the glide backstage to slow down your stroke, and take time to exert more pressure during the bent-arm pull in order to push more still water back.

5. Double-arm Backstroke: To get a feel for the bent-arm pull by doing it with both arms simultaneously.

Do the backstroke, pulling with both arms together, and pausing at the catch to glide.

- Pull one lap of the double-arm backstroke; then swim one lap of regular backstroke.
- Use the whip kick (or frog kick) (See "Breaststroke," page 150) while pulling.
- Use the dolphin kick (see "Butterfly Stroke," page 160) while pulling.

(This drill can also be used as a stroke variation. Some swimmers find it easier than the alternating-arm windmill backstroke, or useful as a preliminary step in learning the windmill. Since you can't utilize the body roll here, the pull is shallower than in the regular backstroke.)

BACKSTROKE DRILLS: LEGS

∽

Do these drills with or without fins; fins help your ankle flexibility, which is very important in the backstroke kick. You may need to hold on to a kickboard or to support your head with a pull-buoy, but most people will find these unnecessary. Kick drills, done with no arm motion, improve the technique of your kick and strengthen the leg muscles—important in this stroke, since your body position depends on a good kick.

1. Sit and Kick: To get a "feel" for the water by keeping your ankles as loose as possible while kicking from the hip and thigh.

Flutter kick while sitting on the edge of the pool, on steps in the shallow water, or on a ladder rung.

2. Wall Kick: To practice supine kicking and to get a feel for proper body position.

With both hands, hold on to the edge of the pool, the steps in the shallow end, or a ladder. Get comfortable (the corner is the best wall position). Flutter kick in the supine position, trying to make the water just "boil," and kicking from the thigh and hip.

3. Free Kick: To practice good flutter kicking form and body position.

Flutter kick on your back with both arms extended overhead and pressed close to your ears, and with your palms touching. Keep your body as stretched and streamlined as possible, and your head stationary in line with your body. (If you need to at first, place a kickboard above your stomach, holding the edges lightly, as if you were playing a piano.)

4. Kick and Roll: To get a feel for the water in different positions; to practice body roll. (May also serve as a preliminary step in coordinating the arm and leg motions.)

Do the free-kick drill, rotating your body a quarter turn after every ten kicks. Begin in the supine position, then turn onto one side, then onto your back again, then onto the other side, and onto your back once more. Use the bent-arm pull to rotate your body and a sculling motion to raise your head when you need to inhale while you're on your side.

5. Supine Half-turns: To obtain a higher shoulder recovery; to balance body roll; to increase DPS.

Do the free-kick drill with one arm extended overhead in the catch position, the other down at your side with the shoulder raised as during the body roll.

- Kick whole laps, alternating the extended arm for each lap.
- Kick six beats, alternating arms for each set of kicks. (Change arms mid-lap by doing the bent-arm pull with the extended arm and recovering with the other.)
- Change arms after every three kicks. (This can also be a preliminary step in coordinating the arm and leg motions.)

COMMON BACKSTROKE ERRORS AND WHAT TO DO ABOUT THEM

Body Position

Error	Correction
"Sitting" in the water; body position too low, or piked at hips.	Push chest up and arch back, pressing hips closer to surface. Check head position; if too low, body will pike.
Head too far back, too far forward, and/or moving	Tuck chin in so that water barely covers ears; keep head still.

Arms: Bent-Arm Pull

Error	Correction
Flat hand entry at catch	Pinky enters first, four to eight inches under water.
Arms crossing beyond midline of body during entry	Hands should recover and enter along the shoulder line.
Stroke too fast and shallow, missing depth of pull	Do catch-up backstroke drill; concentrate on shoulder roll, pulling 1½ feet below surface and continually pushing "still" water.
Straight-arm underwater pull (thus reducing leverage)	Press "still" water with bent-arm S pull; do catch-up double-arm backstroke drill and one-arm backstroke drill.
Arm bent during recovery	For recovery, arm should be straight and directly over shoulder, close to midline of body. Arm lift natural and relaxed.
Irregular or hesitant pull	Remember opposition of arms while pulling: as one arm pulls, the other recovers.

Legs: Supine Flutter Kick

Error	Correction
Legs too high and/or bent; splashing water	Legs should just make water "boil" or foam at surface.
Stiff knees	Knees should bend slightly on upbeat (power) phase
Shallow kick	Kick should be about 1½ feet deep at lowest point; use fins during kick drills.
Toes turned outward or flexed straight up; ankles stiff	Toes should be turned inward during upbeat to push water backward.
Irregular kick	Let an even, rhythmic kick come naturally (a six-beat kick usually completes one full arm cycle).
Legs and hips too low in water	Arch back slightly and emphasize upbeat of kick.

Breathing

Error	Correction
Water washes over face, making breathing difficult	Check head and body position; keep head still and look diagonally in direction from which you are swimming.
Not exhaling completely or inhaling deeply, causing undue fatigue	Establish and maintain rhythmic inhalation and exhalation that is full and deep.

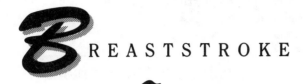

BREASTSTROKE

In its commonly used form, the breaststroke would probably win a worldwide popularity contest, thanks to its most outstanding characteristic—a relatively long, restful glide. The stroke's two other attractions are the natural way that the breathing coordinates with the lift of the head and shoulders, and its excellent visibility. All in all, this is an easy and relaxing stroke when swum slowly.

For the fitness swimmer, the breaststroke is more than a good way to vary the strenuousness and pace of a workout. It's also one of the biggest favors you can do for your inner and outer thighs as well as your inner and upper arms—areas that stubbornly resist toning and trimming during most other forms of exercise. And they don't call it the breaststroke for nothing—the arm motions give your pectorals (the muscles that help support and shape the chest area) a real workout, too. The breaststroke, by the way, is also ideal for swimming in rough water, a busy pool, or water rescues.

Historically, the breaststroke is perhaps the oldest stroke. For many centuries it was the stroke that swimmers learned. It's long been a favorite for recreational and practical purposes, too, especially in Europe. The breaststroke was also the first stroke to be used in competition. Now it's the slowest of the competitive strokes, because of the resistance encountered by the underwater recovery of the arms and legs. But it's still the preferred stroke of many, and actually becomes quite strenuous and surprisingly fast when swum at the competitive level. Anita Nall and Mike Barrowman, 1992 Olympic breaststroke champions and record holders, have demonstrated how powerful and fast this stroke can be swum, using recently developed techniques.

LEARNING THE BREASTSTROKE

~

The conventional breaststroke, which had been around for hundreds of years pretty much unchanged, has recently undergone major revisions. These exciting, speed-inducing innovations have naturally been adopted by successful record-breaking swimmers, but they also make the stroke more effective for swimmers on virtually every level.

The most substantial change has been in the kick. Originally, almost everyone did a wide frog kick, in which the knees lead as they bend and the legs simultaneously sweep outward in a broad curve and finish by squeezing together while fully extended. Now the newer, narrower, and more efficient whip kick is recommended; in this kick much of the propulsion comes from the calf and foot. The arm stroke has also been improved—from an upside-down heart-shaped pull that allows one to press "still" water backward, to using a sculling motion for greater propulsion.

In the breaststroke, the leg motion ideally supplies 50 percent of the forward propulsion. However, if you have a strong whip kick, by all means take advantage of it and allow your legs to supply more than half the power. In the breaststroke, unlike in the freestyle, backstroke, or butterfly, you can't really overkick.

Body Position

As you'll see later, the hips and body (and sometimes the shoulders, too) undulate slightly during the course of the stroke cycle, but basically your body is in a prone, face-downward, streamlined position. At the beginning of the stroke, your arms should be extended straight out in front of you with hands together, palms down, thumbs slanted slightly downward, angled about four to eight inches below the surface. Your legs should be extended with your hips and feet just underwater.

Arm Motion

In the breaststroke, the arms move simultaneously and symmetrically underwater throughout the entire stroke, beginning with arms extended overhead. Both arms moving together trace the outline of an upside-down

The breaststroke.

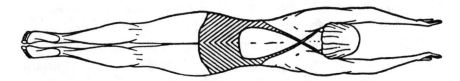

The catch.

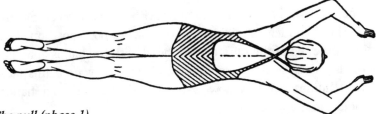

The pull (phase 1).

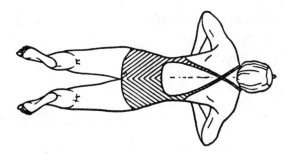

The pull (phase 2).

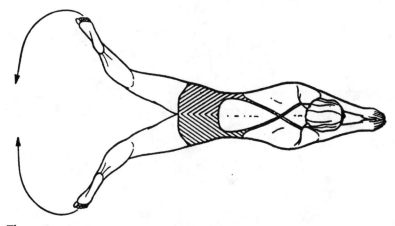

The recovery.

heart shape during the pull: a smooth, outward, and downward pull in phase 1, and an accelerated, inward sculling movement in phase 2. Then both arms extend overhead and straight underwater for the recovery.

Practice just the arm motion, then add coordinated breathing as described later. Work in shoulder-deep water, first just standing, then walking forward as the arm motion propels you through the water. To learn sculling, review the sculling arm motion for treading on pages 68–69.

THE CATCH

Start and end each stroke cycle by reaching with your arms completely extended overhead and legs straight in a streamlined body position. The catch begins at the top of the upside-down heart with the hands approximately shoulder width apart. Turn your hands so that your palms face outward with thumbs pointing downward. You should feel your hands getting a "hold" on the water.

THE PULL

This is the power part of the arm motion. To get the most leverage, keep your elbows higher than your hands throughout.

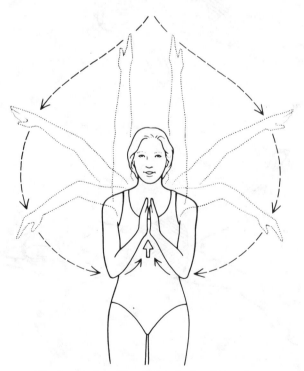

The heart-shaped pull for the breaststroke.

PHASE 1: After the catch, pull by moving your arms diagonally outward, keeping elbows slightly bent. This pull ends approximately at the shoulders.

PHASE 2: Turn your hands inward with thumbs pointing up, bring your forearms inward under your chest, then squeeze your elbows together, completing the bottom of the heart shape. This motion creates a high upper-body position. Your shoulders and head rise up here to allow you to take a breath.

THE RECOVERY

This should be a smooth, natural motion that blends imperceptibly with the end of the pull. With your hands four to eight inches underwater, elbows close to your body, and your arms as parallel to the surface as possible, quickly bring your arms forward into a streamlined position. You can recover your hands with palms together, in a prayer position; or palms up, with little fingers touching; or overlapping, palms either up or down. Use whatever is most comfortable for you. Since this is the recovery, not the power phase of the stroke, the important thing is to keep your arms relaxed to give them a short rest, and to get the hands into a palms-down position as quickly as possible to help streamline your body. During the recovery, your head and shoulders will drop back down in the water to their starting position; as your arms extend fully, you'll be ready for the catch, which begins the next stroke.

Refined Breaststroke Arm Motion

For the competitive breaststroker, the arm pull is often described as a sculling action. At the catch, the arms scull outward, followed by an inward scull. Propulsion is obtained equally from both the outward and the inward scull.

Recovery for some swimmers occurs with hands actually breaking the surface of the water. To achieve this type of recovery, head and shoulders must ride high in the water.

To help perfect this motion, practice sculling drills, such as vertical treading.

Leg Motion

There are two basic leg motions—the frog and whip kicks—that are used when swimming breaststroke. Unlike the flutter kick, these leg motions are simultaneous and symmetrical.

The propulsion from the traditional frog kick comes from the legs sweeping outward and then squeezing together to compress the water. This is basically the same principle that oars use to propel a rowboat. The whip kick, on the other hand, is more like the propeller action that drives a motorboat. It results in a more direct application of backward force, in a faster tempo, and in a more streamlined overall stroke. However, the whip kick requires more flexibility in the knees, ankles, and feet, and may place more of a stress on your knees. (See Swimmers' Shape-ups, page 371.) You might begin with a modified whip kick, in which you separate your knees only slightly beyond the hip width. Then you can gradually work up to the narrow whip described above. Whatever variation of the kick you do, use how your knees feel as an indicator of your kick.

Practice on dry land by lying face down on a bench, or by sitting in a chair (brace yourself with your arms). Next, kick while holding on to the edge of the pool or a step; finally, progress to the kick drills below.

Whip Kick: In the whip kick, with legs extended and together, begin by bringing your heels together up close to your buttocks. Bend your hips as little as possible. Allow your knees to separate to no more than hip width as you rotate your feet outward. Your feet are flexed at this point, and your lower legs form a V. Immediately "whip" your lower legs down, around, and together in an outward and backward semicircle, straightening your knees and pointing your feet during the accelerated snap. This circular, backward motion—with the sole, instep, and calf—presses almost directly back on the water and is the main propulsive force behind the kick. Even though they don't seem to move very much, the power actually comes mainly from the hip and thigh muscles. The kick ends with the legs fully extended and pressed together, toes pointed for maximum streamlining.

Frog Kick: In the traditional frog kick, you begin by separating your knees wider than your hips and bringing them to your chest, so that your legs make a diamond shape. Then you straighten your legs, spread them wide apart, and stretch your feet out to the sides, forming a wide V. Then you squeeze your legs together to complete the kick, extending your legs completely and pointing your toes for a streamlined position.

Breathing

Inhale when the head and shoulders rise together during the sculling phase of the pull. Exhale as your face submerges during the recovery. Ideally, your head should remain still in relation to the rest of your body. Try to have the sensation that your head is motionless and that the water is rising and falling around it. Be careful not to nod your head.

Coordinating Arms, Legs, and Breathing

Although there is some overlap, the basic sequence is: "pull (inhale), kick, and glide." Bend your knees to begin the kick when the arms are just finishing the pull and are under your chest. As your arms are beginning the recovery, your knees are bent to their fullest. Then both arms and legs move simultaneously to finish the stroke, with everything fully extended and streamlined for the catch, during which your body should be rail straight and gliding. Note that your legs remain in the streamlined position a bit longer than your arms do, since the kick begins only after your arms are well into the pull.

CHECKLIST FOR A BETTER BREASTSTROKE

➤

As you practice, remember these tips:

- Keep your head still, with your chin jutting out slightly.
- For the catch, keep your elbows straight with your hands facing outward; your thumbs are pointing down.
- The outward pull goes only to shoulder height.
- Inhale quickly when your head and shoulder rise naturally as a result of the inward scull. Try not to lift your head any farther than you have to.
- Begin the whip kick as your arms start the pull.
- Aim for a narrow kick—when your heels come up toward the buttocks, the knees, ideally, should be no farther than hip width apart. But modify the kick according to your comfort and ability.
- Snap your lower legs and feet together in a downward arc to get a whiplike action that propels water directly backward.

- Be as streamlined and extended as possible during the glide, and hold it for as long as your momentum will allow.

- Try *downstreaming,* a technique used in competitive swimming to gain more speed. Here's how its done: at the end of the kick and the beginning of the glide, squeeze arms covering ears, lift the hips, legs, and feet up to the surface of the water so that they are higher than the hands. This creates a "downstream position"— almost as if you were swimming downhill. Since this follows the rise and fall of the torso during the pull, you move in a wavelike motion, which gets your hips higher and your entire body involved in the stroke. (This is similar to the undulation found in the butterfly stroke, in which your body is alternately piked and arched.)

- Remember your coordination: pull (inhale), kick, and glide.

BREASTSTROKE DRILLS: ARMS

～

These drills may be done with or without a pull-buoy for support, and, for the more advanced swimmer, with or without additional resistance devices such as hand paddles (see page 329). Pull drills are done with just the arms; use your legs where indicated.

1. Vertical Treading: Stand in chin-deep water and review sculling arm motion for treading. Create a figure 8 with each arm simultaneously, keeping arms at chest level (see treading, page 68). Scull outward with thumbs down and scull inward with thumbs up. Bend your knees to keep your feet off the bottom and support your body with the sculling arm motion only.

2. Progressive Sculling: To work toward the breaststroke heart-shaped arm motion with coordinated breathing.

First standing, then walking, in shoulder-deep water, extend your arms straight out in front of you, palms facing out, and begin to make small outward circles with your wrists, flexing them downward while pushing outward, then sculling them inward. Gradually progress to a larger pull, but don't bring your hands farther than shoulder height.

3. DPS (Distance Per Stroke):   To maximize the efficiency of your stroke.

Count the strokes you need to complete a lap while only pulling, or while swimming. On succeeding laps, try to decrease the number of strokes needed.

BREASTSTROKE DRILLS: LEGS

These drills may be done with or without a kickboard; you'll obtain better body position without one. During the drills, do the frog, whip, or modified whip kick, whichever you prefer, unless specified otherwise. In kick drills, only the legs are used; this allows you to improve your leg strength and to concentrate on your kicking mechanics.

1. Sit and Kick: To get a "feel" for the kick.

Sit on the pool deck, a step, or a ladder rung, your legs extended to the water's edge. Do the frog kick or whip kick, analyzing your form. Pay particular attention to the position of the feet during the whip, as this is the trickiest part of the action to master.

2. Wall Kick: To practice good kicking form.

In supine position: Hold on to the wall with your back toward it, your arms extended to either side. Practice kicking, paying close attention to your form.

In prone position: Facing the pool edge, grasp the gutter with one hand and press the other hand flat against the wall, fingers pointed downward, approximately two feet below the water line. Practice your kick, being careful not to break the surface.

3. Free Kick: To practice kicking form; to increase the power of the kick; to get the feel of correct body position.

In prone position: Extend your arms straight in front of you, with or without a kickboard, and kick several laps. If you use a kickboard, either keep your head above water and breathe normally or coordinate the inhalation and exhalation with the kick. If no kickboard is used, scull outward with your hands to raise your shoulders and head when you need to inhale.

In supine position: Support yourself by holding a kickboard over the abdomen, your fingers resting lightly on the sides. Kick several laps.

4. *Prone and Supine Heel Touch:* To develop flexibility and power in your whip kick; to balance and narrow the stroke.

Do the whip kick with your hands resting on your buttocks, trying to touch your heels to your hands. Inhale as your knees come up to your hands.

5. *Vertical Kick:* To strengthen the kick.

With arms motionless in the water or above the surface (the higher the arms, the harder the drill), practice the whip kick while in a vertical position. As a variation, try the egg-beater kick described on page 378.

BREASTSTROKE DRILLS: COORDINATION AND BODY POSITION

～

Because of the nature of this stroke, the coordination of the arm and leg motions affects the body's position in the water. The drills that include the dolphin kick help you to get the feel of the wavelike action called *downstreaming,* where the hips and legs lift up.

1. *Pull with Dolphin Kick:* To get a wavelike action in the body (downstreaming).

Alternate one breaststroke pull, then one dolphin kick for an entire lap. Swim the next lap with the regular breaststroke, using the whip or frog kick, and trying to incorporate the wavelike action into your stroke.

2. *Double-arm Backstroke with Kick:* To coordinate the kick with a double arm motion without rhythmic breathing.

For the first lap, do the double-arm backstroke (both arms pulling together) with the whip or frog kick. For the next lap, swim the regular breaststroke.

3. *Pull-Pull-Kick or Pull-Kick-Kick:* For variety; to help you get a feel for the undulating body motion; to concentrate on the pull.

- Alternate two arm pulls with one whip kick or frog kick for one lap; then swim the next lap normally.
- Alternate one arm pull with two whip kicks or frog kicks for one lap; then swim the next lap normally.
- Do one arm pull, then one whip kick, then one dolphin kick, and so on, for one lap; then swim the next lap normally.

- Another variation is to alternate one pull with two whip kicks followed by two dolphin kicks.

4. Push-off: To check streamlining; to slow down the parts of the stroke in order to feel each one better.

Push off the wall of the pool underwater and see how far you can go with one slow pull-kick-glide.

BREASTSTROKE DRILL: BREATHING
❧

Breathing during the breaststroke occurs as the head and shoulders naturally lift out of the water as a result of the inward arm motion (phase 2 of the pull). So practice the coordination during the arm, leg, and body position drills described earlier. To increase your breathing capacity, try this one.

Coordinated Breathing: Stand in chest-deep water. In slow motion, practice coordinating each breaststroke arm pull with a breath. Be certain to inhale and exhale fully.

COMMON BREASTSTROKE ERRORS AND WHAT TO DO ABOUT THEM
❧

Body Position

Error	Correction
Body not streamlined	Stretch and extend the body during the glide; practice push-off drill for "downstreaming" effect.
Body position too low	Accentuate upward hip motion; practice breaststroke arm pull with dolphin kick.
Hips too high	Straighten body line at waist. Arch lower back to raise upper body.
Body off center, tipped to one side	Contract the muscles slightly on alternate sides of body to help shift and balance body position; do pulling and kicking drills to even out stroke.

Arms: The Heart-Shaped Pull

Error	Correction
Pull too long	Pull outward just to shoulder level; do progressive-sculling drill.
Hands pointed upward, losing leverage and "slipping" through the water	Elbows should be higher than hands; palms face outward for catch of stroke; do DPS and vertical treading drills.
Recovery of hands is forced; or hands are flexed upward so that they push water forward	During recovery, hand position should be natural, with fingertips slightly downward. Experiment to find what feels best for you.
Elbows bend outward during recovery, increasing water resistance	Keep elbows close to rib cage, forearms squeezed together, as arms drive forward in a streamlined position.
Arms move too fast or too flat, thereby "slipping" through the water	Do vertical treading and progressive sculling drills.
Hesitation between pull and recovery	Keep entire arm stroke smooth and continuous. Exhale with face underwater immediately after inhalation.

Legs: The Whip Kick

～

Error	Correction
Feet break surface of water during recovery	Increase hip flexion slightly and lift head upward to keep feet just below surface.
Feet slide through the water rather than catching water to push it backward	Flex ankles so that soles of feet "catch" water as power phase of pull begins; do sit-and-kick drill.
Toes turned inward	Turn and flex feet outside of knees; do sit-and-kick drill.

Error	Correction
Knees move outside hip, and legs are too wide	Knees should be parallel to each other at approximately hip width; do sit-and-kick, wall-kick drills.
One leg "hooks" higher than the other; one foot breaks surface (This is illegal in competition.)	Legs should move simultaneously and parallel to each other; practice wall-kick drill.
Legs too low, kick drags	Lift hips and feet at end of kick (dolphinlike hip action).

Breathing

Error	Correction
Head lifts and lowers (nods) independently of shoulders	Keep head forward and moving in relation to water level; head and shoulders should move as one.
Holding breath and keeping head underwater	Lift head during every stroke; breathe rhythmically. Do coordinated breathing drill.

Breaststroke Coordination

Error	Correction
Breathing too early or too late	Head lifts for inhalation as arm pull finishes and leg kick begins; do progressive sculling and coordinated breathing drills.
Lack of power and smoothness during propulsion phases	Practice pull-pull-kick and pull-kick-kick drills.
Arms and legs move continuously, eliminating glide	Shorten pull to shoulder line; keep arms and legs still during glide. Begin with progressive sculling drill.

Error	Correction
Components of stroke out of sequence	Isolate and practice arm and leg movements separately before combining them; remember, pull (inhale), kick, glide.

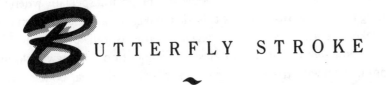

BUTTERFLY STROKE

The butterfly can be the most exciting and graceful stroke to swim and to watch: where else can you find such sinuous, flowing movement combined with an exhilarating sense of power? Although the "fly" is usually considered the most difficult stroke to master, you can actually learn it fairly easily by applying the basic S pull used in the crawl or freestyle. There's no denying that the butterfly is a strenuous stroke, though—even well-trained "fliers" stick to swims of a relatively short distance. (You'll notice that when it's introduced in the workouts you rarely swim the butterfly continuously for more than twenty-five yards or meters, whereas you do many times that distance for every other stroke.)

The butterfly has much in common with the breaststroke, from which it is derived, in that both arms and legs move simultaneously and symmetrically. But swimmers and coaches had long realized that the resistance caused by the underwater arm recovery of the breaststroke slowed the stroke down. In 1933 Henry Meyer had the idea of trying an over-the-water recovery. The resulting hybrid stroke was still within the rules for competitive breaststroke swimming, but a new and superior stroke was born with the substitution of the dolphin kick for the whip or frog kick. In 1952 the "butterfly," as the new stroke was called, was accepted as an official competitive stroke, and by 1956 it was a part of the Olympics. Mark Spitz, winner of seven Olympic golds in 1972, brought the "fly" into the limelight, as did 1988/1992 Olympic Champion Matt Biondi and 1992 Olympic wonder Pablo Morales.

During its short life, the butterfly hasn't undergone quite as many refinements as the other, older strokes have. Back in the early days, the frog kick was used; in fact, some people still prefer it, especially when first learning the stroke. But because this kick makes for a rather uneven overall stroke, eventually swimmers developed the fishtail, or dolphin kick, which is now required in all but Masters competition. The new kick, used in conjunction with the S-pattern underwater pull that has done so much for the other strokes, makes the butterfly very fast, and its popularity has soared.

LEARNING THE BUTTERFLY

◄

Yes, the butterfly has earned the reputation of being "the hard stroke." And it is true that many swimmers experience frustration when first learning it—even those who eventually learn it well enough to do it in competition. But there must be some reason why so many people keep trying until they get it right. And the butterfly isn't really all that difficult once you've learned the basic mechanics and can relax and get into the rhythm of it. If you keep at it, the day will come when you find yourself doing the "fly."

The "fly" requires a different kind of stamina than the other strokes, which makes it a superb cardiovascular conditioner. That's because there's none of the alternating motion of the freestyle or backstroke, in which one arm rests during the recovery while the other works during the pull phase. You also need more overall flexibility for the butterfly, especially in the shoulders, hips, ankles, and feet, as well as greater upper-body strength. So weight training and stretches (see "Swimmers' Shape-ups," page 371) are definite aids to learning and practicing the "fly."

The buterly shares with the breaststroke the simultaneous underwater pull. In addition, the kick, which usually accounts for 30 percent of the stroke's power, helps to set up an undulating, dolphinlike motion through the body that resembles in part the downstreaming used in the breaststroke. The butterfly has so much in common with the breaststroke, in fact, that it may be wise to master the breaststroke as a preliminary to learning the "fly." (And once you've mastered the butterfly, you'll be rewarded with a better breaststroke!)

Another general tip when training in the butterfly is to stick to distances that allow you to maintain a semblance of the stroke. When your stroke begins to deteriorate, it's a sure sign that you should go on to something else.

The butterfly stroke.

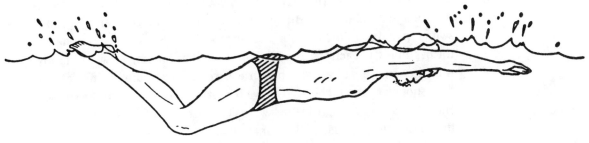

The catch.

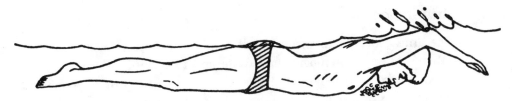

The pull (phase 1).

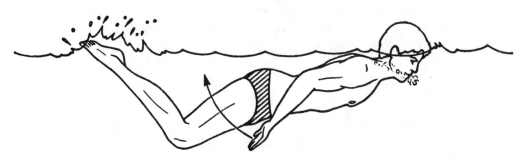

The pull (phase 2).

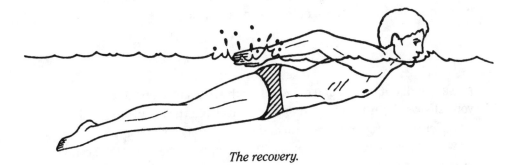

The recovery.

Body Position

In the butterfly, as in the breaststroke, your body sets up a wavelike motion that adds grace and efficiency to the stroke. In general, your body swims in a streamlined, prone position, with arms and legs extended at the beginning of each stroke cycle. You should be looking forward slightly, with the water about even with your eyebrows (except during inhalation). Your shoulders should be high above the water and parallel to the surface. Hips are generally high in the water. (Women, by the way, tend to find this part easier because of their anatomy.)

Arm Motion

The arms move simultaneously and evenly in a mirror image of each other, with each arm moving underwater in an S-shaped pattern.

Since the arms move simultaneously, however, the stroke resembles an hourglass or keyhole. Also, since there's no side-to-side body roll, the underwater pull is shallower and the overwater recovery is wider and lower. As in the other strokes, keep your elbows higher than your hands to get the best leverage.

Practice the arm stroke on land, then in shoulder-deep water (first just standing, then walking); next, when the arm motion alone is comfortable, begin to work on coordinating it with the breathing.

THE CATCH

Hands enter the water together, shoulder width apart: your elbows are up and your thumbs are down, as in the crawl/freestyle. Slide your hands forward, outward, and downward at a 30- to 45-degree angle from the water's surface, to a depth of four to eight inches. This is the "catch," during which you should get a good "hold" on the water. You have only a moment to do this, because of the timing of the kick.

THE PULL

PHASE 1: Pull out, down, and back with both arms simultaneously, bending your elbows slightly and rotating your arms from the shoulders. End this phase with your forearms vertical and palms facing back toward your feet, no wider than shoulder width apart. This completes the top of the keyhole or hourglass shape.

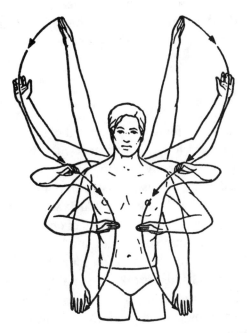

The keyhole-shaped pull for the butterfly stroke.

PHASE 2: This is the acceleration phase of the pull. Begin by bringing your hands together under your abdomen so that your elbows bend at about 90 degrees; then press outward and back toward your feet, as for the crawl stroke, accelerating the movement begun in phase 1. Continue pressing water directly backward, until your arms are almost fully extended and your hands are just past your hips. (This will begin to raise your shoulders out of the water and is the time to inhale, as described later.)

THE RECOVERY

As your hands emerge from the water, swing them around to the sides and front. The elbows are higher than the hands, and the arms are rounded, with the fingertips skimming just above the surface. At the start of the recovery, your hands trail behind, and your elbows lead the swing; about halfway, the hands take over the lead as the forearms extend in front of you just prior to the catch. During the initial part of the recovery, your arms should be relaxed, but they should move quickly, using the power generated by your upper back and shoulders during the acceleration phase of the pull. Then the momentum continues to carry your arms forward, to begin the catch again. Your shoulders are higher in the water during the recovery than at any other point; as the hands come forward, the shoulders return to their lower position. This shoulder undulation contributes to, and coordinates with, the wavelike motion of the hips and legs.

Leg Motion

The dolphin kick accounts for about 30 percent of the power of the overall stroke and must be carefully coordinated with the arm motion, the breathing, and the wavelike body motion.

The aim of the dolphin kick is to push a column of "still" water backward quickly and forcefully. It's a two-beat kick, with both legs moving up and down together twice, during the course of one arm cycle. It's similar to the flutter kick except that your knees and hips bend a bit more, and of course, both legs move in unison. Bring your hips up during the downbeat so that your buttocks just break the surface, and bring them down during the upbeat—this results in a sinuous, undulating motion that adds to your forward power by getting your whole body, not just your limbs, involved in the stroke.

On the downbeat of the kick, the feet should be pointed to help them direct the water backward, not downward, and to continue the undulation that began in your hips. On the upbeat, your feet should just break the surface. Practice while sitting on a chair on dry land, then proceed to the kick drills described later.

Breathing

For maximum streamlining and efficiency, the ideal breathing pattern is to inhale on every other stroke (alternate breathing). However, because of the intense, explosive action of the butterfly, you may find that this is not enough. So establish and stay with a breathing pattern that is comfortable for you. This might be a breath on every stroke, or you might alternate a single breath with a double breath—i.e., stroke, stroke (breathe); stroke (breathe); stroke, stroke (breathe); and so on.

Practice coordinating the breathing with the arm motion, first on land, then while standing in shoulder-deep water, and finally during the drills that follow.

Inhale at the end of phase 2 of the arm pull, just as the arms are beginning to recover and your shoulders are at their highest. Extend your chin slightly forward—just enough to get your mouth out of the water. As you lift, look forward and take a big bite of air. Then lower your head immediately to restore the streamlined body position. (Some people prefer to turn the head to one side during the inhalation because in this position the "bow wave" from the head allows them to get a breath while keeping the cheek closer to the water.)

Coordinating Arms, Legs, and Breathing

The common kick cycle is two beats per arm stroke. The downbeat of the first kick begins when your hands are shoulder width apart and have entered the water for the catch. This kick is completed during phase 1 of the pull and is followed by a quick upbeat when your arms are between phase 1 and phase 2, at the narrowest point of the keyhole or S. Then the downbeat of the second kick synchronizes with the explosive finish of phase 2 of the arm motion. There is a second, relaxed upbeat kick during the arm recovery of the stroke.

To coordinate breathing, begin inhaling at the completion of your arm stroke, so that your mouth clears the water as your arms recover.

To coordinate your entire stroke, swim in the following sequence: catch and kick, pull and kick, inhale and recover. Most simply, this coordination can be thought of as a downbeat kick at the beginning and at the end of each arm stroke, with inhalation taking place at the start of the recovery. Use the drills that follow to help you get the timing.

CHECKLIST FOR A BETTER BUTTERFLY STROKE

～

- Hands enter thumb first at a 30- to 45-degree angle from the water surface; it's essential to "grab hold" of the water immediately at the "catch" of the stroke.

- At entry, hands should be approximately shoulder width apart; elbows are bent and higher than the hands.

- During phase 1 of the pull, your hands should pull shoulder width apart, outward and downward. The phase finishes with your forearms in a vertical position.

- During phase 2, accelerate the pull, pushing water backward toward your feet.

- The ideal breathing pattern is one inhalation every other arm stroke, but adapt this to your own needs; inhale when your shoulders are highest, at the end of phase 2 of the pull; raise your head just high enough for your mouth to clear the water.

- Economize on the recovery—your arms should barely clear the water. Keep the arms relaxed, elbows turned slightly upward.
- The ideal kick cycle is two beats per arm stroke. The first kick occurs during the "catch" and phase 1 of the arm pull; the second kick occurs during phase 2 of the arm pull.
- Get a whipping action by pointing your toes during the downbeat. Relax your feet during the upbeat of the kick.
- To coordinate the stroke elements, remember: catch and kick, pull and kick, inhale and recover.

BUTTERFLY DRILLS: ARMS

These drills may be done with or without pull-buoys for support. To build upper body strength during the arm drills, the more advanced swimmer can use resistance devices such as an inner tube, or "donut," around the ankles, or pull-buoys between the ankles.

1. Progressive Pulling: To first learn the keyhole arm pull without becoming fatigued by the overwater recovery; to gradually develop strength and flexibility in order to do the overwater recovery.

Practice the butterfly arm pull, but recover arms under the water, as in the breaststroke. See how far you can glide after each pull—the greater the distance, the more efficient your stroke.

When this drill is comfortable and your pull is strong, switch to the overwater recovery, breathing whenever necessary; practice first while standing, then while walking, in shoulder-deep water.

- Do two butterfly pulls with the overwater recovery; then complete the lap using the underwater recovery. Continue practicing, trying to use the overwater recovery for longer and longer distances.
- Another variation is to alternate four pulls with overwater recovery and four pulls with underwater recovery.

2. Free-fly Pull: To keep pull balanced on both sides; to practice coordination of stroke and breathing; to experiment with your own breathing pattern and stroke coordination.

Alternate keyhole butterfly pull with catch-up freestyle pull (see page 125).

- Variation 1—two butterfly pulls
    one catch-up freestyle pull—*right* arm
    two butterfly pulls
    one catch-up freestyle pull—*left* arm
    and so on

- Variation 2—one butterfly pull
    one catch-up freestyle cycle (*right and left*)
    one butterfly pull

- Make up your own variations. But begin with one pattern and stay with it throughout the drill.

Throughout the drill, as always, inhale during the catch-up freestyle with your head turned to the side. During the butterfly, you may inhale with your face either forward or to the side, whichever is more comfortable (the forward breathing style is more common).

3. DPS (Distance Per Stroke):   To develop maximum stroke efficiency for the advanced butterflier.

Count the number of pulls you need per lap, trying to decrease the number each time by streamlining your stroke. To do this, pause momentarily at the catch position and take advantage of the glide. (Remember, though, this is a *drill*; while swimming the actual stroke, the catch position is held for a shorter time, keeping the glide to a minimum.)

BUTTERFLY DRILLS: LEGS

➤

Some of these drills may be done with a kickboard or other flotation device. They may be done with or without fins. Fins are especially recommended for practicing the dolphin kick, because they help you get a feel for the whipping motion that you're trying for. Fins also give you added propulsion, and they help you to build up your leg strength by increasing the resistance of the water.

1. Stand and Kick: To get a feel for the wavelike body motion initiated in the lower-back muscles.

While standing on dry land or in chest-deep water, do a half knee bend. From this bent-knee position, tilt your hips out to the back; then press your hips and lower back forward forcefully as you straighten and stand. Also practice this kick in deep water, with your body in vertical position.

2. Sit and Kick: To help you learn the bent-knee action of the dolphin kick.

Sit on the edge of the pool, with hips forward. Bend your knees so that your heels drop and touch the wall beneath the surface of the water. From this position, extend your legs again, feeling the water roll off the front of your foot.

3. Wall Kick: To get the feel of doing the kick in the water; to help you get your lower back arched slightly while practicing the kick.

In supine position: Hold on to the wall with your back against it, your head resting on the trough and your arms extended out to either side. Practice the dolphin kick, watching your form carefully to make sure that your legs just break the water surface.

In prone position: Facing the wall, pull on the gutter with one hand and press the other hand flat against the wall, fingers pointed downward, one to two feet below the surface. Practice the dolphin kick, including the undulation that travels from the lower back and hips toward the legs and feet.

4. Free Kick: To help streamline your body during the stroke; to develop good kicking form; to increase the strength of your kick.

Floating in a prone position, dolphin kick with your arms extended overhead so that they cover your ears. To inhale, scull momentarily and lift your head out of the water (either straight forward or to one side). Or, if you like, keep your arms at your sides so that you can concentrate on the kick. If you use a kickboard, try the two-beat kick. You can either keep your head up and breathe normally or coordinate the inhalation with every other kick. You may also practice this drill in a supine position.

5. Side Kick: To help develop the wavelike motion of the hips and legs as well as the body undulation during the dolphin kick.

Dolphin kick while on your side, your lower hand extended overhead, holding a kickboard, and your top arm resting on your thigh. To inhale, scull or pull underwater with the extended arm and lift your head slightly to get a breath; if you use a kickboard, coordinate the breathing and kicking as in the free-kick drill. Alternate sides.

6. Kick and Roll: To practice the wavelike motion of the kick; to practice coordinating the arm and leg motions.

Do the side-kick drill, changing positions after every ten kick cycles.

Start on one side; then rotate your body a quarter turn to kick in the prone position; then rotate another quarter turn to kick on your other side; then rotate to the prone position again, and so on.

7. Body Wave: To get the feel of the undulating body motion that comes from the dolphin kick; to help develop breath control.

Pushing off from the pool bottom, your arms extended overhead, dive over the surface of the water, arching your back and bringing your body into a "hole" created by your arms (like a porpoise or dolphin). Submerge and touch your hands to the bottom, then draw your knees up to your chest in a tuck position. Plant your feet firmly on the bottom and spring up, arms extended overhead, to repeat the drill.

- Under-under Variation: Dolphin kick underwater, arms either extended in front of you or down at your sides, for as long as you can.
- Under-over Variation: Do this drill in deep water without touching bottom. Dolphin kick underwater for as long as you can, then resurface, inhale, and do four kick cycles on the surface. This drill can be done in pyramid pattern (i.e., two kick cycles above, two below; four above, four below; six above, six below; four above, four below; two above, two below; etc.)

BUTTERFLY DRILLS: COORDINATION
➤

1. Single-arm Pull with Single-beat Kick: To develop coordination of arms, legs, and breathing.

Do one dolphin kick with each arm stroke. Begin by inhaling on every stroke, then work up to alternate breathing.

2. Two-beat Kick with Delayed Pull: To further coordinate the double-beat dolphin kick with the butterfly pull.

Do one butterfly pull with one dolphin kick; keep your arms extended forward in the catch position as you complete the second kick. Make the glide gradually shorter at the start of each stroke.

3. Progressive Pull with Two-beat Kick: To isolate coordination of the two-beat kick at the beginning and end of the pull.

Practice the butterfly pull, but recover your arms underwater, and kick at the beginning and at the end of the pull. See how far you can glide after each pull-and-kick cycle before recovering your arms underwater.

4. Butterfly Pull with Breaststroke (Whip) Kick: To get a feel for the overall stroke; a preliminary step in coordinating arms, legs, and breathing.

Do one butterfly pull for each whip kick. Begin the kick as the hands enter the water for the catch of the stroke. When both pull and kick have finished, glide a moment before beginning the next cycle.

This stroke variation can be used either as a drill or as a stroke itself. Some people also find that this variation helps them to get the flexibility needed for the dolphin kick. So before skipping over the butterfly stroke, try this variation—you might like it, especially since the glide gives you a momentary rest between stroke cycles.

5. Double-arm Backstroke with Whip or Dolphin Kick (Double-arm or Inverted Butterfly):   To develop the flexibility needed for the overwater arm recovery; to practice phase 2 (acceleration phase) of the pull while breathing normally.

On your back, do the double-arm or inverted butterfly arm motion with either a single whip kick or a single- or double-beat dolphin kick.

Butterfly Drills: Breathing

～

Since breathing for this stroke coordinates naturally with the arm motion, as you practice the pulling drills you'll be practicing breathing as well. As your pull and kick become stronger, your head will lift high enough out of the water for inhalation. To help increase your lung capacity and help you get a "second wind," the body-wave drill (page 169) and its variations are also especially useful.

1. Pull-and-breathe Drill: To develop an inhalation pattern with the butterfly arm motion.

Begin by standing in place and coordinating a single breath with the pull; then walk forward while adding the alternate breathing pattern. Concentrate on exhaling during phase 2 of the pull and inhaling immediately after the arm recovery begins.

2. Freestyle Pull and Dolphin Kick: To develop an alternate breathing pattern and a sense of timing.

Do the freestyle arm motion, dolphin kicking as you execute phase 2 of each pull. Inhale to the side, as in the freestyle, as you begin the recovery of every other arm cycle (every four strokes).

COMMON BUTTERFLY ERRORS AND
WHAT TO DO ABOUT THEM
❧

Body Position and Breathing

Error	Correction
Head stays up too long during inhalation	Return head to downward position immediately after inhalation.
Early or late inhalation	Lift head to inhale toward end of phase 2 of pull, just prior to recovery.
Head lifts too high during inhalation	Lift your head only high enough for your mouth to clear the water. Keep your chin forward.
Holding breath; or sporadic breathing pattern	Be certain to inhale and exhale fully and continuously. Do freestyle pull and dophin-kick drill.
Stiff body position	Add undulating body-wave action to stroke; do body-wave drill.

Arms: Keyhole Pull

Error	Correction
Arms pull straight back, "slipping" through the water	Isolate two-stage keyhole arm motion, always pressing "still" water back; do DPS drill.
Arms cross, or enter too far to sides, during catch	Arms should enter water shoulder width apart.
Arms are too low during recovery	Lift elbows to clear arms from water during recovery; do progressive-pull drill.
Hands splash excessively during entry	Slice hands into water at 30- to 45-degree angle, thumbs downward.
Arms aren't moving together during recovery	Move arms simultaneously throughout pull; do free-fly pull drill.

Legs: The Dolphin Kick

Error	Correction
Body wave is absent and body remains stiff during the two-beat kick	Practice body-wave action in the side-kick drill; do body-wave drill.
Knees bend without body-wave action	On the downbeat of each kick, lift your hips; on the upbeat lower them; do stand-and-kick, wall-kick drills.
Legs lift above water; knees bend too much	Just break water's surface; extend legs backward; do free-kick drill.
Legs move water up and down rather than backward	Try to feel the water slide backward off your feet as you kick; practice with fins to get a feel for this whipping action.

Coordination

Error	Correction
Unintentional "flutterfly" stroke done in several possible variations (i.e., butterfly pull with flutter kick, freestyle pull with fly kick)	Isolate and practice components: move both arms together and both legs together.
Too long a glide or a "dead" spot in stroke after hands enter for "catch"	Begin downbeat of first kick as you start the pull, when momentum of the stroke begins to slow.
First kick occurs too early or late	Downward beat of first kick begins during catch of pull; do progressive pull with two-beat-kick drill.
Second kick occurs too early or late	Downbeat of second kick begins with phase 2 of pull; do progressive pull with two-beat-kick drill.

Error	Correction
Coordination of stroke components out of sequence	Isolate and practice each part separately. Then combine entire stroke to: pull and kick, catch and kick, inhale, and recover.

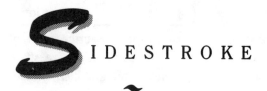

SIDESTROKE

*T*he sidestroke, which grew out of the breaststroke and the elementary backstroke, was used in competition during the nineteenth century. Although it's no longer a competitive stroke, the sidestroke is nevertheless a handy skill to have. It's easy to learn and master, and the long glide and underwater recovery make for a graceful, restful stroke useful for long, relaxing swims. It is one of the fundamental transitional strokes for synchronized swimmers. This is the preferred stroke of many recreational swimmers, especially in open water, because the face remains above the surface at all times, making breathing easy and visibility constant. For these reasons, the sidestroke is also widely used in water rescues.

Since the sidestroke is the least strenuous of the strokes, it isn't quite as effective as the other four in improving your physical fitness. However, the sidestroke is ideal for varying the pace of your workouts, or when you aren't up for so strenuous a swim.

LEARNING THE SIDESTROKE

The sidestroke differs from all the other strokes in several ways. First, you do it on your side. (Therefore, we'll be referring to the top and bottom arm or leg instead of to the right or left.) Second, it is asymmetrical— neither leg and neither arm does exactly the same thing, either simultaneously or alternately. The stroke incorporates elements from the elementary backstroke (see page 85) and the breaststroke (see page 145), so if

174

you know either of these strokes, you will recognize several similarities, including the aforementioned prolonged glide, the whiplike leg action, and several elements of the arm movement. When learning or reviewing the sidestroke, try to do it on both sides. One will probably feel more natural, but with practice, both sides can become comfortable. (Swimming the same distance on each side results in more balanced muscle development and body conditioning.)

Another way the sidestroke is unique is that there are so many variations. There are two types of arm motions and two types of leg motions, which may be combined in four different ways. When you also consider that you can do these four variations on either your right or your left side, that adds up to a total of eight variations. So try them all! You can use several in the same workout, or even in the same lap, to add variety to your swims.

Body Position

Your body is in a horizontal position on one side. One cheek rests on the water, and your neck is curved up slightly—just enough for your mouth to clear the surface. You may look upward and forward, out to the side, or slightly down and back toward the direction from which you are swimming (the last is most common).

During the glide, your body is in a straight, stretched, steamlined position. Your lower arm is extended straight ahead, covering your lower ear and continuing the line of your body; the palm is down. Your upper arm is extended and resting along your upper side, palm on your thigh. Your legs are fully extended and together, one on top of the other, in line with your body; your toes are slightly pointed.

Arm Motion

In both types of arm motion, the functions of the arm alternate: while the bottom arm is pulling, the top arm is recovering, and vice versa. The regular arm motion, in which both arms pull and recover underwater, is most common and so is described first. The action in both variations is similar to reaching overhead to pick an apple from a tree, then transferring the apple to your other hand, and throwing it down toward your feet as your "picking" arm reaches for the next apple. Unlike other strokes, the sidestroke is best understood as a *two-phased stroke* with a glide after each phase, rather than as a two-phased arm pull. (Each arm motion, though, still has a catch, a pull, and a recovery.)

The sidestroke.

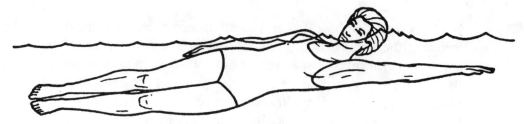

The glide.

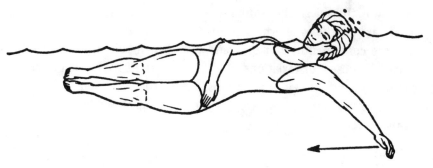

Phase 1. The bottom arm pulls as the top arm recovers.

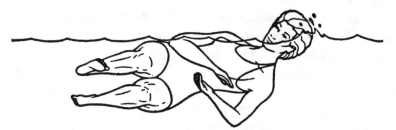

Arms meet at chest level.

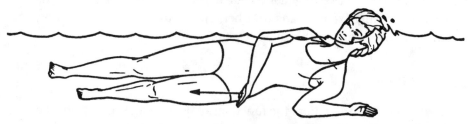

Phase 2. Top arm pulls as bottom arm recovers.

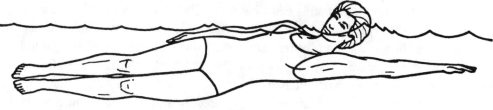

The glide.

176

Practice while standing on dry land first. Then progress to shoulder-deep water, first standing, then walking sideways, with the bottom arm extended underwater in the direction in which you are moving.

Bottom Arm (extended overhead in the glide position): To begin the catch, slide your hand four to eight inches under the surface to get a good hold on the water. To begin the pull (phase 1), bend your elbow and begin to push water straight back with your palm and inner forearm, keeping the elbow higher than the hand. When your hand and arm have reached a point just past the shoulder line, accelerate the movement and continue to press water back down toward your feet. The pull for this arm stops at chest level, and your elbow stays close to your body the whole time.

To begin the underwater recovery (phase 2), pull your elbow in closer to your chest, and rotate your forearm so that the thumb leads the movement back toward your shoulder. Keep your arm as close to your body as possible in order to minimize resistance. When your forearm is as parallel to your torso as possible, extend your arm forward and overhead back to the starting position. Hold this extended position for the glide phase of the stroke.

Top Arm: While your bottom arm is pulling, your top arm (resting along your upper side, palm on thigh) does an underwater recovery (phase 1). Slide your hand, thumb leading, up toward your shoulder; it meets and crosses your lower hand, which is just completing its pull, at approximately chest level. To begin the catch with the top arm, rotate your forearm so that the palm faces your feet. For the pull (phase 2), simply press water directly backward toward your feet, using your palm and the inside of your forearm and making sure that your elbow is higher than your hand. When your arm is completely extended, place it on your thigh and hold this position for the glide. (At this point, your bottom arm has recovered and is extended overhead.)

Overarm Variation: This is a more efficient variation in which the top arm recovers *over* the water, similar to the crawl-stroke recovery. From its extended position on the thigh (glide), raise your top arm above the surface (elbow high), then slide your hand into the water at a 30- to 45-degree angle in front of your face (catch). As your arm extends slightly, it's now ready to pull (phase 2) as usual.

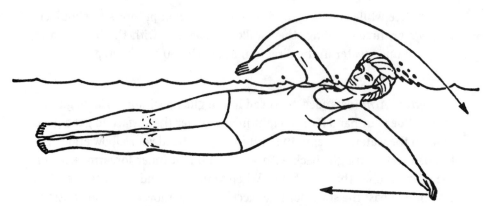

The overarm variation of the sidestroke.

Leg Motion

The leg motion used in the sidestroke is called the scissors kick because the legs separate, then come together, cutting through the water much like the blades of a pair of scissors. As with the arm stroke, there are two variations. The first described is the regular scissors kick, which is the most common.

Practice while sitting down, bracing yourself with your hands, leaning to first one and then the other side. Or, if you want, practice while lying on your side on the floor.

Begin in the glide or extended position, with your legs together and the toes pointed. Recover your knees by bringing them toward your chest, your hips flexing back slightly (phase 1). Then separate and straighten your legs, the top one moving forward and the bottom one moving backward. Separate them as much as possible, forming a wide V. Your top foot should be flexed and the lower one extended with the toes pointed behind you (catch of the feet). Next squeeze your legs together to push water backward (phase 2). As your legs meet, point your top foot—the alternate flexion and extension resembles pedaling a bicycle. Hold this position, legs together, body extended and streamlined, for the restful glide. Make sure that your legs move parallel to and stay under the surface of the water during the entire kick, and try to open each leg the same distance from the midline of your body.

Inverted Scissors Kick Variation: This is done in the same manner as the regular kick, except that the bottom leg moves forward and the top leg moves back. This kick is often used in water rescue carries for greater mobility and comfort for both the rescuer and victim.

Breathing

Your breathing should be regular and continuous. Inhale during phase 1 as your bottom arm pulls and your top arm and your legs recover. Begin exhaling during phase 2 as your lower arm recovers, your legs snap together, and your top arm pulls; continue to exhale during the glide.

Coordinating the Arms and Legs

Remember, this stroke can be simplified into two phases. Think of phase 1 as ending in a tight contraction, as everything in your body bends and comes together at once at your midpoint. Think of phase 2 as a return to a stretch as everything straightens and extends to its fullest; hold this for the *glide*. Everything begins to happen at once, but imagine the bottom arm as the crank that starts the action.

PHASE 1: From the glide position, your bottom arm bends and *pulls* down toward your chest to initiate this phase, as your top arm and your legs bend. This phase ends when your hands and knees meet at chest level. (It helps if you remember that the hand of your top arm moves together with your top leg.)

PHASE 2: As your bottom arm extends to *recover*, your top arm *pulls* while your legs straighten and squeeze together. Arms and legs remain extended for a moment for the *glide*, during which you can rest and allow the momentum of the stroke to propel you through the water. When the momentum begins to slow, it's time to begin the stroke cycle again.

CHECKLIST FOR A BETTER SIDESTROKE

~

- Remember to keep your body stretched and streamlined. Keep your top shoulder and hip toward the ceiling and your body perpendicular to the surface of the water.
- Keep the arm stroke in a vertical plane; avoid moving your arms too far out in front or too far behind you.
- For greatest streamlining, make sure that the top arm stays close to your body during the recovery.
- Legs should bend toward the chest, extend smoothly outward, then snap together quickly; hold for the glide.

- Keep your legs close to the surface of the water but don't break the surface.

- As your front leg bends, flex that foot; then point it during the snap to get the foot to contribute to forward propulsion and streamlining. Try to keep the motion fluid, as though you were pedaling a bicycle.

- Breathe continuously and rhythmically; time your inhalation to coincide with the pull of the lower arm (and the recovery of the top arm and the bending of the legs). Exhale during the recovery of the bottom arm (and the pull of the top arm and the straightening of the legs). Continue to exhale during the glide.

- Between phases 1 and 2, all four limbs come together at mid-body. Then all four extend for the glide. Hold this glide until the momentum begins to fade.

- Remember, begin and end stroke in the extended glide position. Here's the sequence: phase 1, tuck; phase 2, straighten and glide.

SIDESTROKE DRILLS: ARMS

～

Unless you're very buoyant, you'll need a flotation device to help support your body during these drills.

1. One-arm Pull: To practice each arm motion separately, and thereby to acquire a feel for the two-phase stroke.

To practice the top arm motion, hold a kickboard in front of you with your bottom arm; your arm is straight, with your hand gripping the front of the board, and the back end of the board is braced with or near your armpit. Float on your side, practicing the pull and the recovery of the regular and/or overarm sidestroke with your top arm.

To practice the bottom arm motion, hold on to the kickboard with your top hand and place it on your top hip.

- Pull one lap of the regular sidestroke with the top arm; then, on the same side, pull one lap of the regular sidestroke with the bottom arm.

- Repeat, swimming on your opposite side.

- Repeat the drill, using the overarm sidestroke, first on one side, then on the other. Sidestroke for one lap, alternating four strokes of the regular sidestroke with four of the overarm sidestroke. Repeat on the opposite side.

2. Stroke and Roll: To use the elementary-backstroke arm motion (see page 85) to lead up to the sidestroke pull.

In a supine position, do the elementary-backstroke arm motion for four strokes; when you're in the glide of the fourth stroke, with your arms at your sides, press one shoulder down toward the pool bottom and raise your bottom arm overhead (this is a 90-degree or quarter turn). Do the sidestroke (regular or overarm) on this side for four strokes. Then return to the supine position and do four more elementary backstroke pulls; rotate a quarter turn onto your other side and practice the sidestroke arm motion again. Repeat until comfortable.

3. Two-arm Pull: To isolate and practice the sidestroke arm motions.

Using a flotation device such as a pull-buoy, practice the regular or overarm sidestroke pull, using both arms together.

- Pull one lap on one side using the regular arm stroke; pull the next lap on the other side using the regular arm stroke.
- Pull one lap on one side using the overarm pull; pull the next lap on the other side using the overarm pull.
- Pull for one lap, alternating four regular pulls with four overarm pulls.

SIDESTROKE DRILLS: LEGS

⌐

You may need a flotation device to help support you during some of these kicking drills.

1. Sit-and-Kick Progression: To use the supine whip kick (used in the elementary backstroke; see page 96) to lead up to the regular or inverted scissors kick.

Begin by sitting on a bench or the edge of the pool deck; review the supine whip kick. Then lie down on your side and practice either the regular or the inverted scissors kick. Rotate back to a sitting position to practice the whip kick again; then turn onto your other side to practice the scissors kick once more.

2. Wall Kick: To get a feel for the scissors kick in the water.

Use the bracket position (see page 29) to float on your side. Practice the regular scissors or the inverted scissors kick, making sure that your legs don't break the surface. Then turn around and practice on the other side.

3. Free Kick: To practice the regular or the inverted scissors kick while in proper swimming position; to develop leg power.

Use a kickboard (as described in arm drills) if necessary.

- Using the regular scissors kick, kick one lap on one side, the next lap on the other side.
- Using the inverted scissors kick, kick one lap on one side, the next lap on the other side.
- Kick one lap, alternating four regular with four inverted scissors kicks.

4. Kick and Roll: To use the supine whip kick (see the elementary backstroke, page 96), lead up to the scissors kick.

This is the same idea as the stroke-and-roll drill (page 181) except that instead of alternating the elementary backstroke pull and the sidestroke pull, you alternate four supine whip kicks with four scissors kicks. If necessary, use a kickboard (as described in the arm drills) or small sculling motions to support your upper body.

5. DPK (Distance Per Kick):   To measure the efficiency of your scissors kick.

Kick one lap, counting the number of kicks you need. Then try to lower the number of kicks (of same kind) on each consecutive lap.

SIDESTROKE DRILLS: COORDINATION

～

1. Bend and Straighten: To coordinate simultaneous movements of arms and legs.

Standing first on dry land, then in shoulder-deep water, practice the various sidestroke combinations in the following form: as your arms meet at your chest, bend your knees; as the arms extend for the glide position, straighten your legs. Repeat until the coordination comes easily.

2. Grapevine Walk: To practice coordinating the eight variations of the sidestroke.

Next, walk sideways as you coordinate the arm and leg motions by doing an alternating crossover side step. For the *regular scissors kick* (top leg moves forward): as your arms meet at your chest, bend both legs and cross the "top" leg in front of the "bottom" leg. As your arms extend for the glide, straighten both legs and bring your back foot around to meet the front foot, uncrossing your legs and ending with feet together. For the *inverted scissors kick* (top leg moves backward): as your arms meet at the chest, bend both legs and cross the "top" leg *behind* the "bottom" leg. As your arms extend for the glide, straighten both legs and bring your front foot to meet your back foot, uncrossing them and ending with feet together.

Practice walking each of the eight variations, first on land, then in shoulder-deep water:

1. Regular arm stroke, regular scissors kick (right side)
2. Regular arm stroke, regular scissors kick (left side)
3. Regular arm motion, inverted scissors kick (right side)
4. Regular arm motion, inverted scissors kick (left side)
5. Overarm motion, regular scissors kick (right side)
6. Overarm motion, regular scissors kick (left side)
7. Overarm motion, inverted scissors kick (right side)
8. Overarm motion, inverted scissors kick (left side)

3. One-arm Pull with Kick: To coordinate the top and bottom arms individually with the scissors kick.

Do the one-arm-pull drill (see page 180), adding the kick. Practice all eight variations listed above.

Common Sidestroke Faults and What to Do about Them

～

Body Position

Error	Correction
Loss of balance; rolling too far forward or backward	Maintain your balance on your side by keeping the center of your top shoulder and hip toward the ceiling.
Poor body alignment; body not streamlined, bent at waist	Press your hips forward; increase joint extension and muscle stretch.
Head too high; legs too low or too deep	To help raise the legs, lower your head so that the water is at ear level; reduce the length of your glide.

Arms: 2-Phase Arm Motion

Error	Correction
Arms slip through water and lose their leverage	Keep the elbows of both arms higher than the hands during pull phases.
Arms drag through water or break the surface during recovery	Keep your elbows close to the body; recover your hands underwater.
Top arm splashes water during overwater recovery	Lift top arm as in crawl-stroke recovery, elbow high.
Difficulty in recovering arm at the end of the pull, resulting in a lowering of body	Avoid pulling arms beyond your chest.

Legs: Regular and Inverted Scissors Kick

Error	Correction
Front or back foot breaks surface at beginning of power phase	Practice sidestroke leg drills to keep the top hip from rotating forward or backward.
Lack of power; forward foot not flexed	Increase the speed and force of the squeezing action; alternately flex and point forward foot during the kick, as in pedaling a bicycle.
Uneven leg motion; off-center line of movement	Extend and separate both legs an equal distance from the midline of the body.

Breathing

Error	Correction
Head moves forward and backward; face drops below water level so that mouth is submerged	Keep your head still; keep the top of the head facing in direction in which you are swimming.
Holding your breath or breathing irregularly, causing fatigue	Establish continuous inhalation (during phase 1) and exhalation (during phase 2) cycle for each stroke.

Coordination

Error	Correction
Being one-sided; doing only one variation	Try all eight variations of the sidestroke, so that both sides, both arms and both legs, are used equally.
Lack of power and smoothness during propulsive phases of stroke	Begin the pull of the lower arm as the top arm and leg recover, so that the transition is balanced and smooth.

Error	Correction
Continuous arm and leg movement; no glide	Concentrate on relaxation and extension of the body, with no arm or leg movement during the glide.
Breathing not coordinated with stroke	*Inhale* during phase 1 (recovery of legs and top arm, pull of lower arm); body should end in tuck position. *Exhale* during phase 2 (power phase of kick and pull of top arm, recovery of lower arm); continue to exhale during glide.

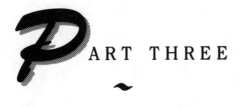PART THREE

STARTS, DIVES, AND
TURNS

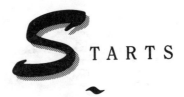

S TARTS

here are two ways to begin a swim: *in-the-water starts,* which are discussed here, and *out-of-the-water starts,* or *dives,* which are discussed later. The object of any start is to use the firm resistance of the pool wall or bottom to give you a speedier, more efficient send-off.

STARTING TIPS

All starts have these basic principles in common:

- You should push off aggressively; timidity will get you nowhere.
- The power for the push-off comes from the legs. (Jumping jacks and light weight training will improve your starts.)
- Your body should be streamlined and stretched, with your legs straight and your toes pointed, muscles tight; your head should be in line with your body and your arms should cover your ears during the glide.

CRAWL/FREESTYLE IN-THE-WATER START

Stand in the water with your knees bent and your back foot braced against the wall. Extend your arms straight out in front of you in the glide posi-

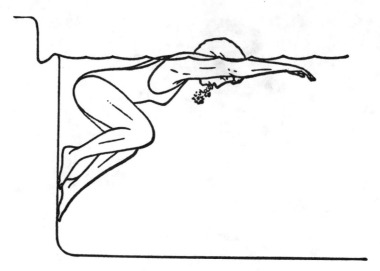

Crawl/freestyle in-the-water start.

tion and take a bite of air. Immediately drop underwater, brace your other foot against the wall, and straighten both legs as forcefully as you can. During the glide, keep your body stretched and streamlined and your toes pointed. When you begin to lose momentum, start flutter kicking and you will rise to the surface. Begin your first pull with the arm opposite your breathing side. Then, as you recover the other arm, take your first inhalation.

A variation is the one-arm side-standing position. Hold on to the gutter with one hand, elbow bent; extend the other arm forward in the direction in which you will be swimming, so that your side is facing the pool wall; rest your cheek on the surface before pushing off.

BREASTSTROKE IN-THE-WATER START

~

Similar to the freestyle start, but the push-off is deeper because here you'll take one underwater pull and kick before coming up for your first inhalation.

BUTTERFLY IN-THE-WATER START
∾

A little deeper than the freestyle in-the-water start, but shallower than the breaststroke start. While still underwater, take one dolphin kick to help bring you back to the surface.

SIDESTROKE IN-THE-WATER START
∾

Similar to the freestyle start, except that the push-off is shallower so that the body barely submerges. (The one-arm push-off variation is best for this stroke.)

BACKSTROKE START
∾

Grasp the gutter, or the bar on the backstroke starting block if there is one (in competition, this occurs at the signal "Swimmers"). Place your feet against the wall just below the water surface (one slightly higher than the other, if you find that easier), and bend your knees, bringing your body into a tucked position. Bend your elbows and pull your body up so that the surface of the water approaches hip level (when the starter says, "Take your marks"). To push off (at the signal "Go"), swing your arms around to the sides in a wide, sweeping motion, your head tilted slightly backward. Arch your back and stretch your body as you push off with your legs, so that you spring back in a sort of upside-down swan dive.

Your arms should cover your ears. Ideally, your shoulders, hips, and legs should clear the water's surface. Exhale forcefully through your nose and mouth as you glide below the surface in a streamlined position. Keeping arms extended overhead, while still underwater, begin to flutter kick or dolphin kick. Once your torso has entered the water, bend slightly at the hips, this action will begin to propel you toward the surface. Before losing momentum, your face should emerge from the water by taking your first alternating arm pull (not recovery) and leaving the other arm in the overhead "catch" position.

The dolphin kick is most effective before arms begin stroking. Once your arms begin pulling, switch to the flutter kick. (This underwater dolphin kick technique for starts and push-offs was revolutionized by back-

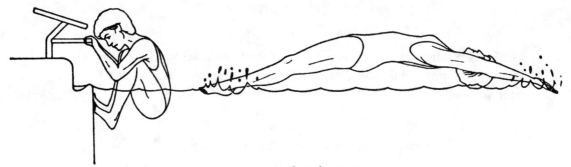

Backstroke start.

stroke 1988/1992 Olympian David Berkoff, who exploded off his start with the Berkoff Blast-off for thirty-five meters underwater! The rules currently allow only fifteen meters to be swam beneath the surface.)

DIVES

A dive is really an out-of-the-water start—it begins on land but ends in the water. As with the in-the-water starts, the object is to use the resistance of a stationary object (in this case, the pool deck or a starting block) to give you more distance. Since dives are faster than in-the-water starts, most races (except for backstroke events) begin this way. But even if you're not aspiring to be like multi-Olympic diver Greg Louganis, you will probably appreciate the thrill of diving and want to learn this useful skill.

PRACTICE/PREPARATION

The idea of soaring through the air in a smooth, graceful arc may make you a bit nervous at first. After all, it's a different sensation to enter the water head first, even though your arms are stretched out to protect you. So, to keep the fun and excitement in, and the pounding heart and shaky knees to a minimum, it's important that you learn how to dive correctly and in gradual stages. In the step-by-step progression that follows, what you learn in one dive becomes the foundation for what you learn in the next.

Begin by practicing the shallow surface entry and the sitting dive entry (Lessons 7 and 8, pages 81 and 88). Next, do surface, or "porpoise," dives (see page 81) in waist-deep water: imagine you're diving over a barrel floating on the surface without touching it. Then you will learn the kneeling dive, the semi-standing, and the standing dive. And if you find that you really like diving, go on to learn the racing dives—whether you plan ever to compete or not.

DIVING TIPS
～

All dives share these five components:

1. Stance: Once you are sitting, kneeling, or standing, with toes curled around the edge of the pool, your body is balanced, poised, and ready for takeoff.

2. Takeoff: The energy comes from the legs; the push-off is aggressive and assertive; your eyes look diagonally forward and downward.

3. Flight: The body extends and arcs smoothly through the air; your position is taut and streamlined.

4. Entry: The arms are extended and enter the water first; the head is tucked down between them, ears covered.

5. Recovery: You ascend to the surface in a smooth arc by lifting your chin and angling your hands and arms upward.

For Safe Diving

- Check pool regulations for safe diving.
- Be sure you dive into water that's deep enough. Depending on the height of pool edge and your height, the water should be at least nine feet deep.
- Check pool markers and ask the lifeguard to determine safe depth.
- If there are no markers, enter feet first initially to test depth. This is especially important in an open water environment.
- Review and practice diving skills in a safe progression.
- Extend your arms over your head during every dive.
- If you wear goggles, you'll have to make the strap a bit tighter than usual to keep them on as you enter the water.
- Do not use competitive starting blocks or platforms unless supervised.

KNEELING DIVE

～

To assume the *stance,* kneel at the edge of the pool, with your weight on one knee and the toes of your other foot curled securely around the edge for traction. (If it's uncomfortable to kneel, raise the weight-bearing knee off the ground slightly.) Tuck your chin to your chest and extend your arms straight out in front of you with your biceps tight against your ears. The most common diving error is raising the head during entry. Since the body follows the path of the head, lifting the head is what makes for so many belly whops. Also remember to keep your eyes open throughout the dive—since you'll be landing in the water head first, you want to see where you're going. To keep your arms straight and your hands together, hook your thumbs, or grasp one wrist with the other.

To begin the takeoff, lean forward so that your hands almost touch the water. Keep leaning farther and farther, gradually shifting your weight forward until your rear foot lifts off the deck and your body begins to "fall" toward the surface. Bring your legs together as you enter the water. Don't give in to the temptation to raise your head. And as you practice, start to push off with the forward leg, so that instead of falling into the water you spring with energy. Also, point your hands downward at a 45-degree angle on entry and point your toes and tighten your leg muscles to obtain a streamlined position.

Begin to exhale a second before you hit the surface. Once in the water, continue to exhale slowly, and stretch and streamline your body as it glides through the water in a downward arc.

To *recover,* point your fingers upward. Arch your back slightly, lifting

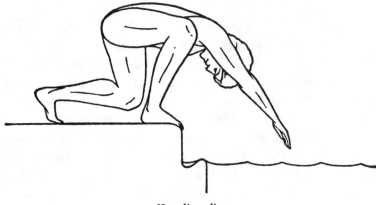

Kneeling dive.

your chin and raising your head and arms toward the surface. You may begin to kick, or simply assume a prone float, prior to recovering to a stand.

SEMI-STANDING DIVE ("TIP-IN" DIVE)
～

Once you are comfortable with the kneeling dive, learn to dive from a slightly higher stance. Stand with one foot in back of the other (with the toes of the forward foot curled securely around the edge of the deck so that you don't slip). Bend (*pike*) at the waist with your head tucked down (looking forward or toward the bottom) and your arms extended overhead and hugging your ears. Then press your head and arms downward, while your back leg presses upward. Lean forward, lifting the back foot off the deck and shifting all your weight onto your front leg, until you "fall" toward the surface. As you enter, fingertips leading, straighten your legs and bring them together, toes pointed. Make an arc underwater, as you did for the kneeling dive, and remember to keep your head tucked down and your arms close to your ears until it is time to recover to the surface.

STANDING DIVE
～

Stand in a piked position with your knees bent slightly, both feet together, toes curled around the pool edge. Again, your arms are extended straight in front of you at a 45-degree angle to the water, your head is down, and your biceps are covering your ears. Think of your body as a seesaw with your hips as the fulcrum. Bend your knees further, then straighten them during takeoff to give the dive a spring and therefore more height. As you push off, lift your hips, tighten your legs and extend them up and straight behind you, and point your toes. As your skill improves, gradually straighten your body out of the piked position during the flight. Keep your head down and your arms extended as you stretch and spring up and over, traveling in a smooth, graceful arc before entering the water. Since the higher stance of the standing dive increases your distance from the water, you will enter faster and deeper than with the kneeling or semi-standing dives. This may result in a longer recovery, so remember to exhale slowly until you've surfaced.

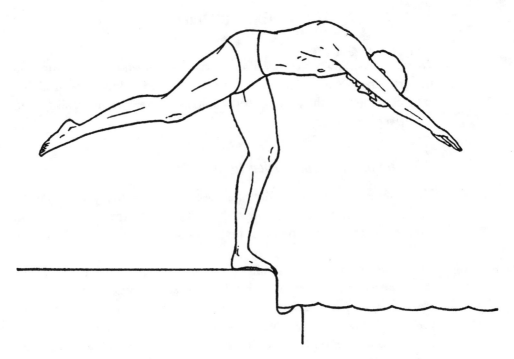

Semi-standing dive.

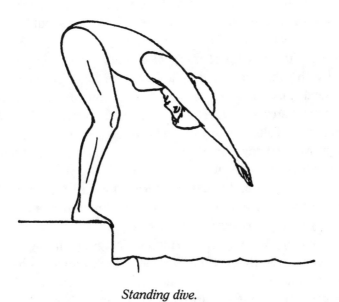

Standing dive.

RACING DIVES

～

There are basically two competition starts, the conventional wind-up, and the grab start. You can vary starts and entries according to your ability and needs, but the shallower entry should be mastered before going on to the newer piked entry.

Wind-up or Arm-swing Dive (with Shallow Entry)

The conventional wind-up dive has been used for many years for all strokes swum in the prone position. Even if you're a fitness swimmer, you too may prefer to enter the water for a workout using this clean and fairly shallow dive.

In competition, the dive takes place off a starting block thirty inches above the water's surface. The object is to create as much *horizontal* forward propulsion and as little resistance as possible. In order to do this, you create a "hole" in the water for your body to enter. This is also termed a nonresistance entry because the body enters the water cleanly, through a vacuum that it has created for itself.

Before learning the dive, get the feel of the "hole" by practicing this drill in waist-deep water. Push off forcefully from the bottom of the pool, diving over the surface of the water. During the over-the-water arc, extend your arms overhead, arch your back, and lift your head. Then, as you enter the water, drop your head and round your shoulders, so the rest of your body passes through the "hole" created by your shoulders and arms.

To begin the wind-up dive (in competition, at the signal "Swimmers"), step forward to the edge of the pool or onto the starting block. Stand straight with your toes curled tightly over the edge, feet about hip width apart. Bend your knees (at the signal "Take your marks"), and let your arms hang wherever they feel comfortable and balanced. Your weight is forward, on the balls of your feet, and your eyes are looking ahead.

To push off (at the signal "Go"—a gun, whistle, horn, beeper, etc.), drop your head, round your shoulders, and swing your arms vigorously backward and upward. As your body leans forward (or "overbalances"), swing your arms back down and around to the front in a semicircle. Begin to extend your legs to initiate the takeoff.

Continue to push off, straightening your legs and lifting your head to look at your target. By the time your feet lift off, your arms have stopped their swing and are straight ahead of you, pointed forward and downward at a shallow angle. Your legs are as stretched and streamlined as possible.

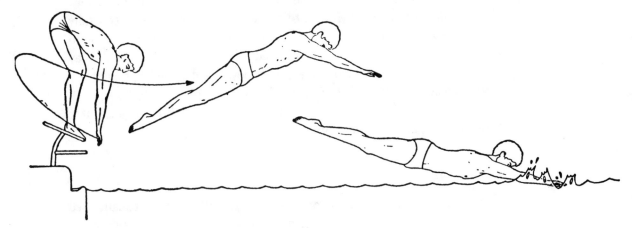

Wind-up racing dive with shallow entry.

Once you're completely extended over the water, drop your head downward to try to get your body to pass through the "hole" made by your hands. Your entry should be relatively flat, at about a 10- to 20-degree angle.

After you've entered the water, glide, holding your streamlined position, until you begin to lose momentum; then initiate the kick, followed by the arm motion.

Grab Start (with Shallow Entry)

This is a newer variation of the racing dive. Although it is similar to the wind-up start in many ways, it usually gets you into the water faster.

Stand at the edge of the pool or on the starting block (at the call of "Swimmers"), your feet hip width apart and your toes curled around the edge. Bend forward at the waist (at the signal "Take your marks") and grasp the gutter of the pool or the platform or bar of the starting block. Your hands are usually between your feet at this point, but you can also place them outside your feet. The grab position should allow you to balance your weight forward over the starting block. At the signal "Go" overbalance your body by pulling and stretching your shoulders and head down. Then release the platform or bar as your torso goes forward. This levels off your trajectory as you leave the starting block in much the same way that the wind-up arm swing of the conventional racing dive does, but the grab start takes less time.

As your hands release, look up toward the end of the pool and swing your arms up and forward. Follow through with your body and straighten your knees to begin the forward thrust. As your arms extend completely, at a 45-degree angle downward to the water, let your legs extend fully behind you, completing the takeoff. Your hips should pike in the air to help your body enter the "hole" created by your arms. Your hands may overlap for the entry, which is at a greater downward angle (approximately 30 to 45 degrees) than that of the shallow entry.

To recover, lift your head and arch your back slightly. Begin flutter kicking and, as you surface, initiate the arm stroke.

Pike Entry

This is a newer version of the racing-dive entry. Although it's usually used with a grab start, you can also use it with the wind-up dive. The pike entry is faster than the more shallow entry because it takes advantage of the whipping action of your legs and hips during the flight to give you additional propulsion.

Assume your stance, looking diagonally forward and down. As you push off with your legs, spring up into the air. Lift your head as your hands drive forward to lift your hips higher than your original standing position. Then bend your hips to assume a partial jackknife position. Enter the water hands first with head dropped between your arms; then, as your shoulders enter, straighten your hips and pull them down into the "hole" that your arms have made. Since your body position is deeper here than in other racing dives, begin your kick early to help you rise to the surface quickly. If you've done it correctly, you'll know it—compare your distance with that from the other dives.

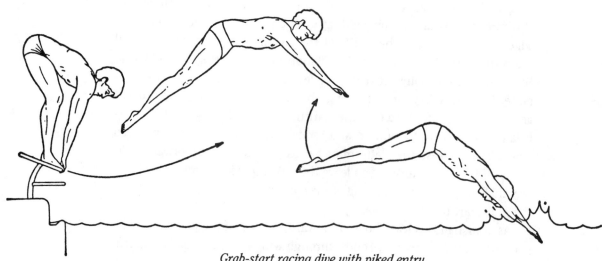

Grab-start racing dive with piked entry.

COMMON DIVING ERRORS AND WHAT TO DO ABOUT THEM
☙

A dive can go wrong anywhere along the way. If your diving isn't all you'd like it to be, check for these common errors.

Stance:

Error	Correction
Body falls forward; off balance	Grasp edge firmly with your toes for support while maintaining your balance with your arms; hips serve as center of gravity.
Arms too far back overhead	Keep arms below shoulder level to protect head.

Takeoff:

Error	Correction
Weak push-off	Review porpoise dive push-off.
Legs hit edge of deck	Push off aggressively, pointing your toes as you take off; be certain to curl toes over edge during stance.

Flight:

Error	Correction
Body loses stream-lined position	Press legs up while arms direct downward motion; keep body extended. Stretch and maintain streamlined body position; keep arms and legs together.

Entry:

Error	Correction
Belly whop; head and chest enter the water first	Keep chin tucked to chest; use arms to protect head and for streamlining; enter hands first.

Error	Correction
Body crumples on entry	Keep arms extended overhead until hips and feet have entered the "hole" made by hands.
Water enters the nose and/or mouth	Begin exhaling a moment before head enters water.

Recovery:

Error	Correction
Water enters nose and/or mouth	Continue to exhale to counteract water pressure.
Body pops up to surface too soon	Delay recovery until forward and downward momentum have slowed; then begin kick.

TURNS

If you swim laps in a pool, you should have at least some idea about what to do when you get to the other end. Just how *do* you turn your body around in an efficient, graceful way in order to begin the next lap? *Turns* are the answer. They also add variety to your swimming workouts, and the push-off stage is an effective way to condition your legs.

The turns are slightly different for each stroke, but all have the same purpose: to use your body's momentum to make a 180-degree turn—and to do it with no wasted effort and no pause. There are two basic types of turns. In ascending order of speed, efficiency, difficulty, and impressiveness, they are the *open turn* (used in all strokes, along with the *closed-turn* variation used in the crawl) and the *flip turn* (used in crawl and backstroke). Fitness swimmers should learn at least the open turn for each stroke, but there's no need to stop there. The closed crawl turn will come easily as your fitness, breath control, and confidence increase. Before long you may be tempted to try the flip turn—and you'll be able to do it, too, by following the step-by-step progression explained below. In addition, there are *transitional turns* used to change from one stroke to another, as when you go from swimming the freestyle to swimming the breaststroke.

TURNING TIPS

Remember, there are five components to any kind of turn:

1. The Approach: Timing is important here. In order to begin the turn at just the right moment, you must be able to judge the distance between your body and the end of the pool, so that you will be in proper position as you near the wall. Use your momentum to accelerate as you approach the wall.

2. The Turn: During the 180-degree turn, you shift your body so that your feet are planted on the wall and your torso is facing the new direction. Just before push-off, your body should be tucked, or coiled, as tightly as possible, ready to spring into action.

3. The Push-off: Be aggressive during this phase. Push off forcefully with your legs, as though the wall of the pool were the floor and you were trying to jump as high into the air as possible. Don't hesitate; the idea is to hit the wall and ricochet off it like a bullet.

4. Glide: Extending and streamlining your body, glide through the water on the momentum from the explosive push-off.

5. Recovery: When the glide begins to slow, resurface and immediately initiate the stroke so that you don't lose the momentum. Usually you resume kicking first, then add the arm motion.

In general, you should be sure of your open turns before attempting the closed turn; once you have the closed turn, you can move on to the flip turns used in the crawl and backstroke. Practice each turn in shallow water first, if possible, before trying it in deep water. Always practice turning to both sides an equal number of times; try not to favor one side over the other. This is especially important in the crawl and the backstroke, which have alternating arm movements—you never know which arm will be leading when you reach the wall. But it's important in the other strokes, too, because the top leg tends to exert more force than the bottom leg during the push-off. So turning to both sides helps to balance muscle development as well.

OPEN TURNS
～

This is the easiest type of turn, and you should learn it before attempting the more advanced ones. There are two important things to remember:

the first is to keep your body as low in the water as possible during the inhalation; try to let just your head come up out of the water—not your shoulders. The second thing to remember is the principle of opposing hands—the hand that contacts the wall is *opposite* the side to which you are going to turn. For example, if your left arm touches the wall, you turn to the right.

Crawl-stroke/Freestyle Open Turn

Approach the wall with your eyes open and your face in the water; look slightly forward so that you can see the marker on the bottom and/or on the wall (in the absence of either of these, look for the line at which the bottom meets the wall). Try to maintain your normal stroke as you arrive at the wall with one arm extended in the catch position; try not to shorten your stroke or to glide too much. As you approach the wall, "kick in" if necessary rather than overstroking.

To begin the turn, grasp the gutter with your extended hand (in the absence of a gutter, press your hand against the wall at water level to stabilize your body). As your hand touches, flex your elbow, bring your head and body in close to the wall, allow your opposite shoulder to drop, and rotate 180 degrees so that you're facing the new direction. As you rotate, bend your knees and swing your feet and hips under your body. Lift your head just enough to inhale quickly as your weight shifts. As your feet contact the wall, let go with your hand and swing it over your shoulder and drop it about one foot beneath the surface to join your other arm, which stays extended away from the wall throughout. Both arms are now stretched over your head and pointing toward the opposite end of the pool, your feet are still pressed against the wall, and your entire body is slightly on its side.

Next, push off forcefully from the pool wall by extending your body and straightening your knees. Keep your body streamlined, arms stretched overhead, knees locked and toes pointed. As you begin your glide, rotate back into a fully prone position and continue the glide toward the surface.

As you begin to lose the momentum of the push-off, start to flutter kick. As you surface, add the arm stroke, pulling first with the arm opposite your breathing side; as you complete the pull on your breathing side, take your first inhalation.

The crawl-stroke/freestyle open turn.

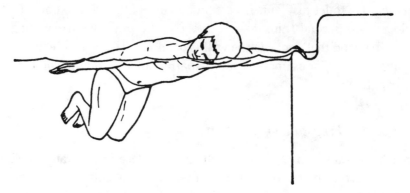

The approach.

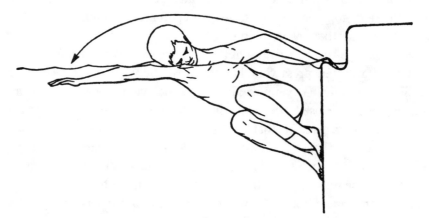

The turn.

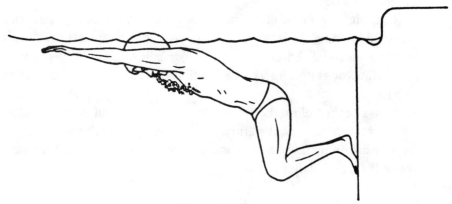

The push-off.

PRACTICE: Learn the open turn in gradual steps:

- In shallow water, practice the in-the-water start, the push-off, the glide, and the recovery and stroke initiation.
- Next, add the turn. Start by grasping the gutter or touching the wall with one hand, leaving the other arm extended toward the opposite end of the pool. Place your feet on the wall in the push-off position, with your head resting on your free arm, which remains extended about one foot below the surface toward the opposite end of the pool. Inhale, drop underwater, and push off. Practice on each side of your body.
- Walk toward the wall with one arm extended and practice the entire open turn first with one hand, then the other. Repeat, this time kicking toward the wall with one arm extended.
- Finally, swim toward the wall and do the open turn.

Crawl/Freestyle Closed Turn

The closed turn is faster than the open turn because the transition is smoother and more efficient. Learning the closed turn is also an intermediate step in learning the freestyle flip turn, and it helps to develop your controlled breathing. The closed turn is done exactly like an open turn except that your face stays underwater. Just before your forward arm touches the wall, take a big bite of air; then return your face to the water.

Backstroke Open Turn

In this stroke, although you can't see the approaching wall, you can still use your momentum to advantage. To begin the turn, grab the gutter or deck edge with one hand (or press the hand to the wall at water level, palm flat and thumb up). Bend and drop your elbow to bring your head and body close to the wall as you turn toward your contact arm. Tuck your knees in close to your chest and, keeping your free arm extended in the direction you just came from, turn 180 degrees on your back so that you end up facing the wall with your feet touching it. Inhale as you bring the contact arm overhead to meet the extended one.

To initiate the push-off, stretch your arms and upper body as you straighten your knees. Keep your head tucked between your arms, slightly underwater; as you glide, approach the surface at a slight angle, exhaling continually.

Backstroke open turn.

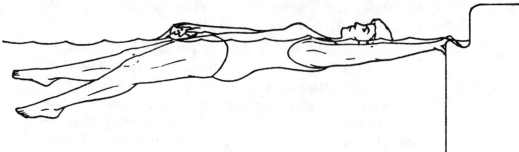

The approach.

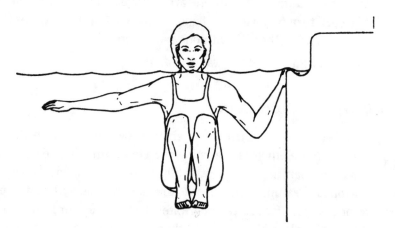

The turn.

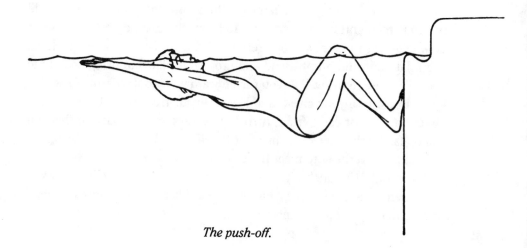

The push-off.

To recover to the surface, begin to flutter kick as your momentum from the push-off decreases. Take a pull with one arm just as you reach the surface, keeping the other arm extended in the catch position for the best streamlining. Inhale when your face clears the water. When the first arm begins to recover, pull with the other arm.

Instead of turning your head continually to take a peek at the approaching wall (thus losing momentum), you can use some sort of stationary reference point (such as the flags strung width-wise across some pools five yards from each end, or even a ladder) to warn you of your arrival. Just remember the number of strokes needed to reach the end from this point. As you arrive at the wall, keep one arm extended overhead in the catch position and kick in, with the other arm remaining in the direction from which you came.

PRACTICE: Learn the open turn in gradual steps:

- Practice in shallow water, beginning with the in-the-water push-off, the glide, the recovery and stroke initiation.

- Walk backward toward the wall with one hand extended to it and the other hand facing the opposite end of the pool. When your hand contacts the wall, make an open turn. Repeat, contacting with the other hand.

- Next, flutter kick toward the wall on your back, with one hand extended behind you; practice the open turn first on one side, then on the other.

- Finally, backstroke to the wall and do the open turn (remember to check for your landmark as you approach the wall).

Breaststroke Open Turn

Approach the wall with your eyes open, looking slightly forward so that you can see it coming. Try to maintain your speed and rhythm, and try to arrive at the wall in full stroke, both arms extended underwater in front of you, parallel to the water surface and to each other.

To begin the turn, touch the wall at surface level with both hands. As you touch the wall, immediately inhale and turn toward one side by driving that shoulder into the water at a 90-degree angle and drawing the same elbow to your side. As you turn, swing the other arm of the driving shoulder away from the wall, and pivot 180 degrees, being certain to complete your inhalation before your head drops. Release the other hand from

Breastroke and butterfly open turn.

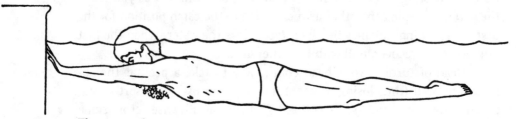

The approach.

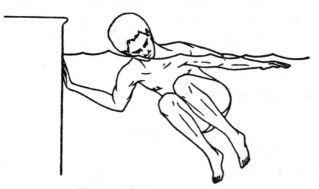

The start of the turn.

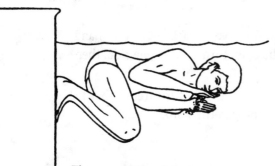

The completion of the turn.

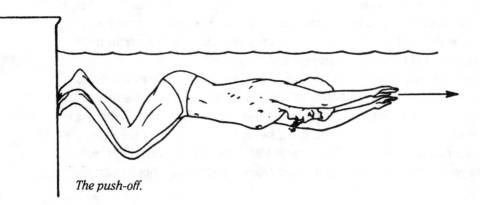

The push-off.

the wall as you pivot; then bend your legs and bring them under your body, planting your feet on the wall, one higher than the other. (As your turn improves, you may notice that during this exchange there is a moment when no part of your body is touching the wall.) Extend both arms in front of you; your body is still slightly tilted or rolled on the driving shoulder side. (Some competitive swimmers attempt to obtain additional streamlining by crossing their feet and hands during the turn.)

Push off by straightening your legs and extending your body into a streamlined, fully prone position. Also, push off at a slightly downward angle (hips higher than head and arms) to take advantage of this extra bit of speed. During this deeper push-off, you should feel as if you are going downhill for a moment ("downstreaming"). As you begin to lose the momentum from the push-off, take one underwater pull (see "Breaststroke In-The-Water Start," page 190). Make this pull as powerful as possible and don't stop at shoulder level as usual—extend the pull by bringing the hands under your chest and abdomen and pushing all the way under the thighs. As you recover the arms, take one kick, moving the hips up to get the dolphin body wave (see page 154). Then, as you surface, begin to take your second arm pull to continue the breaststroke. In competition, you are allowed only one pull and one kick before your head must break the surface.

PRACTICE: Practice this turn in stages, on each side of your body.

- Practice the in-the-water start (the push-off, the glide, and the recovery and stroke initiation) in shallow water.

- Add the turn, grasping the wall with both hands to negotiate the exchange. Try to increase your distance each time you practice.

- Walk to the wall with both arms extended and practice the turn. Next, kick to the wall with both arms extended and make the turn.

- To get more speed in the turn, you can lift your head as you contact the wall, then start the rotation immediately.

Butterfly Open Turn

Like the breaststroke turn, the butterfly turn is a two-hand touch. However, do not push off at as deep an angle as in the breaststroke push-off. During the glide, extend your body into a streamlined, fully prone position and keep your arms extended in front of you. (Unlike the breaststroke turn, there's no underwater pull.) The glide is followed immediately by one or more dolphin kicks to help you surface.

Breastroke pull-out.

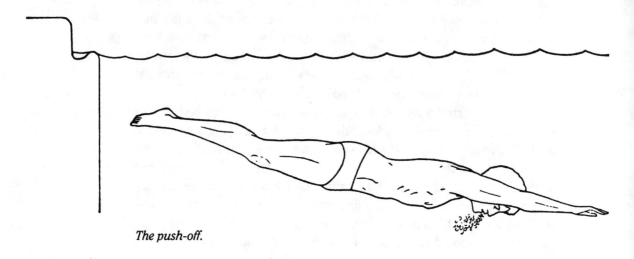

The push-off.

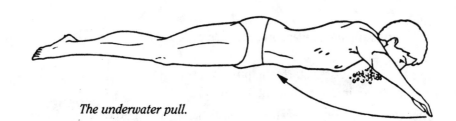

The underwater pull.

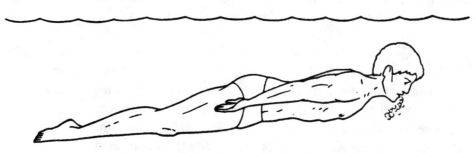

The recovery to surface.

Sidestroke Open Turn

Use a variation of the crawl-stroke open turn. Touch the wall with the leading arm, shift your weight, bringing your feet around to touch the wall and driving the shoulder of the free arm into the water at a 90-degree angle. Push off and initiate the stroke, swimming on the side opposite the one you used during the previous lap.

FLIP TURNS

~

Flip turns may be done during the freestyle and backstroke. The flip (which is like a somersault combined with a twist for the crawl, and actually more like a swivel for the backstroke) adds speed and power to the turn.

Freestyle Flip Turn

Approach the wall, looking forward and, if necessary, accelerating your stroke. When your leading arm is two to four feet from the wall, tuck your chin to your chest, pull with your extended arm (so that both arms are at your sides), and do a dolphin kick (see page 164) to initiate the flip.

The timing of the turn is very important. In general, it's best to judge the distance conservatively (i.e., to give yourself more room than you need to execute the turn) than to cramp the turn and possibly hit your heels on the deck. Just prior to beginning your flip, when you take your last rhythmic breath, be certain to get a big bite of air (because you will not take another breath until you surface after the flip).

To begin the flip, back water (scoop water from your hips toward your face) with the arm opposite the side to which you are going to turn. To lift your hips and legs up out of the water, bend your upper body forward and push water toward your abdomen with your leading arm. Then tuck your body and bend your knees, as the lower part of your legs come out of the water.

As your feet flip over your head, twist your trunk to one side. (It may help to make a little circular motion at this point with the hand on the side that you are turning toward; e.g., if you turn to the right, circle with your right hand.) As you complete the flip, begin to straighten out of the tuck; plant your feet on the wall and begin to extend both arms in front of you.

On the push-off, continue to twist and extend your body during the glide so that you finish face down in a fully prone position.

Recover to the surface (as in the other turns) by lifting your head and arching your back (hyperextending your body) to streamline your body before beginning to flutter kick.

PRACTICE: Practice the flip turn in gradual steps:

- First get accustomed to somersaulting in water. Practice this from a standing position while walking and then while swimming in shallow water.
- Next practice the closed turn, contacting your extended hand lower and lower on the wall (hand flat, fingers pointed downward), and gradually lifting your hips and legs higher and higher out of the water.
- When your hand makes contact about two feet below the water surface, add the full somersaulting and twisting action.

Freestyle flip turn.

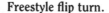
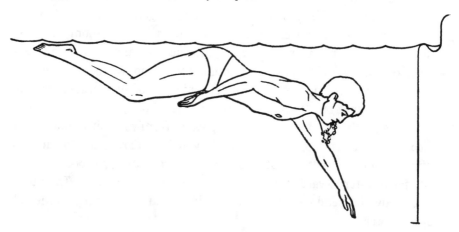

The approach. Chin tucks to chest, extended arm pulls, legs dolphin kick.

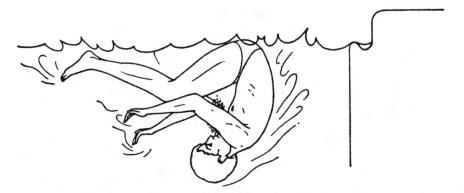

The tuck. Backwater, lift hips out of water, bend upper body forward; tuck body and bend knees.

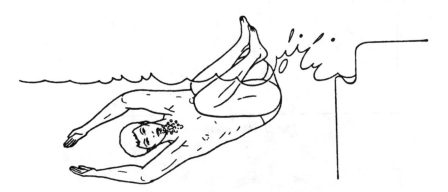

The flip. Trunk twists while feet contact wall.

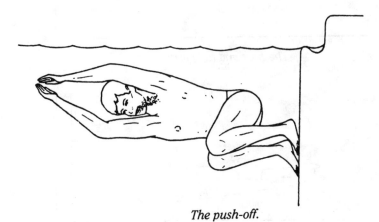

The push-off.

Backstroke flip turn.

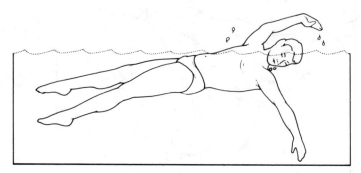

The roll during approach.

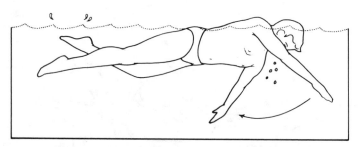

The pivot to prone position.

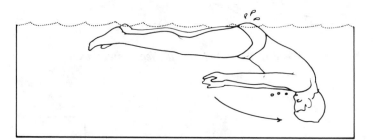

The tuck and flip position.

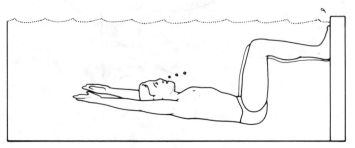

The push-off position.

Backstroke Spin Turn

This is similar to the open turn, but you'll contact the wall with the palm of your extended hand, fingers pointing downward. Arch your arm, cocking your wrist just prior to contacting the wall. As you touch, continue to kick in, bending your elbow, bringing your head and body close to the wall, and taking a bite of air. Bend your knees, legs together, so that they emerge from the water. As your head tucks down to your chest and your upper body drops below the surface, your lower body spins 180 degrees in a sideways position.

Quickly spin your legs and hips over the shoulder of your extended arm, so that your feet land on the wall, ready for push-off. To help you turn, use your free arm, which initially is near your hips, to back water (to push water up toward your face). As you turn, the free arm ends up back overhead, where it continues to back water.

As you plant your feet on the wall, extend both arms overhead for maximum streamlining. Push off, glide, recover, and initiate the stroke as you would for the backstroke open turn.

Practice the backstroke spin by mastering the open turn first. As you turn, gradually lift your legs and hips higher and higher, still keeping your upper body in an arched position, chest up. The lower your contact hand, the more leverage you will have to spin your legs around.

Backstroke Flip Turn

This is similar to the freestyle flip turn. As you approach the wall, roll onto your arm that is extended overhead into a prone position, and pull both arms under your body. Both arms are now at your sides so you can begin to flip. Turn your palms to face the bottom of the pool. Scoop them overhead, flipping your legs out of the water so that your feet then contact the wall. Push off from this tuck position, staying on your back, and resume a streamlined backstroke push-off.

TRANSITIONAL TURNS (USED IN INDIVIDUAL MEDLEY)
~

Occasionally you will want to change from one stroke to another, so you will have to modify the turns somewhat. This occurs, for instance, in the competitive event called the Individual Medley (or IM), where one goes from swimming the butterfly to the backstroke, to the breaststroke, to the freestyle—without stopping. For instance, 1992 Olympian swimmer Summer Sanders utilized transitional turns in her medal-winning swims. IMs, naturally, are often incorporated into fitness workouts because they're a great way to add variety to your swimming, no matter what your level.

Butterfly to Backstroke

Touch the wall with both hands and tuck your body, bringing your feet to the wall. Inhale at this point. Then push off as you would for the backstroke start. A faster variation is to drop one shoulder after touching the wall, pushing off sideways to avoid your own wake and being certain both arms are extended overhead before push-off.

Backstroke to Breaststroke

To accomplish this as an open turn, begin the open backstroke turn, bringing your knees toward your chest as your body rotates (with the hips as the fulcrum) from a supine to a prone position. Inhale at this point. You will now be facing the new direction. Let go of the wall and swing your arm to meet the leading arm, which has remained in place during the turn. Drop your head and push off.

To do this as a flip turn, begin by taking a quick bite of air. Bring your knees directly overhead and rotate to a prone position, ending up facing in the new direction. Push off as usual.

Breaststroke to Freestyle

As you touch the wall with two hands, immediately release one arm and bring it around over the water in the same direction that you will turn. Inhale as you pivot and swing the other arm to meet the first; push off on one side and during the glide gradually untwist to end up in a fully prone position.

TURNING WITH EQUIPMENT

～

You're not a show-off if you turn while using equipment—it's actually easier to do some turns this way. If you're wearing a combination of equipment, combine the following techniques as applicable.

Kickboards

Reach for the wall with one hand while the other holds on to the kickboard. Turn 180 degrees in either direction as the leading edge of the board approaches the wall, as for the open turn. Keep your arms extended and your body streamlined as you come out of the turn.

Pull-buoy

You may do a flip or an open turn (eventually, a flip will be the easiest). For either of them, be certain that your legs are pressed together, so that you don't lose the pull-buoy. As you approach the wall with your forward arm, execute the turn of your choice, bend your knees into a tucked position, and press your thighs together as tightly as possible. As you come out of the turn, initiate your stroke with a pull (or you can do a dolphin kick).

Fins

Since you swim faster with fins, you'll need to anticipate the wall earlier than usual. During the open, closed, or flip turn, begin to tuck your knees to your chest as you approach the wall. Be certain to *flex* your feet toward your shins, the fins hitting the wall as flat as possible, so that you don't "trip" on them.

Hand Paddles

Since you can't grasp the gutter while wearing hand paddles, approach the wall with your forward hand flexed (even if you're doing an open turn and usually grasp the gutter). Plant your forward hand on the wall sideways, your fingers pointing in the direction of the turn, below water level. Continue the turn as usual, recovering with your hands on, next to, or on top of each other—paddles pointed downward. Using hand paddles won't interfere with your flip turn.

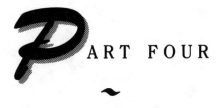

PART FOUR

SWIMMING-FOR-FITNESS PROGRESSIVE WORKOUT PROGRAM

THE TRAINING EFFECT

It's all because of Milo. He's the wrestler who walked around ancient Greece all day with a calf draped over his shoulders. Every day, as the calf grew larger, Milo grew stronger from bearing the increasing weight. Today, Milo's method would draw more than a few snickers even from warm-up-suit-clad fitness freaks. But in a manner of speaking, we too carry growing calves on our shoulders when we "work out" regularly: all training is based on the age-old principle of gradual overload and our body's adaptation to it.

All the components of total fitness—endurance, strength, flexibility, and speed—depend upon this basic principle: by overloading your body, by making demands on it that are just a bit more than it can handle comfortably, you force it to adapt. This marvelous adaptation is known as the "training effect." Your body will, of course, protest a bit ("no pain, no gain"), and can only adjust to a certain amount of strain without injury. But if you train sensibly and increase the workload gradually, it will reward you with the capability to work harder and perform better under all conditions.

In a well-designed, all-round fitness program, you become stronger because initially your muscle fibers break down under the strain and use the diminishing supply of oxygen and nutrients less and less efficiently (that's why you get tired and perhaps a bit sore). Then they regenerate and, in the process, become stronger and more efficient (just as scar tissue is tougher than unscarred skin, and a fracture, once healed, is stronger than the rest of the bone). Muscle fibers also become permanently elongated, giving you greater flexibility. At the same time, your cardiovascular system eventually comes to supply blood and oxygen more efficiently, giving you greater endurance.

223

How fit you become depends upon your inherited physical capabilities, how much time you spend training, how far your enthusiasm carries you, and what your goals are. For example, you might set one or more of these goals for yourself:

Distance:	1 mile
Speed:	50 yards in 1 minute
Weight Loss:	10 pounds
Skills:	learn the butterfly; master the crawl
Competition:	win one 50-yard race
Appearance:	lose 1 inch off hips; firm up thighs and chest

WHY FOLLOW A WORKOUT?

~

A swimming workout is a specific length of time (for most swimmers from one half to one hour is about right) during which you develop your swimming ability and improve your physical condition. If you're interested, a workout will also prepare you for competition. A good workout does not mean that you jump into the water and start swimming as fast as you can for as long as you can. For one thing, that's dangerous; for another, it's boring; for yet another, it won't improve your swimming or your fitness all that much. To be effective, there must be a method to your training. Some competitive swimmers train under the watchful eyes of a swim coach, whose job it is to devise their workouts. By following the workouts in this section, you too will have your own coach—on paper.

FOLLOWING THE WORKOUTS

~

There are four phases to the following fitness program. (I) Beginner, (II) Intermediate, (III) Advanced, and (IV) Super (geared toward people who want to compete, or at least to be as physically fit as competitive swimmers).

Where you begin the program depends on how fit you are now (as indicated by how far you can swim without stopping) and how many skills you've already mastered. Where you end is up to you—if you want to be a competitive swimmer, it should be phase IV; but if you just want to be reasonably fit, that would be the end of the Intermediate phase.

The program is progressive. Each phase has ten workouts—along with tips on how to vary them—that are designed to increase your fitness and your skills gradually. Once you've found your level, repeat each workout at least three times before going on to the next. If you work out:

Once a week: Your skills will improve; your fitness will improve somewhat; and you will enjoy the relaxing and therapeutic benefits of water.

Three times a week: You will also improve your physical condition, help to control your weight, and improve your muscle tone. (Studies have shown that it takes twelve to twenty weeks working at a minimum of three days per week to affect your cardiovascular conditioning; alternating days of training with rest days gives your body time to recover.)

Every day: You will progress even faster and become even more fit. (Actually, you should work out only six days in a row at the most, and give your body a rest on the seventh.) Studies have shown that during the first ten weeks of a conditioning program the training effect is similar whether you exercise three days a week or more; but after that, exercising five or six times a week will result in faster and greater progress.

However often you choose to work out, don't skip any level, and wait until you feel you're ready before you go on to the next stage. Strive for a balance between taking it too easy and pushing yourself too hard and too fast. Listen to your body. Physical fitness, like Rome, isn't built in a day. (See "Watch Out!" below.) After a workout, you should feel exhilarated yet pleasantly tired. Your body should feel more relaxed, yet stronger, more flexible, and more alive.

WATCH OUT!

➤

My program is a step-by-step progression. Don't skip any level—in your enthusiasm, you may be tempted to overdo it. Be on the lookout for any of these danger signals that mean you're doing too much too fast. If any occurs, reduce the intensity, frequency, and/or duration of your workouts; if it persists, consult a physician. Moderation is the key; heed the following:

- Tightness or pain in your chest/skipped heartbeats
- Severe breathlessness
- Dizziness or nausea
- Loss of muscle control
- Joint pain
- Fatigue during the day; difficulty sleeping at night

To help prevent them, follow these tips:

- If you have any doubt as to your physical condition, have a checkup before you begin.
- Maintain a balanced diet.
- Warm up thoroughly before the main set of your workout, and cool down afterward.
- Monitor your pulse to make sure you don't exceed your target rate.
- Make sure you're comfortable at your present level before you proceed to the next.
- Don't swim when you're injured, sick, or very tired. Use your judgment here—even if you're not up to a full workout, you may be able to take a short swim, practice a few skills, or do some water exercises.

TRAINING CONCEPTS
～

You get the training effect when you overload your body by increasing the intensity, frequency, and duration of your swims. There are a number of ways to accomplish this, and you don't have to be a competitive swimmer to use these tried-and-true training methods. All of the following concepts we used in the workouts that follow. You can also use these underlying principles to create your own workouts or individualize those on pages 239 through 318. Depending on your goals, your pool facility, and your mood, you may choose to emphasize some over others. By incorporating them all into your swimming program, though, you're sure to keep your workouts interesting and challenging, and to subject your body to different types of stress.

Marathon, or Distance, Swimming: This is swimming for a relatively long distance without stopping for a rest. You can either swim easily without regard to the clock, or time the swim or some part of it. Without some sort of timing, though, most people tend to take it too easy and swim too slowly (pulse rate remains under the target rate) to get much conditioning. You'll still burn up calories, and it's an excellent way to swim if you're tired. The term "garbage yardage" is popularly used to describe long, easy swims that aim for quantity instead of quality. Even if you don't use the clock, you can still vary your pace—just swim parts a little faster, some a little slower. Or you can try to pace the entire swim; this offsets the tendency to start too fast, wear yourself out, and limp the last few laps home. Marathon swims are used primarily to improve your endurance; your heart rate doesn't climb that high (about 50–60 percent of maximum); but it stays at that level for the duration. Although you might not have thought so, this type of swim is often used as a warm-up before the main set. Every time you swim marathon-style, try to increase your distance by at least a few laps; common goals are 400 yards/meters (about a quarter mile), 800 yards/meters (about half a mile), or 1,600 yards/meters (about one mile). To keep track of your marathon swims, enter them on one of the Red Cross 50-mile swim charts that are posted at many pools.

Fartlek Training: Long a favorite training technique in Sweden (especially for running), this method breaks a swim into alternating slow and fast laps. It not only makes a long swim (for instance, 500 yards/meters or more) more interesting, it's a great way to develop speed and endurance simultaneously, because the slow laps, at about 50 percent of your maximum heart rate, enable you to exert yourself more during the fast laps, during which you swim at 80 percent of your maximum. You can modify the Fartlek technique by varying the number of laps swum at each speed. For instance, you can swim pyramid style: 1 fast, 1 slow; 2 fast, 2 slow; 3 fast, 3 slow; 2 fast, 2 slow; 1 fast, 1 slow. Make up your own patterns.

Interval Training: In this method, which was introduced into competitive swimming workouts during the 1940s, you do a series of repeat swims of the same distance, each within a specified length of time. The amount of rest you have after each swim is determined by how fast you go. For instance, if the *interval set* is four 50-yard swims in 1 minute and 15 seconds each (4 × 50 on 1:15), and you take 1 minute to swim the first 50, you have 15 seconds' rest before beginning the next 50-yard swim; if you swim the 50 yards in 45 seconds, you have 30 seconds to rest.

Competitive swimmers swim at slower speeds in a workout than dur-

TRAINING CONCEPTS CHART

This chart is geared mainly to serious fitness and competitive swimmers. Distances, rest intervals, and target pulse rates will vary, depending on the swimmer.

TYPE OF TRAINING	EXAMPLES OF DISTANCE (Yards/Meters)	APPROXIMATE REST TIME	ENDURANCE DEVELOPMENT RATIO	SPEED	TARGET PULSE RATE (Percentage of Maximum Pulse Rate)
Marathon	1,000–3,000	0	95%	5%	60%
Fartlek	500–1,000	0	35%	65%	80% (Hard)
Interval	8 × 100 or 15 × 50	15–30 sec.	55%	45%	70%
Repetition	4 × 100 or 8 × 50	1–2 min. (rest = swim time)	25%	75%	90%
Sprint	3 × 50 or 4 × 25	5 min.	5%	95%	100%

ing the actual competiton, but the intervals are still pretty fast—100s on 1:30 is typical at this level.

Usually, intervals are designed to give swimmers a short rest period relative to the length of time spent swimming. This way, you don't allow the heart rate to drop too much, but the short rest lets you push yourself harder during each swim, which results in greater cardiovascular benefits. Interval swimming, therefore, is the best all-round training method for developing speed and endurance. This method should get your heart rate up to approximately 70 percent of your maximum during the swim, and the rest period should be short enough so that your heart rate doesn't recover all the way down to your resting rate. Intervals are widely used as part or all of the main set of a workout.

It's easiest if you begin each interval set on the 60-second mark: if the interval were 1 minute (1:00), you would begin the second swim when the second hand hit the 60-second mark. If the interval were on 1:15, you would begin the first swim on the 60-second mark, the second on the 15-second mark, the third on the 30-second mark, and so on. (Another type of interval training may be used, too, in which the amount of rest is held constant—say, 10 seconds after each 50 yards/meters—regardless of the time it takes you to do each swim.)

Repetition, or Repeat, Training: These are sets of swims of the same distance done at close to maximum effort (up to 90 percent of your maximum heart rate), but with a long rest period after each swim (usually equal to the swimming time) that allows the heart rate to come back down to nearly normal. This type of swimming develops your speed and anaerobic capacity (the ability to work at intense levels, by using stored oxygen, for moderate periods of time); since it is fatiguing, this method is used sparingly, usually to prepare competitive swimmers for peak performances, and only after a thorough warm-up.

Sprints: These are short, fast swims done at maximum speed (up to 100 percent effort) to simulate the conditions of a race. The amount of rest is usually very long, and allows the heart rate to approach the resting rate. Because of the increased resistance encountered while moving faster, sprinting gives you more muscle power and strength than endurance; like repetition swimming, it also improves your anaerobic capacity.

COMPONENTS OF A WORKOUT
～

All of the workouts are composed of three parts: the warm-up, the main set, and the cool-down.

Warm-up: Swimming strenuously without being properly prepared results in discomfort, a poor performance, and possibly injury. So initiate each workout with a warm-up, which increases your body temperature slightly, gets the blood flowing to where it will be needed, and begins to raise your heart rate. Usually you should do some sort of warm-up on land: for example, light calisthenics such as those suggested in "Swimmers' Shape-ups," page 371. (Many of these exercises may also be done in shallow water, if you prefer.) If you have the time and inclination, you may choose to do some more serious activity, such as working out with resistance devices (freeweights, stretch cords, or Nautilus or Universal weight machines) or some light jogging, before a swim.

Regardless of what you do on land, there's always a water warm-up of some sort—when you just swim in an easy, relaxed manner. This not only raises your body temperature, it also gets you in "the groove" for swimming, the way pitchers throw a few practice balls, tennis players rally, and singers practice the scale before plunging into the real thing. To make the warm-up interesting, you can, for example, break it up into several pull, kick, swim sets. The point is to ease the body into the main set of the workout. The warm-up should take at least five minutes, or about 20 percent of the total workout time or distance, whichever is greater.

Main Set: This is usually a swimming set (meaning that you use your arms and legs together), and should be the most demanding part of the workout. Most main sets consist of one long set or several subsets with short breaks between. Advanced swimmers might do these against the clock (interval or repetition swims) to get their heart rate up to 70 percent of their maximum. Sometimes a main set consists of a marathon swim; in this case the heart rate doesn't get all the way up to 70 percent, but you improve your endurance. The duration of the main set will vary according to the overall workout, but, in general, it is at least 50 percent of the total time/distance.

Cool-down: This consists of a few laps at the end of the workout to relax and loosen the body. It's also a way of letting your heart rate return

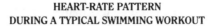

HEART-RATE PATTERN
DURING A TYPICAL SWIMMING WORKOUT

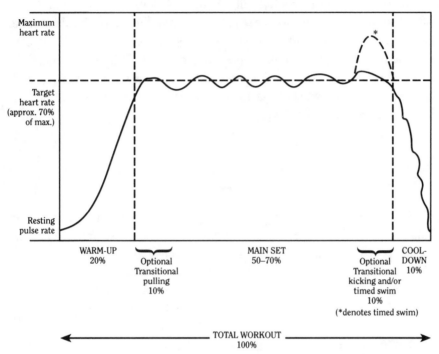

gradually to your resting rate. A cool-down is about 10 percent of the total workout, or about half the distance of the warm-up. You might want to add a post-cool-down on land. This should consist of gentle static stretches to keep your muscles loose. (See "Swimmers' Shape-ups," page 371, for suggestions.)

Transitions: At higher levels, where you are swimming longer distances, some coaches add two transitional stages to the workout. When used, each transition accounts for about 10 percent of the total workout. The first comes between the warm-up and the main set, and often consists of pulling in a descending fashion. For example, you might do 5 × 50 (50 yards/meters five times), where each 50 is pulled faster than the previous one. In this way, by the end of the pulling set you have gradually brought your heart rate up to 70 percent of maximum (the target rate), thus completing the warm-up process and setting yourself up for the more strenuous work of the main set.

The second transition comes between the main set and the cool-down. This transitional phase should be less demanding than the main set, both psychologically and physiologically. It usually consists of a kicking set. After the main set, your arms are probably tired, but there should still be plenty of energy in your legs. Occasionally, the end of a workout can include something challenging, like a timed sprint. This sprint shouldn't be done every day, though: if it becomes a habit it will get boring, and besides, your body needs time to recover. When done, it should be followed by a few easy laps.

WORKOUT TERMS
~

As you progress from phase to phase, you'll also begin to learn a new language—the language of swimming. Like all sports, swimming has its special terms and verbal shortcuts. Here are a few to get you started.

Distance Notation: The first new terminology you'll need in the workouts is the most basic: how distances are indicated. For instance:

1 × 50 means swim 50 yards or meters 1 time
2 × 50 means swim 50 yards or meters 2 times (with a rest after each 50)
1 × 100 means swim 100 yards or meters

Pulling,   or using the arm motion without kicking, helps you learn or practice a stroke and to build upper body strength. Pulling drills are good for your warm-up. Mixed with kicking and swimming laps, they can add variety to your main set, too. During pulling drills, you can use training devices such as pull-buoys to help support your lower body, or hand paddles and/or "donuts" to improve your technique and to increase the resistance.

Kicking   means using only the leg motion of a stroke. Recently there's been some debate as to how much of it should be done and where in the workout it should come. On the one hand, the arms—not the kicking—should generate most of the power of the stroke. On the other hand, it's important to practice your kicking, since it's central to the stability, timing, and coordination of your stroke, and to the development of your stomach and chest muscles, and your legs. Since the legs contain large muscles, they require a great deal of oxygen; therefore, kicking hard during a workout helps to improve your cardiovascular efficiency. So kicking *is* important, but more so in training than when you're swimming normally. Also, kicking is often used as a transitional set between the main set and the cool-down. You can do kicking drills and use training devices such as swim fins and kickboards to help you learn or improve a kick, or increase in strength and power.

Pull-Kick-Swim Set: Here you pull the first lap, kick the next lap, swim (use arms and legs together) for the last lap. By isolating each component first, you refine and improve the whole stroke.

Controlled Breathing: As you improve your cardiovascular fitness you may need to take fewer breaths as you swim the freestyle. In the freestyle, inhaling on every third pull is called bilateral breathing. By breathing on both sides and by taking fewer breaths you may improve the efficiency of your strokes.

When you take fewer breaths as you swim, you increase your body's ability to function efficiently with less oxygen. By training your body to do more with less, you increase your cardiovascular fitness and your ability to get a "second wind." In the freestyle, controlled breathing is usually introduced by inhaling on every third pull (*bilateral breathing*); eventually you can work your way up to swimming an entire lap without inhaling.

Broken Swims: These are timed swims that are interrupted by short rests of a specified length (e.g., ten seconds). After completing the entire swim, you subtract the total resting time from the final time to determine your swim time.

Build-ups: In this training technique, you begin each lap slowly and gradually build up speed as you reach the wall. This allows you to establish your technique and maintain it as you build up speed.

Crescendo Set: This is several swims of regularly increasing distances (for example: 1×25, 1×50, 1×75).

Pyramid Set: This is several swims of regularly increasing, then regularly decreasing, distances. (For example, 1×25, 1×50, 1×75, 1×50, 1×25.) This is also known as an ascending/descending set.

Stroke Counting: Here you count the number of strokes needed to complete a certain distance (usually one lap, or 25 yards/meters), then try to lower the count the next time you swim it (while maintaining your speed). Do a stroke count periodically to check your improving efficiency and power.

Paced Swims: Try this so that you don't go all out during the first half of your swim and fade out toward the end. By timing yourself for both halves of a swim, and approximating the same time for each, you get a feel for pacing yourself. This is known as *even splitting.* If the second half is faster than the first, it's called *negative splitting;* you can do this by concentrating on your pulling in the beginning and gradually increasing the intensity of your kicking. You can apply this principle to all swims 100 yards/meters and longer. Pacing yourself also gets you accustomed to reading the clock while you swim and thus prepares you for interval swimming.

Pulse Rates and Pulse Check: Checking your pulse immediately after a main set or timed swim is one way of determining whether you're overdoing it or not doing enough. It will eventually be a way of measuring your progress, because the lower your resting rate the more efficient your cardiovascular system.

To take your pulse, press the inside of your wrist firmly with the fingertips of the other hand. (Using the thumb will not give you an accurate reading, because it has its own pulse.) Or feel for your pulse on your throat, just below the angle of the jaw. Count the beats for 6 seconds; then add a 0 to the end to give you the per-minute rate.

First take your *resting rate,* which is best done in the morning before you've exercised or drunk any coffee (caffeine stimulates the heart and would influence the reading). Write it down somewhere (perhaps in the spaces allocated in the workouts, or in your Swimmers' Log). The average resting rate is 72 beats per minute, but athletes' pulse rates are often lower.

Next, calculate your *maximum heart rate (MHR).* To approximate this, subtract your age from a base of 220. Therefore, if you are thirty-five years old, your MHR will be about 185. The next figure to be concerned with is your *target rate (TR).* To calculate your TR, multiply your MHR by approximately 70 percent. So, if your MHR is 185, your TR would be about 130. To improve your cardiovascular capacity, your heart rate should average your TR during the main set of your workout.

Be aware that, as you train and improve your cardiovascular conditioning, it will take more effort (i.e., you'll have to swim faster) to obtain your target heart rate.

Recent research indicates that your heart rate may be lower in the water compared to exercising on land by 10 to 15 percent.

Timed Swim and Pulse Check: For this, you time yourself as you swim a particular distance, comparing your performance to your previous times. Afterward, you check your pulse rate to see if you have approached your 70 percent target rate (usually you do this by swimming fast, but not "all out"—the latter would elevate your pulse to 100 percent of its maximum rate, which is rarely desirable). A timed swim in conjunction with a pulse check gives you a feel for what working at this level of effort is like. You also get accustomed to referring to the clock, which will figure into your workouts more and more as you progress. (All swims, except for warm-ups, cool-downs, and other specified easy swims, should be done at an average of about 70 percent effort.) You can do a timed swim (with or without a pulse check afterward) during any workout; it should be near the end of the main set so that you're nicely warmed up for a fast swim. Timing yourself lets you see the progress you're making, makes the workout more interesting, and helps you determine your time interval for interval swims.

VARIETY IS THE SPICE OF SWIMMING, TOO
～

The workouts will improve your fitness gradually and safely. But won't just swimming a little farther each time do that? Yes, but that would be boring.

In these workouts, on the other hand, you'll be doing a variety of strokes; you will alternately swim (use your arms and legs together), pull (use only your arms), and kick (use only the legs); you'll swim varying distances; in addition, you'll be using different pieces of equipment. All this adds up to a tremendous variety. And as you progress you can swim against the clock (intervals, repeats, sprints, paced swims) to make things even more interesting.

The workouts on the following pages do this, and more: they are also learning workouts during which you may add to your repertoire of skills. (If you're not up to learning a new skill, substitute practicing something you do know and want to improve in order to get the same amount of working out.) But if you want to learn something new, it's there for you to take advantage of, presented in a logical sequence and in the context of a workout that contains other related skills to make learning easier and more understandable.

REMEMBERING THE WORKOUTS
～

The more involved you become in swimming, the more you'll realize that it's a mental as well as physical discipline. Swim teams are lucky enough to have a coach telling (yelling at!) them exactly what to do for every phase of their workout—and, in addition, the day's workout may be written on a large blackboard near the pool. For those of you who are following these workouts solo, it's a different story: you don't have anyone to rely on except yourself.

The simplest solution is to memorize the workout. To do this, read it over several times before you go to the pool. Go over every one of the exercises, drills, and swims in your head. The purpose here is to remember the workout. If any new skills are involved, be sure to practice them on dry land first so that by the time you get to the water you're pretty well familiar with them.

If you have a swimming buddy, you can help each other to remember.

If memorizing the workouts doesn't come easily to you, there are several alternatives. First, you could enclose the entire book in plastic and take it to the pool with you. (The clear zip-up bags used to store food are ideal for this.)

Better yet, you could rewrite the day's workout on a small piece of paper. Use a heavy pencil or a ballpoint pen and, at the pool, dip the paper into the water and slap it either onto the wall just above the water line or on the deck. (Wetting it keeps the paper from flying away, and the ink doesn't run as much as you'd expect.)

Or you could write each workout on an index card, then, for instant waterproofing, simply return the card to the plastic wrapper that the pack came in. You could also make each workout waterproof by encasing the card in transparent plastic with a self-stick, peel-off backing. A fringe benefit of this method is that you'll end up with your own set of permanent workout cards that you can take with you anywhere.

WORKOUT TIPS AND REMINDERS
➤

- If the specified distances for the continuous swims are too long for you at first, swim as far as you can, gradually increasing the distance each time you do the workout until you can swim the specified distance without stopping.

- If you find that the specified rests are more than you need, decrease them accordingly.

- Try to swim at least three times a week, and repeat each workout at least three times, preferably every other day, before progressing to the next level. If you begin a new workout every week, it will take you approximately two and a half to three months to complete each phase of your fitness program and to advance to the next phase. At that rate, if you start the program as a Beginner, by the end of about a year you will have progressed through the Super Swimmer phase.

- To learn or refine a new skill, practice the motions on dry land before you get to the pool (they're explained in "The Techniques of Swimming," pages 109–86). And once you've learned them, you should generally incorporate them into your swimming from then on. For instance, once you've learned the S-pattern crawl stroke, the body roll, or the flip turn, use them whenever you swim.

- Use the different training concepts to create your own workouts and to add variety to your swims. For instance, use Fartlek training during a long swim; or do a pull-kick-swim series instead of just swimming; or time yourself; or do a stroke count periodically.

- If you're swimming every day, try to avoid doing the same kind of workout. For example, about twice a week concentrate on practicing skills and techniques that you know need improvement. (Refer to the checklists and the catalog of common errors found in "The Techniques of Swimming" and do the suggested drills.) On other days, go for quantity as well as quality.

- If you like, record your workouts in the Workout Log on page 394—especially if you're doing workouts in addition to those in this book.

- Record your times in the Timed Swim Log on page 396.

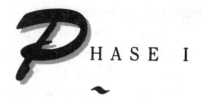

PHASE I

BEGINNERS' WORKOUTS

WHO'S A BEGINNER?

You're a Beginner swimmer if you:

- Can swim 10–25 yards/meters without stopping and using any combination of strokes.
- Know at least "The Fundamentals of Swimming" taught in Part One of this book (crawl stroke, elementary and windmill backstrokes, treading, sculling, sitting and kneeling dives).

If you are a more advanced swimmer, you can still use these workouts when, for some reason, you can't follow your regular workout.

BEGINNER SKILLS AND TERMS

The crawl stroke term is used starting in the Beginners' workout. With each progressive workout and phase, you will be refining these techniques. This refined crawl stroke is popularly termed "freestyle" and therefore the terms "crawl" and "freestyle" are often interchangeable.

In these workouts you'll practice the following skills (explained in "The Techniques of Swimming") and use the following terms (explained in "Workout Terms," page 232):

- S-pattern crawl/freestyle arm motion
- Windmill backstroke body roll
- Sidestroke
- Breaststroke
- Open turns for crawl and backstroke
- Crescendo set

Your level of fitness will improve with each workout:

- You'll be swimming longer and longer distances without stopping (from 25 yards/meters in Level 1 to 75 yards/meters in Level 10).
- You'll get gradually less rest between swims (from one minute in Level 1 down to 30 seconds).
- You'll be swimming longer total distances (from 100 yards/meters in Level 1 to 300 yards/meters in Level 10).

Each workout begins at the shallow end of the pool and lasts about 30 minutes, depending on how fast you swim. About half the workout time is devoted to the warm-up and cool-down combined, and half to the main set, which is the most strenuous. The warm-up is about 10 minutes, the main set is about 15 minutes, and the cool-down is 5 minutes. The warm-ups usually include some Swimmers' Shape-ups (see page 371), which may be done on dry land or in the shallow end of the pool; it also includes shallow-water practice of any skills highlighted in the workout. The cool-down also usually includes a few Swimmers' Shape-ups, which may be done in the shallow end of the pool or on dry land.

SPECIAL TIPS FOR BEGINNING SWIMMERS

➤

- Notice that when a specific stroke is highlighted the total distance swum doesn't increase. The distance is held steady so you can devote your energies toward learning and practicing the new skill.
- Ideal pool size is 20 or 25 yards/meters. If the length differs much, alter the workouts accordingly. First, find out how long the pool is by checking the pool markers (or ask the lifeguard, pool manager, or other swimmer). Otherwise, the handiest way to approximate the length is by pacing it off; walk the length, placing one foot directly in front of the other, and count each pace as one foot. Then

divide the number by three to get the approximate yardage. Once you have the yardage, adjust the workouts accordingly. For instance, if the pool is 15 yards long, you can just double the number of laps: for a 25-yard swim, do two laps, or 30 yards. If it's a much longer pool, determine the 25-yard mark and stop there to rest before resuming the workout.

- If there's no clock with a second hand, or you don't have a waterproof wristwatch you can approximate your rest times by counting off the seconds in your head.

TO VARY THE WORKOUTS
～

If you choose to stay at the Beginner level, or to take longer to progress to the Intermediate phase, you'll be repeating each workout more than three times. In order to add more variety to them:

- Begin to use some of the equipment described in that level.
- Choose different Swimmers' Shake-ups (see page 371) for warm-ups and cool-downs.
- Add more distance to the main set (but not to exceed a total of forty-five minutes in the water). You might even repeat the entire main set.
- Change the pace over the course of the workout. Each workout lasts approximately twenty-five to thirty minutes. Leave the warm-up and cool-down intact, but vary your speed during the main set; take longer or shorter rests between laps.
- Stress the skills that you need to brush up on. Ask a friend to help you check your form. Don't hesitate to go back and repeat an earlier workout in order to review certain skills.
- Try to increase the amount of continuous swimming you do. Aim for 300 consecutive yards/meters for each stroke that you know.
- If you get really itchy for a change, it's a definite sign that you are ready to go on to the Intermediate phase, which will add to your skills and improve your fitness even more.

BEGINNERS' LEVEL 1

～

Highlights: Reviewing the fundamentals of swimming (sculling, treading, crawl stroke, elementary backstroke, and sitting dive) in the form of a workout

Total Distance: 100 yards/meters

Warm-up

5 minutes Swimmers' Shape-ups
1 minute each: bobbing: with breathing
                 supine flutter kick: on wall
                 prone flutter kick: on wall
                 rhythmic breathing: on wall

Main Set (1 minute rest after each)

1 × 25 crawl stroke
1 minute bobbing: with breathing
1 × 25 crawl stroke
1 minute bobbing: with breathing
1 × 25 sculling
1 × 25 elementary backstroke

Cool-down

1 minute treading in place: rest when needed
3 × push-off into prone glide
3 × sitting dive
1 minute Swimmers' Shape-ups: stretches

BEGINNERS' LEVEL 2

～

Highlights: S-pattern crawl stroke (see page 119)

Total Distance: 100 yards/meters

Warm-up

Skill practice: catch-up S-pattern crawl stroke on land
3 minutes Swimmers' Shape-ups
1 minute each: bobbing: with breathing
     catch-up S-pattern crawl stroke: standing in place in
      shallow water
     catch-up S-pattern crawl stroke: walking with head up
      (two pool widths or about 25 yards/meters)
     catch-up S-pattern crawl stroke: walking with rhyth-
      mic breathing (two pool widths or about 25 yards/
      meters)

Main Set (1 minute rest after each)

1 × 25 catch-up S-pattern crawl stroke: with flutter kicking
1 × 25 elementary backstroke: with flutter kicking
10 cycles catch-up S-pattern crawl stroke: standing in place in shallow
 water
1 × 25 S-pattern crawl stroke: with flutter kicking (no catch-up)
1 × 25 sculling: with flutter kicking

Cool-down

1 minute each: bobbing: with breathing
     catch-up S-pattern crawl stroke: walking with rhyth-
      mic breathing
     treading: in place
Push-up exit from pool
1 minute Swimmers' Shape-ups: stretches

BEGINNERS' LEVEL 3

～

Highlights: Crawl-stroke open turn (see page 205); swimming the crawl stroke continuously for 50 yards/meters

Total Distance: 150 yards/meters

Warm-up

3 minutes Swimmers' Shape-ups
1 minute each: catch-up S-pattern crawl stroke: on land
                  prone flutter kicking: on wall
                  catch-up S-pattern crawl stroke: standing in place in shallow water
                  open crawl turn: walking toward wall in shallow water (alternate contact arms)
                  catch-up S-pattern crawl stroke: walking with rhythmic breathing (two pool widths or about 25 yards/meters)

Main Set (1 minute rest after each)

1 × 50 S-pattern crawl stroke: with flutter kicking, using open turn
1 × 25 sculling: with flutter kicking
½ minute treading: in deep water (with or without assistance)
1 × 25 elementary backstroke
1 × 50 S-pattern crawl stroke: with flutter kicking, using open turn (other hand, if possible)

Cool-down

1 minute open crawl turn: walking toward wall in shallow water (alternate contact arms)
½ minute treading
Push-up exit from pool
3 × sitting dive/push-up exit
1 minute Swimmers' Shape-ups: stretches

Beginners' Level 4

~

Highlights: Windmill backstroke body roll (see page 137)

Total Distance: 150 yards/meters

Warm-up

3 minutes Swimmers' Shape-ups for arms and shoulders

1 minute each: bobbing: with breathing

supine flutter kick: on wall, or with kickboard across width

catch-up S-pattern crawl stroke: walking with rhythmic breathing (two pool widths or 25 yards/meters) using open turn

windmill backstroke: standing in place with body roll

windmill backstroke: with body roll, walking backward in shoulder-deep water (two pool widths or 25 yards/meters)

Main Set (1 minute rest after each)

1×25 sculling or elementary backstroke: with flutter kicking

½ minute treading: in deep water (with or without assistance)

1×25 windmill backstroke: with body roll and flutter kicking

1×50 S-pattern crawl stroke: with flutter kicking, using open turn

1×25 windmill backstroke: with body roll and flutter kicking

½ minute treading: in deep water (with or without assistance)

1×25 windmill backstroke: with body roll and flutter kicking

Cool-down

1 minute each: treading, alternating with prone float rest

windmill backstroke: standing in place with body roll

windmill backstroke: with body roll, walking backward in shoulder-deep water (two pool widths or 25 yards/meters)

3 minutes Swimmers' Shape-ups: arm and shoulder stretches

BEGINNERS' LEVEL 5

～

Highlights: Backstroke open turn (see page 207); swimming the backstroke continuously for 50 yards/meters

Total Distance: 150 yards/meters

Warm-up

3 minutes Swimmers' Shape-ups
1 minute each: catch-up windmill backstroke: on land or in place in shoulder-deep water
backstroke open turn: walking toward wall in shallow water (alternate contact arms)
bobbing: with breathing
supine flutter kick: on wall
backstroke open turn: walking toward wall in shallow water (alternate contact arms)

Main Set (½ minute rest after each)

1 × 50 windmill backstroke: with flutter kicking, using open turn
1 × 25 elementary backstroke
½ minute treading: in deep water (with or without assistance)
1 × 25 S-pattern crawl stroke: with flutter kicking
½ minute treading
1 × 50 windmill backstroke: with flutter kicking, using open turn

Cool-down

1 minute each: backstroke open turn: walking toward wall in shallow water
sculling: alternating with treading
whip kick: in supine position on wall or with kickboard
push-up exit from pool
2 × sitting dive/push-up exit
2 × kneeling dive/push-up exit

BEGINNERS' LEVEL 6

～

Highlights: Swimming the crawl and backstroke continuously for 50 yards/meters

Total Distance: 200 yards/meters

Warm-up

3 minutes Swimmers' Shape-ups
1 minute each: bobbing: with breathing
                prone flutter kicking: on wall with rhythmic breathing
                S-pattern crawl stroke: in shoulder-deep water, using open turn (two pool widths or about 25 yards/meters)
                windmill backstroke: in shoulder-deep water, using open turn (two pool widths or about 25 yards/meters)
                push-up exit from pool

Main Set (1 minute rest after each 50; 1 minute treading after each 25)

1×50 continuous swim: sitting dive, 1×25 crawl, open turn, 1×25 windmill backstroke
1×25 elementary backstroke
1×25 crawl
1×25 sculling: with flutter kicking
1×25 elementary backstroke
Push-up exit
1×50 continuous swim: kneeling dive, 1×25 crawl, open turn, 1×25 windmill backstroke

Cool-down

1 minute each: whip kick: on wall in supine position
                whip kick: on wall in prone position
                prone flutter kick: on wall
2 minutes Swimmers' Shape-ups: stretches

BEGINNERS' LEVEL 7

Highlights: The breaststroke (see page 145)

Total Distance: 200 yards/meters

Warm-up

2 minutes Swimmers' Shape-ups: arm and shoulder exercises
1 minute each: breaststroke arm motion: on land
        combined breaststroke arm and leg motions: on land
        bobbing: with breathing
        whip kick: in prone position, on wall or with kick-
          board
        breaststroke arm motion: while standing in place in
          shoulder-deep water
        breaststroke arm motion: with walking and breathing
          (two pool widths or about 25 yards/meters)
        combined breaststroke arm and leg motions: sitting
          or standing

Main Set (½ minute rest after each 50 and 25)

1 × 50 continuous swim: backstroke, open turn, crawl
1 × 25 breaststroke pull: (kicking and equipment optional)
½ minute whip kick: in prone position on wall
1 × 25 breaststroke swim: (arm and legs combined)
Push-up exit
1 × 50 continuous swim: kneeling dive, crawl, open turn, elementary
  backstroke with whip kick
1 × 25 breaststroke swim
½ minute treading
1 × 25 breaststroke swim

Cool-down

1 minute each: whip kick: on wall in supine position
        combined breaststroke arm and leg motion: standing
          in place
        whip kick: on wall in prone position
2 minutes Swimmers' Shape-ups: stretches

BEGINNERS' LEVEL 8

～

Highlights: Breaststroke, crawl stroke, open turns, backstroke, treading, and diving

Total Distance: 250 yards/meters

Warm-up

5 minutes Swimmers' Shape-ups
1 minute breaststroke arm motion: with coordinated breathing, standing in shoulder-deep water
½ minute each: bobbing: with breathing
  whip kick: in supine position, on wall or with kickboard
  breaststroke arm motion: with coordinated breathing walking in shoulder-deep water
  combined breaststroke arm and leg motions: standing in place

Main Set (½ minute rest after each 50; 1 minute treading after each 25)

1 × 50 continuous swim: backstroke, open turn, crawl
1 × 25 breaststroke
1 × 25 sculling
Push-up exit
1 × 50 continuous swim: sitting dive, crawl, open turn, elementary backstroke with whip kick
2 × 25 breaststroke
Push-up exit
1 × 50 continuous swim: kneeling dive, crawl, open turn, stroke of your choice

Cool-down

1 minute each: whip kick: in prone position, on wall or with kickboard
  prone flutter kicking: on wall or with kickboard
2 minutes Swimmers' Shape-ups: stretches

BEGINNERS' LEVEL 9
～

Highlights: The sidestroke (see page 174)

Total Distance: 250 yards/meters

Warm-up

1 minute each: regular sidestroke arm motion: (each side) on land
sidestroke overarm variation: (each side) on land
scissors kick: (each side) on land
bobbing: with breathing
scissors kick: on wall or with kickboard (each side)
regular sidestroke arm motion: while walking across
pool width or swimming with kickboard (each side)
overarm sidestroke variation: while walking across
pool width or swimming with kickboard (each side)
your choice of combined sidestroke arm and leg motions: while standing in place (each side)

Main Set (½ minute rest after each)

1 × 50 elementary backstroke: with whip kick, open turn, breaststroke
1 × 25 sidestroke: on right side (with or without assistance)
1 × 25 sidestroke: on left side (with or without assistance)
1 × 50 continuous swim: sculling with flutter kicking, open turn,
crawl
1 × 25 sidestroke: on right side
½ minute treading
1 × 25 sidestroke: on left side
Push-up exit
1 × 50 continuous swim: kneeling dive, crawl, open turn, backstroke

Cool-down

1 minute each: whip kick: in supine position, on wall or with kickboard
scissors kick: with kickboard (each side)
combined sidestroke arm and leg motions: while
standing in place (each side)
2 minutes Swimmers' Shape-ups: stretches

Beginners' Level 10
~

Highlights: Swimming two crescendo-type sets of 25, 50, and 75 yards/meters

Total Distance: 300 yards/meters

Warm-up

1 minute each: windmill backstroke arm motion
crawl-stroke arm motion: standing in place
elementary backstroke arm motion: standing in place
breaststroke arm motion: standing in place
sidestroke arm motion: (your choice of regular or overarm—each side), standing in place
bobbing: with breathing
flutter kick: (prone or supine) on wall or with kickboard
whip kick: in supine position, on wall or with kickboard
sidestroke arm motion: walking across pool or with kickboard (your choice—each side)
combined sidestroke arm and leg motions: standing in place (your choice—each side)

Main Set (½ minute rest after each)

Repeat 2 ×
1 × 25 sidestroke
1 × 50 continuous swim: catch-up crawl, open turn, regular crawl
1 × 75 continuous swim: backstroke, open turn, breaststroke, open turn, sculling

Cool-down

1 minute treading: alternating with prone or supine float
2 minutes Swimmers' Shape-ups: stretches
Push-up exit
2 × kneeling dive/push-up exit

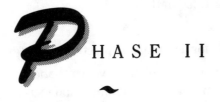

$\mathcal{P}$HASE II

INTERMEDIATE WORKOUTS

WHO'S AN INTERMEDIATE?

You're an Intermediate swimmer if you:

- Can swim at least 75 yards/meters without stopping.
- Know the skills taught in "The Fundamentals of Swimming" (crawl stroke, elementary and windmill backstrokes, treading, sculling, sitting and kneeling dives), plus the skills and terms included in the "Beginners' Workouts": S-pattern crawl-stroke arm motion, windmill backstroke body roll, sidestroke, breaststroke, open turns for the crawl and backstroke, crescendo set. If you need to, learn or review these skills before beginning the following workouts.

INTERMEDIATE SKILLS AND TERMS

As an Intermediate swimmer, you'll practice these skills (explained in "The Techniques of Swimming") and become more familiar with the terms (explained in "Workout Terms" and "Training Concepts"):

- Backstroke start
- Butterfly stroke
- Crawl/freestyle body roll

- Individual Medley (IM)
- Stroke counting
- Stroke drills for learning and practicing skills
- Using equipment to isolate movements and/or increase resistance, in order to improve your technique and increase your strength
- Pull-kick-swim series and variations: kick-swim series, pull-swim series, kick-swim-kick series
- Timed swim and pulse check
- Pyramid sets—ascending/descending

Your fitness will continue to improve:

- You'll progress from swimming 50 consecutive yards/meters in Level 1 to 250 yards/meters in Level 10.
- You'll get less rest between swims.
- Your total workout distance will increase from 300 yards/meters in Level 1 to 1,000 yards/meters in Level 10.

Each workout lasts between thirty and forty-five minutes, depending on how fast you swim, and on how long and how often you need rest. The warm-ups include some Swimmers' Shape-ups, which may be done on land or in shallow water, and to which you might want to devote more time on your own; the warm-ups also include dry-land or shallow-water practice of any new skills highlighted in the workout. It's also advisable to add some stretches from the Swimmers' Shape-ups to your cool-down.

Since Levels 1–5 highlight a number of skills during the warm-up, the distances actually swum in this part of the workout are shorter than they ordinarily would be. During Levels 6–10, though, the warm-up distances become increasingly longer because the number of review skills decreases. By Level 10, you'll be doing 150 yards/meters as a warm-up, and 50 yards/meters as a cool-down, with 800 yards as a main set.

SPECIAL TIPS FOR INTERMEDIATE SWIMMERS

～

- By now make the effort to swim in a 20- or 25-yard/meter pool. Since the workouts are based on a 25-yard/meter lap, alter the workout slightly if your pool measures only 20 yards/meters: swim 1 × 20 instead of 1 × 25; 1 × 40 (two laps) instead of 1 × 50; and

1×80 (four laps) instead of 1×75. For 1×100 swims, you can swim five laps instead of four to obtain the same total. (Make similar adjustments if your pool is a different size.)

- If you're in a long-course (50-meter) pool, you'll be making fewer turns and so getting a more strenuous workout. Therefore, if you need to, arrange to swim in an outside lane, which will enable you to stop and rest mid-lap, especially during 25- or 75-yard/meter swims. Another thing—most long-course pools do not have an end shallow enough to allow you to practice skills. If this is the case in your pool, practice new skills first on dry land as best you can, or try to find a pool more suitable for such practice.

- If you've no clock or watch with a second hand, approximate the seconds by counting to yourself, or by bobbing at the rate of one bob per second; get a feel for the rhythm by practicing with a clock first. If you do timed swims, though, you need a more accurate way of measuring time.

- If you find that you're having trouble with a new stroke at first, substitute another, more familiar one (such as the crawl/freestyle) for part of the swim. But don't forget about the new stroke completely.

- The Individual Medley is a combination of the four competitive strokes in a particular sequence. Here's how I remember the order: First you do the butterfly, which takes the most energy; then you turn over to do the backstroke because you're dying for air from the butterfly; next comes the breaststroke to let you rest and stretch some more if you need to; then you end with the fastest stroke, the crawl/freestyle.

INTERMEDIATE LEVEL 1

～

Highlights: Single-beat dolphin kick (see page 164); use of fins (optional); timed 50-yard/meter swim and pulse check

Total Distance: 300 yards/meters

Warm-up (50 yards/meters)

3 minutes: Swimmers' Shape-ups
1 minute each: prone flutter kicking: with rhythmic breathing on wall
      new skill practice: dolphin kick in supine position on wall (in corner if possible)
      catch-up S-pattern crawl stroke: while standing in shoulder-deep water (see page 139)
      new skill practice: dolphin kick in prone position, on wall or across pool width
1 × 50 easy swim: kneeling dive, crawl stroke or your choice

OPTIONAL: Introduction to use of fins. Review the supine and prone flutter kick, then the dolphin kick in the supine and prone positions. Use fins (kickboard optional) during the rest of the workout and in subsequent workouts if you're having a problem with any kicking.

Main Set (200 yards/meters)

3 × 50 kick-swim series (½ minute rest after each 50):
  1 × 50 continuous kick-swim: 1 × 25 dolphin kick, 1 × 25 crawl
  1 × 50 continuous kick-swim: 1 × 25 backstroke flutter kick, 1 × 25 backstroke
  1 × 50 continuous kick-swim: 1 × 25 dolphin kick, 1 × 25 crawl; rest as needed
1 × 50 timed swim: kneeling dive, crawl/freestyle or swimmer's choice
Pulse check
(Record timed swim and pulse check in Timed Swim Log.)

Cool-down (50 yards/meters)

2 × 25 easy swim
  1 × 25 sculling
  1 × 25 elementary backstroke
New skill review: 1 minute dolphin kick on wall or across pool width;
  5 × push-off into prone glide with dolphin kick across pool width (use crawl/freestyle to complete width if needed)
2 minutes Swimmers' Shape-ups (stretches)

INTERMEDIATE LEVEL 2

Highlights: The butterfly pull and coordinating it with the single-beat dolphin kick (see page 160)

Total Distance: 300 yards/meters

Warm-up (50 yards/meters)

3 minutes Swimmers' Shape-ups
5 minutes skill practice (1 minute each):
    butterfly pull, standing in place
    butterfly pull with breathing, walking across width of pool
    single-beat dolphin kick on wall
    combined butterfly pull and kick, standing in place
    butterfly pull with breathing, walking in shallow water
1 × 50 easy swim: crawl/freestyle

Main Set (200 yards/meters; 2 × 25s alternating with 50s)

2 × 25 with ½ minute rest after each 25:
    1 × 25 butterfly
    1 × 25 crawl/freestyle or breaststroke
1 × 50 swim: crawl/freestyle; use catch-up S-pattern pull for first half
  of each 25
½ minute rest
2 × 25 butterfly swim with ½ minute rest after each 25
1 × 50 swim: crawl/freestyle

Cool-down (50 yards/meters)

2 × 25 easy kicking:
    1 × 25 dolphin
    1 × 25 whip
Skill review: 1 minute butterfly pull with breathing, standing in place;
    5 × push-off into prone glide with dolphin kick across pool width
2 minutes Swimmers' Shape-ups: stretches

INTERMEDIATE LEVEL 3

~

Highlights: The double-beat dolphin kick (see page 162); learning how to use pull-buoys (optional—see page 328); swimming a 250-yard/ meter pyramid set

Total Distance: 350 yards/meters

Warm-up (50 yards/meters)

2 minutes Swimmers' Shape-ups
3 minutes skill practice (1 minute each):
    double-beat dolphin kick in supine position on wall
    combined butterfly pull and kick, standing in place
    butterfly pull with breathing, walking in shallow water
1 × 25 easy swim: breaststroke
1 × 25 double-beat dolphin kick (kickboard optional)

OPTIONAL: Introduction to use of the pull-buoy. Review the crawl/ freestyle, backstroke, breaststroke, and butterfly pulls, using pull-buoys. Use them from now on whenever you want to isolate and practice a pull.

Main Set (250 yards/meters)

1 × 250 pyramid swim (½ minute rest after each swim):
    1 × 25 butterfly (double-beat kick)
    1 × 50 backstroke
    1 × 75 crawl/freestyle
    1 × 50 breaststroke
    1 × 25 butterfly (double-beat kick)
    1 × 25 crawl/freestyle

Cool-down (50 yards/meters)

Skill review:
    1 × 50 easy dolphin kick
    1 minute butterfly pull in shoulder-deep water walking across pool width
    5 × push-off into prone glide with dolphin kick across pool width
    1 minute Swimmers' Shape-ups: stretches

INTERMEDIATE LEVEL 4
～

Highlights: Practicing the four competitive strokes in the Individual Medley (IM) order by doing a pull-kick-swim set; learning open turns for each (page 204)

Total Distance: 400 yards/meters

Warm-up (50 yards/meters)

½ minute each pull in IM order (butterfly, backstroke, breaststroke, crawl) in shoulder-deep water

Skill practice: each pull in IM order, walking across pool width, using open turns

½ minute each kick in IM order (dolphin, supine flutter, whip, prone flutter) on wall

1 × 50 easy swim: sculling or elementary backstroke

Main Set (300 yards/meters)

4 × 75 pull-kick-swim series in IM order (½ minute rest after each 75):
   1 × 75 butterfly: 1 × 25 pull, 1 × 25 kick, 1 × 25 swim
   1 × 75 backstroke: 1 × 25 pull, 1 × 25 kick, 1 × 25 swim
   1 × 75 breaststroke: 1 × 25 pull, 1 × 25 kick, 1 × 25 swim
   1 × 75 crawl/freestyle: 1 × 25 pull, 1 × 25 kick, 1 × 25 swim

Cool-down (50 yards/meters)

1 × 50 easy swim: sculling or elementary backstroke
2 × kneeling dive
3 minutes Swimmers' Shape-ups: stretches

INTERMEDIATE LEVEL 5

～

Highlights: Backstroke start (see page 191); swimming 100 continuous yards/meters; semi-standing dive (see page 196)

Total Distance: 500 yards/meters

Warm-up (50 yards/meters)

3 minutes Swimmers' Shape-ups
1 minute bobbing: go as high and bend as deeply as possible
Skill practice:
    5 × backstroke push-off with flutter kick
    3 × backstroke push-off with dolphin kick
1 × 25 sculling: start with backstroke push-off
1 × 25 elementary backstroke: start with push-off

Main Set (400 yards/meters; 2 × 50s alternating with 100s)

2 × 50 backstroke with ½ minute rest after each 50 (use backstroke push-off)
1 × 100 crawl
1 minute rest
2 × 50 backstroke with ½ minute rest after each 50 (use backstroke push-off)
1 × 100 in IM order (rest between 25s if needed):
    1 × 25 butterfly
    1 × 25 backstroke
    1 × 25 breaststroke
    1 × 25 crawl/freestyle

Cool-down (50 yards/meters)

1 minute double-beat dolphin kick: in supine position on wall
1 × 25 double-beat dolphin kick
1 × 25 kick: swimmer's choice
2 × kneeling dive
Skill practice: 2 × semi-standing dive
1 minute Swimmers' Shape-ups: stretches

INTERMEDIATE LEVEL 6

Highlights: Timed 50-yard/meter swim and a pulse check

Total Distance: 600 yards/meters

Warm-up (100 yards/meters)

2 minutes skill practice (½ minute each):
   pull in IM order (butterfly, backstroke, breaststroke, crawl/free-style) while standing in shoulder-deep water
   kick in IM order (dolphin kick, supine flutter kick, whip kick, prone flutter kick) on wall
1 minute bobbing with breathing
1 × 100 swimmer's choice of stroke and equipment (rest between 25s if needed)

Main Set (450 yards/meters)

1 × 100 crawl/freestyle
1 minute rest
4 × 50 in IM order with ½ minute rest after each 50:
   1 × 50 butterfly (rest between 25s if needed)
   1 × 50 backstroke
   1 × 50 breaststroke
   1 × 50 crawl/freestyle
1 × 100 crawl/freestyle (rest between 50s only if needed)
Rest as needed
1 × 50 timed swim: semi-standing dive, crawl/freestyle or swimmer's choice
Pulse check

Cool-down (50 yards/meters)

1 × 50 easy swim: sculling or elementary backstroke
1 minute dolphin kick on wall
2 × semi-standing dive
3 minutes Swimmers' Shape-ups: stretches

INTERMEDIATE LEVEL 7

~

Highlights: Stroke count for 25-yard/meter crawl/freestyle and back-stroke swim

Total Distance: 700 yards/meters

Warm-up (150 yards/meters)

4 minutes Swimmers' Shape-ups
3 × 25 easy crawl/freestyle pull-kick-swim series (rest and equipment optional):
  1 × 25 pull
  1 × 25 kick
  1 × 25 swim
3 × 25 backstroke pull-kick-swim series (rest and equipment optional):
  1 × 25 pull
  1 × 25 kick
  1 × 25 swim

Main Set (500 yards/meters; 50s alternating with 100s)

1 × 200 pyramid swim (½ minute rest after each swim):
  1 × 50 crawl/freestyle (count strokes for first 25)
  1 × 100 swimmer's choice
  1 × 50 backstroke (count strokes for first 25)
1 × 100 in IM order (rest between 25s only if needed):
  1 × 25 butterfly
  1 × 25 backstroke
  1 × 25 breaststroke
  1 × 25 crawl/freestyle
1 × 200 pyramid swim (½ minute rest after each swim):
  1 × 50 crawl/freestyle (count strokes for first 25)
  1 × 100 swimmer's choice
  1 × 50 backstroke: count strokes for first 25

Cool-down (50 yards/meters)

1 × 25 easy swim: swimmer's choice
1 minute treading: in deep water
1 × 25 easy swim: swimmer's choice
2 minutes Swimmers' Shape-ups: stretches

INTERMEDIATE LEVEL 8

➤

Highlights: Refining the crawl/freestyle by learning how to roll the body; learning to use hand paddles (optional—see page 329); swimming 150 continuous yards/meters

Total Distance: 800 yards/meters

Warm-up (150 yards/meters)

2 minutes Swimmers' Shape-ups
2 minutes: skill practice (1 minute each): catch-up S-pattern crawl/
          freestyle with body roll, walking in shoulder-deep water
            prone flutter kick: with rhythmic breathing, on wall
3 × 50 easy swim-pull-swim series:
    1 × 50 sculling
    1 × 50 pull: crawl/freestyle
    1 × 50 swimmer's choice

Main Set (600 yards/meters; two ascending sets of 50-100-150)

1 × 50 crawl/freestyle with body roll (use catch-up for first 25)
½ minute rest
1 × 100 in IM order (rest between 25s only if needed):
    1 × 25 butterfly
    1 × 25 backstroke
    1 × 25 breaststroke
    1 × 25 crawl/freestyle
1 minute rest
1 × 150 crawl/freestyle with body roll: use catch-up for first, third, and
    fifth 25 (paddles optional)
1–2 minutes rest
REPEAT MAIN SET

Cool-down (50 yards/meters)

1 × 50 easy kick in IM order:
    1 × 25 prone dolphin, changing to supine flutter at halfway mark
    1 × 25 prone whip, changing to prone flutter at halfway mark
Review skills
    catch-up S-pattern crawl/freestyle with body roll, standing in
        shoulder-deep water
    catch-up S-pattern crawl/freestyle with body roll, walking in
        shoulder-deep water
1 minute Swimmers' Shape-ups: stretches

INTERMEDIATE LEVEL 9

～

Highlights: Swimming the four competitive strokes in reverse Individual Medley (IM) order; repeating stroke count to see how body roll makes stroke more efficient; swimming 200 consecutive yards/meters

Total Distance: 900 yards/meters

Warm-up (150 yards/meters)

2 minutes Swimmers' Shape-ups

3 × 50 pull-kick-swim series with 30 seconds rest after each 50 (swimmer's choice of stroke or combination of strokes):

    1 × 50 pull

    1 × 50 kick

    1 × 50 swim

Main Set (700 yards/meters)

1 × 200 crawl: use catch-up crawl/freestyle for every other length, and body roll throughout

30 seconds rest

1 × 50 crawl/freestyle: count strokes for first 25

30 seconds rest

1 × 100 in IM order (rest between 25s only if needed):

    1 × 25 butterfly

    1 × 25 backstroke

    1 × 25 breaststroke

    1 × 25 crawl/freestyle

30 seconds rest

1 × 50 backstroke: count strokes for first 25

30 seconds rest

1 × 100 in IM order:

    1 × 25 butterfly

    1 × 25 backstroke

    1 × 25 breaststroke

    1 × 25 crawl/freestyle

30 seconds rest

1 × 50 crawl/freestyle: count strokes for first 25

30 seconds rest

1 × 100 in reverse IM order:

    1 × 25 crawl/freestyle

    1 × 25 breaststroke

    1 × 25 backstroke

    1 × 25 butterfly

30 seconds rest
1 × 50 backstroke: count strokes for first 25

Cool-down (50 yards/meters)

1 × 50 easy swim: swimmer's choice
3 minutes Swimmers' Shape-ups: stretches

INTERMEDIATE LEVEL 10

～

Highlights: Timed 50-yard/meter swim and pulse check to compare with the last one; swimming a descending series as the main set, starting with a 250-yard/meter swim and totaling 750 yards/meters

Total Distance: 1,000 yards/meters

Warm-up (150 yards/meters)

2 minutes Swimmers' Shape-ups
1 × 150 easy swim: sculling, elementary backstroke, or any combination of the two

Main Set (800 yards/meters; descending series)

1 × 250 easy crawl/freestyle (rest once during swim if needed)
1 minute rest
1 × 200 in reverse IM order (rest only when needed):
    1 × 50 crawl/freestyle
    1 × 50 breaststroke
    1 × 50 backstroke
    1 × 50 butterfly (rest between 25s if needed)
1 minute rest
3 × 50 crawl/freestyle or swimmer's choice: pull-kick-swim series
    1 × 50 pull
    1 × 50 kick
    1 × 50 swim
30 seconds rest
1 × 100 in IM order:
    1 × 25 butterfly
    1 × 25 backstroke
    1 × 25 breaststroke
    1 × 25 crawl/freestyle
1 minute rest
1 × 50 crawl/freestyle

Rest as needed

1 × 50 timed swim: semi-standing dive, crawl/freestyle or swimmer's choice

Pulse check

Cool-down (50 yards/meters)

1 × 50 easy swim: swimmer's choice

2 minutes Swimmers' Shape-ups: stretches

TO VARY THE WORKOUTS

If you decide to maintain your fitness at the Intermediate level, you'll probably want to vary the basic 1,000-yard/meter workout. In general, you should follow the pattern established in Level 10:

Total distance: 1,000 yards/meters

Warm-up: 150 yards/meters (easy, relaxed swim)

Main set: 800 yards/meters (variety of strokes, distances)

Cool-down: 50 yards/meters (easy, relaxed swim)

Using these guidelines, you can mix and match strokes and skills:

- In the warm-up, alternate different strokes: swim 50s of your best stroke alternating with 25s of your worst.
- Add drills to the warm-up to practice newly acquired skills or to refine familiar ones (see "The Techniques of Swimming"). Add pulling for more variety.
- In the cool-down, use sculling or the elementary backstroke for easy swimming, or tread in place, or use water exercises from "Swimmers' Shape-ups." Add kicking for variety.
- Repeat Levels 1–9, adding distance to bring each workout up to a total of 1,000 yards/meters.
- Do your IMs in reverse order.
- Do a stroke count in all your strokes every once in a while—try to lower your count.
- If you haven't been using any equipment, consider doing so.
- On one day a week, or for one week, tackle a stroke or skill that you've been avoiding or feel uncomfortable doing.
- Do a timed swim and a pulse check occasionally.
- Make up your own main sets consisting of a total of 800 yards/

meters. (This is about half a mile, so why not begin to log your distance either in your own personal log—see Appendix D—or on the American Red Cross 50-mile log that's posted at many pools?) Here are ten sample 800-yard/meter main sets to get you going:

1. 2 × 200 crawl/freestyle
    4 × 50 swimmer's choice
    4 × 50 alternating 25s crawl/freestyle pull with backstroke kick

2. 2 × 75 pull-swim alternating with 1 × 50:
    2 × 75 crawl/freestyle (1 × 75 pull; 1 × 75 swim)
    1 × 50 easy supine flutter kick with sculling
    2 × 75 backstroke (1 × 75 pull; 1 × 75 swim)
    1 × 50 easy supine whip kick with sculling
    2 × 75 backstroke (1 × 75 pull; 1 × 75 swim)
    1 × 50 easy supine flutter kick with sculling
    2 × 75 sidestroke or swimmer's choice (1 × 75 pull; 1 × 75 swim)
    1 × 50 easy supine whip kick with sculling

3. Descending set
    1 × 200 crawl/freestyle
    1 × 100 backstroke
    1 × 50 breaststroke
    1 × 25 butterfly
    1 × 25 sidestroke
    REPEAT

4. 150s alternating with 50s:
    1 × 150 crawl/freestyle: pull-kick-swim series
    1 × 50 easy sidestroke or sculling
    1 × 150 backstroke: pull-kick-swim series
    1 × 50 easy swim—swimmer's choice
    1 × 150 breaststroke: pull-kick series
    1 × 50 easy elementary backstroke or sculling
    1 × 150 crawl/freestyle: pull-kick series
    1 × 50 easy swim—swimmer's choice

5. Pyramind set; one stroke or any combination of strokes:
    1 × 50
    1 × 100
    1 × 150
    1 × 200
    1 × 150
    1 × 100
    1 × 50

6. 150 swims alternating with 150 kick sets:
    1×150 crawl/freestyle
    3×50 kick set: crawl flutter, dolphin, backstroke flutter
    1×150 backstroke
    3×50 kick set: crawl flutter, dolphin, backstroke flutter
    1×150 crawl/freestyle
    1×50 easy kick—swimmer's choice

7. 200s alternating with 100 IMs:
    1×200 crawl/freestyle
    1×100 IM
    1×200 swimmer's choice
    1×100 IM
    1×200 sidestroke or swimmer's choice

8. Butterfly workout:
    1×150 swimmer's choice: pull-kick-swim series
    1×150 crawl/freestyle
    1×25 butterfly
    1×100 crawl/freestyle
    1×25 butterfly
    1×50 backstroke
    1×25 butterfly
    1×100 backstroke
    1×25 butterfly
    1×150 crawl/freestyle

9. IM workout: (In 50-meter pool, change strokes at half-lap marker)
    1×100 pull IM
    1×100 kick IM
    1×100 swim IM
    1×200 swim—swimmer's choice
    1×100 pull IM
    1×100 kick IM
    1×100 swim IM

10. 4×200 mixed strokes:
    1×200 crawl/freestyle: 1×50 pull, 1×50 kick, 1×100 swim
    1×200 backstroke: 1×50 pull, 1×50 kick, 1×100 swim
    1×200 breaststroke: 1×50 pull, 1×50 kick, 1×100 swim
    1×200 sidestroke and/or butterfly: 1×50 pull, 1×50 kick, 1×100 swim

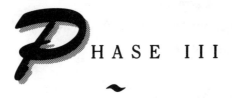

PHASE III

ADVANCED WORKOUTS

WHO'S AN ADVANCED SWIMMER?

You are an Advanced swimmer if you:

- Can swim at least 200 yards/meters without stopping.
- Know "The Fundamentals of Swimming" (crawl stroke, elementary and windmill backstrokes, treading, sculling, sitting dive), the skills and terms taught in the "Beginners' Workouts" (S-pattern crawl/freestyle-stroke pull, windmill backstroke with body roll, sidestroke, breaststroke, kneeling dive, open turns for the crawl/freestyle and backstroke, crescendo swim) plus the skills and terms taught in "Intermediate Workouts" (butterfly stroke, backstroke in-the-water start, crawl/freestyle stroke with body roll, pull-kick-swim series, timed swim and pulse check, Individual Medley (IM), stroke counting, pyramid series. If necessary, learn or review these skills and terms before you begin this phase.

ADVANCED SKILLS AND TERMS

In this phase, you'll learn these new skills (explained in "The Techniques of Swimming") and terms (explained in "Workout Terms" and "Training Concepts" (see pages 232/228).

- Bilateral breathing patterns for crawl/freestyle
- Alternate breathing pattern for butterfly

267

- Backstroke bent-arm pull
- Crawl/freestyle and breaststroke in-the-water starts
- Closed crawl/freestyle turn
- Standing dive
- Easy/hard (Fartlek) swims
- Interval training
- Paced swims

Here's how your fitness will improve:

- You'll progress from swimming 200 continuous yards/meters in Level 1 to 400 yards/meters in Level 10.
- You'll get less rest between swims, and the rest you do get will sometimes be determined by how fast you've just swum (interval training).
- Your total workout distance will increase from 1,000 yards/meters in Level 1 (approximately a half mile) to 1,800 yards/meters in Level 10 (approximately one mile).

Each workout will take about forty-five minutes, depending on how fast you swim and how much rest you take.

The presentation here is more streamlined than in the previous phases.

For instance, there are no Swimmers' Shape-ups indicated for the warm-ups or cool-downs; add your own. And an "easy swim" means that you may use the elementary backstroke, sculling, the sidestroke, or whatever other stroke is relaxing for you.

SPECIAL TIPS FOR ADVANCED SWIMMERS

~

- If you're not swimming in a 25-yard/meter pool, adjust the workouts in the same manner as described for Intermediate swimmers see page 251).
- As an Advanced swimmer, it's important for you to have some sort of clock or watch with a second hand that's clearly visible. The principles of *pacing* and *interval training*, borrowed from competitive swimming, are good concepts for you to put to use at this level. Even though you may be swimming relatively slowly, it's not too early to begin to keep a record of your times—this gives the

workouts more shape, and gives you another set of goals to reach for.

- The *interval swims* are based on the ability of the average fitness swimmer at this level, who can easily swim 50 yards in about 1 minute. Since in this phase resting time should approximate swim time, the average interval (swim time plus resting time) for 50 yards would be 2 minutes ("on 2:00"). If our time is at least 10 seconds faster or slower, adjust the interval by doubling your own time. If you swim a 50 in 45 seconds, your interval would be 1:30. If you hold that time for each 50-yard swim, you get 45 seconds rest between them. As you become able to swim faster you'll be getting more and more rest at that interval and so should reduce your overall interval accordingly. Eventually, you may want to make your resting time shorter than your swim time. (Competitive swimmers' rest times are often far less than their swimming times.) In addition, a meter pool is 10 percent longer than a yard pool, so the intervals would also be 10 percent longer. If your pool is a different size, adjust your intervals accordingly.

- Swim, kick, and/or pull drills in the warm-ups and cool-downs should be done at an easy pace.

- Use equipment such as hand paddles, pull-buoys, and fins to isolate the movements and to help you increase the power of your stroke.

- Try not to rest during the workout except where indicated—gradually reduce your rest each time you repeat a workout.

- Consider joining a swim club or taking part in organized workouts. Many coaches allow noncompetitive fitness-minded swimmers to join in their team's practices. If you do work out with serious swimmers, make sure you're familiar with the appropriate terms, concepts, and pool courtesies beforehand. Often there are lanes designated for faster and for slower swimmers. The lifeguard or coach may ask you to swim in the slower lane. Or you can judge where you should swim by comparing the other swimmers' times, intervals, and distances with your own. The coach may also suggest ways to adapt the workout to your own level and ability. For example, you might do *every other* interval that the team does (if you do this, make sure to stand to the right of the lane, so that the other swimmers may turn.)

- Another tip is to stop swimming when the other members of the workout have stopped swimming, whether you've finished the series or not. Just finish your lap, then go on to begin the next along with the rest of the swimmers.

Advanced Level 1

～

Highlights: Controlled breathing in the freestyle (see page 128). Fartlek training (easy/hard)

Total Distance: 1,000 yards/meters

Warm-up (200 yards/meters)

Skill practice: freestyle with alternate breathing
4 × 50 pull: freestyle; use alternate breathing on odd-numbered 25s; 30 seconds rest after each 50

Main Set (700 yards/meters; descending set)

1 × 200 freestyle: alternate breathing on odd-numbered 25s; 1 minute rest
2 × 100 IM: 1 minute rest after each 100
4 × 50 freestyle: alternate breathing on first 25; 30 seconds rest after each 50
4 × 25 easy/hard: swimmer's choice of stroke

Cool-down (100 yards/meters)

2 × 50 kick: 1 × 50 prone flutter, 1 × 50 supine flutter
Skill review: alternate breathing

Advanced Level 2

～

Highlights: Closed turn for the crawl/freestyle (see page 207); swimming an 800-yard/meter pyramid set

Total Distance: 1,100 yards/meters

Warm-up (200 yards/meters)

Skill practice: closed turn

2×100 swim-pull: freestyle with closed turns; 30 seconds rest after each 100:

1×100 swim with alternate breathing

1×100 pull

Main Set (800 yards/meters)

1×800 pyramid swim: freestyle using closed turn; 15 seconds rest per 50:

1×50 (15 seconds rest)

1×100 (30 seconds rest)

1×150 (45 seconds rest)

1×200 (60 seconds rest)

1×150 (45 seconds rest)

1×100 (30 seconds rest)

1×50 (15 seconds rest)

Cool-down (100 yards/meters)

1×100 kick in IM order

ADVANCED LEVEL 3

～

Highlights: In-the-water starts for all strokes (see pages 189–92); 50-yard/meter timed swim and pulse check

Total Distance: 1,200 yards/meters

Warm-up (300 yards/meters)

Skill practice: in-the-water starts for all strokes
3 × 100 pull-kick-swim series: freestyle or swimmer's choice; use in-the-water start; 30 seconds rest after each 100:
    1 × 100 pull
    1 × 100 kick
    1 × 100 swim

Main set (750 yards/meters)

2 × 200 freestyle: alternate breathing on odd-numbered laps; 1 minute rest after each 200
1 × 100 in reverse IM order
2 × 50 freestyle; 30 seconds rest after each 50
4 × 25 easy/hard freestyle: alternate breathing during easy laps
Rest as needed
1 × 50 timed swim: semi-standing dive; freestyle or swimmer's choice
Pulse check

Cool-down (150 yards/meters)

3 × 50 pull-kick-swim series: easy freestyle or swimmer's choice
Review starts for all strokes (see pages 000–00)

ADVANCED LEVEL 4

~

Highlights: Broken 400-yard/meter swim in two 200-yard/meter paced swims (see page 234); standing dive (page 196)

Total Distance: 1,300 yards/meters

Warm-up (300 yards/meters)

3 × 100 easy swim, 20 seconds rest after each 100:
 1 × 100 backstroke
 1 × 100 breaststroke
 1 × 100 crawl/freestyle, alternate breathing on odd-numbered 25s

Main Set (850 yards/meters)

1 × 400 broken swim:
 2 × 200: standing dive, freestyle, 1 minute rest after each
1 × 50 swimmer's choice
4 × 100 pull-kick series: in IM order; 30 seconds rest after each 100:
 1 × 100 IM pull
 1 × 100 IM kick
 1 × 100 pull
 1 × 100 kick

Cool-down (150 yards/meters)

1 × 150 easy swim: swimmer's choice
3 × standing dive

ADVANCED LEVEL 5

~

Highlights: Swimming timed intervals (see page 227)

Total Distance: 1,400 yards/meters

Warm-up (300 yards/meters)

3 × 100 pull-kick-swim series: swimmer's choice; 15 seconds rest after each 100

Main Set (950 yards/meters; descending set)

3 × 150 swim-pull-swim series: freestyle; 1 minute rest after each 150
1 × 100 easy breaststroke
1 × 100 IM
4 × 50 timed interval: freestyle on 2:00
Pulse check
4 × 25 easy/hard: freestyle; alternate breathing during easy swims

Cool-down (150 yards/meters)

1 × 50 easy kick: swimmer's choice
1 × 100 easy swim: swimmer's choice
3 × standing dive

ADVANCED LEVEL 6

~

Highlights: Breaststroke push-off (see page 204); 100-yard/meter timed swim with pulse check

Total Distance: 1,500 yards/meters

Warm-up (300 yards/meters)

2 × 150 pull-swim: freestyle; 15 seconds rest after each 150:
  1 × 150 pull: freestyle—catch-up S-pattern drill
  1 × 150 swim: freestyle—using alternate breathing on odd-numbered 25s
Skill practice: breaststroke push-off in shoulder-deep water

Main Set (1,050 yards/meters; descending set)

3 × 150 swim: 30 seconds rest after each 150:
  1 × 150 breaststroke, using push-off
  1 × 150 swimmer's choice
  1 × 150 breaststroke, using push-off
2 × 100 IM; 1 minute rest after each 100
4 × 50 timed intervals: freestyle on 2:00
4 × 25 timed intervals: freestyle on 1:00
Rest as needed
1 × 100 timed swim: standing dive, freestyle
Pulse check

Cool-down (150 yards/meters)

1 × 50 kick: frog or whip
1 × 100 easy swim
Skill practice: breaststroke push-off, in shallow water

ADVANCED LEVEL 7

～

Highlights: Backstroke bent-arm pull (see page 134); doing mixed swims during a timed interval

Total Distance: 1,500 yards/meters

Warm-up (300 yards/meters)

1 × 200 easy swim: swimmer's choice
1 × 100 backstroke
Skill practice: backstroke bent-arm pull

Main Set (1,050 yards/meters)

2 × 100 pull-swim: backstroke:
    1 × 100 pull, using bent-arm pull
    1 × 100 swim, using bent-arm pull and flutter kick
3 × 100 pull-swim: backstroke, using bent-arm pull; pull on alternate 50s; 30 seconds rest after each 100
3 × 100 timed interval: mixed swim of 1 × 75 freestyle, 1 × 25 backstroke on 4:00
4 × 50 timed interval: freestyle on 1:45
1 × 50 backstroke, using bent-arm pull

Cool-down (150 yards/meters)

1 × 50 kick: supine flutter
1 × 100 backstroke

ADVANCED LEVEL 8

⌣

Highlights: Alternate breathing for the butterfly (see page 164)

Total Distance: 1,600 yards/meters

Warm-up (400 yards/meters)

4 × 100 reverse IM: 30 seconds rest after each 100
Skill practice: alternate breathing for butterfly

Main Set (1,000 yards/meters)

1 × 200 freestyle: use alternate breathing
4 × 50 mixed swim: butterfly with as much alternate breathing as possible for first 25, breaststroke for second 25
3 × 100 IM: use alternate breathing during butterfly as much as possible
4 × 50 timed interval: freestyle on 1:45
4 × 25 timed interval: freestyle on :45

Cool-down (200 yards/meters)

1 × 100 kick: IM order
1 × 100 easy swim

ADVANCED LEVEL 9

～

Highlights: Descending timed intervals; 200-yard/meter timed swim

Total Distance: 1,700 yards/meters

Warm-up (400 yards/meters)

1 × 300 easy pull-kick-swim set: swimmer's choice
1 × 100 IM

Main Set (1,100 yards/meters)

1 × 300 freestyle or swimmer's choice
6 × 50 timed intervals: freestyle
    2 × 50 on 2:00
    2 × 50 on 1:45
    2 × 50 on 1:30
1 × 150 pull-kick-swim set: swimmer's choice
6 × 25 easy/moderate/hard: freestyle or swimmer's choice
Rest as needed
1 × 200 timed swim: standing dive, freestyle
Pulse check

Cool-down (200 yards/meters)

1 × 100 easy kick: swimmer's choice or combination
1 × 100 sculling or elementary backstroke

ADVANCED LEVEL 10

⮝

Highlights: Doing the whole workout (just over a mile) as a pyramid swim; comparison of two 300-yard/meter timed paced swims; swimming 400 consecutive yards/meters

Total Distance: 1,800 yards/meters

Warm-up (400 yards/meters)

2 × 50 pull: freestyle
1 × 100 pull: IM order
1 × 200 easy swim: swimmer's choice

Main Set (1,200 yards/meters) 1 minute rest after each:

1 × 300 timed swim: freestyle
1 × 400 swimmer's choice
1 × 300 timed swim: freestyle
1 × 200 pull: swimmer's choice

Cool-down (200 yards/meters)

1 × 100 easy kick: IM order
2 × 50 sculling or easy swim

TO VARY THE WORKOUTS

⮝

To vary your fitness program, make up your own workouts, using the following guidelines:

Total distance: 1,800 yards/meters (just over 1 mile)

Warm-up: 400 yards/meters

Main set: 1,200 yards/meters

Cool-down: 200 yards/meters (½ warm-up distance)

- Use the suggestions given in the Intermediate Phase (see page 251) to vary your workouts.

- Mix and match the strokes, skills, and distances found in Levels 1–10.
- You can mix and match the following samples, Chinese-menu style: choose one warm-up, one main set, and one cool-down.
- Include the following freestyle drills in your advanced workouts: fist closed pulling, dig freestyle, and head up freestyle (see page 126).

Samples of 400-yard/meter Warm-ups:

1. 1 × 400 easy swim (any stroke or combination)
2. 2 × 200 easy pull-swim (any stroke or combination)
3. 1 × 200 swim
   1 × 100 pull
   1 × 100 kick
4. 1 × 200 easy swim
   4 × 50 easy pull
5. Swim at an easy pace for 5–8 minutes.

Samples of 1,200-yard/meter Main Sets (Adjust intervals as needed.)

1. 3 × 400 paced swim: freestyle or swimmer's choice; 1 minute rest after each 400
2. 3 × 200 pull-kick-swim set: reverse IM order; 1 minute rest after each 200
   3 × 50 pull-kick-swim set: backstroke; 30 seconds rest after each 50
   3 × 100 pull-kick-swim set: breaststroke; 15 seconds rest after each 100
   3 × 50 pull-kick-swim set: butterfly; rest as needed
3. Descending set (reverse crescendo): freestyle or swimmer's choice; 30 seconds rest per 100
   1 × 400; 2 minutes rest
   1 × 300; 1½ minutes rest
   1 × 200; 1 minute rest
   1 × 150; 45 seconds rest
   1 × 100; 30 seconds rest
   1 × 50; 15 seconds rest
   (This set may also be done in ascending order.)

4.   6 × 100 on 2:00
  1 × 75 freestyle; 1 × 25 butterfly
  1 × 75 freestyle; 1 × 25 backstroke
  1 × 75 freestyle; 1 × 25 breaststroke
  Repeat.
  1 × 200 easy swim
  3 × 100 pull-kick-swim set: freestyle or swimmer's choice; 1 minute rest
  1 × 100 IM

5.   1 × 200 pull: freestyle; alternate breathing on even-numbered 25s; 1 minute rest
  4 × 75 pull-kick-swim set: IM order; 1 minute rest after each 75
  1 × 200 freestyle: alternate breathing on odd-numbered 25s
  4 × 75 pull-kick-swim set: reverse IM order; 1 minute rest after each 75
  1 × 200 freestyle: alternate breathing on even-numbered 25s

6.   4 × 100 freestyle with descending rest periods:
  1 × 100; 1½ minutes rest
  1 × 100; 1 minute rest
  1 × 100; 30 seconds rest
  1 × 100 (no rest)
  1 × 200 easy swim: breaststroke or sidestroke
  4 × 50 freestyle on 2:00
  1 × 200 freestyle: alternate breathing on odd-numbered 25s
  8 × 25 IM on 1:00

7.   Pyramid set: freestyle or swimmer's choice; 15 seconds rest per 50:
  1 × 100; 30 seconds rest
  1 × 150; 45 seconds rest
  1 × 200; 1 minute rest
  1 × 300; 1½ minutes rest
  1 × 200; 1 minute rest
  1 × 150; 45 seconds rest
  1 × 100; 30 seconds rest

8.   Descending set: stroke work; rest as needed
  1 × 100 IM pull
  1 × 400 swim, your best stroke
  1 × 300 swim, your second-best stroke
  1 × 200 swim, your third-best stroke
  1 × 100 swim, your fourth-best stroke

1×100 IM kick

(Or reverse the order—start with your worst stroke for 400 yards/meters and end with your best for 100 yards/meters.)

9. 4×100 swim: swimmer's choice; 1 minute rest after each 100

1×100 easy breaststroke

4×50 freestyle on 1:30

1×50 easy backstroke

4×50 swimmer's choice; 30 seconds rest after each 50

1×50 sculling

4×25 IM order on 1:00

4×25 reverse IM order; 15 seconds rest after each 25

10. 1×250 swimmer's choice; swim as 100-75-50-25; rest 15 seconds after each swim

4×100 freestyle on 2:00; alternate breathing on odd-numbered 25s

1×250 swimmer's choice; swim at 100-75-50-25; rest 15 seconds after each swim

4×50 swimmer's choice on 1:30

1×100 swimmer's choice

Samples of 200-yard/meter Cool-downs:

1. 1×200 easy swim

2. 1×50 easy pull

1×50 easy kick

1×100 easy swim

3. 2×11 easy sculling/sidestroke

4. Easy kick for 5 minutes

5. Tread and bob for 5 minutes (especially if pool is crowded)

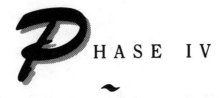

PHASE IV

SUPER WORKOUTS

WHO'S A SUPER SWIMMER?

You are a Super swimmer if you:

- Can swin at least 400 yards/meters without stopping.
- Know all the skills and terms that an advanced swimmer knows (see pages 268–69).
- Want to compete—or be in the same terrific shape that competitive swimmers are in.

SUPER SKILLS AND TERMS

These workouts will fine tune the skills explained in "The Techniques of Swimming" and increase your vocabulary of swimming terms (see "Workout Terms," and "Training Concepts," pages 232 and 228:

- Racing dive
- Descending and/or ascending timed interval sets
- Flip turn
- Controlled breathing
- Grab start
- Even splits

- Time trials
- Build-ups

Your fitness will improve:

- You'll progress from swimming 400 yards/meters to 1,000 yards/meters.
- Your total workout distance will increase from 1,800 yards/meters to 3,000 yards/meters.

SPECIAL TIPS FOR SUPER SWIMMERS

～

- Include your own Swimmers' Shape-ups in your warm-ups and cool-downs. Resistance training (see page 374) is recommended, especially on the days that you don't swim.
- Reading the clock and pacing will be even more important here than during the Advanced Phase. Now that you're doing longer distances—and maybe competing—you should develop a sense of your speed and be able to control it.
- You'll notice that there will be "swim downs" during the main set—because you'll be swimming faster and more strenuously, you will need this rest, but don't swim so slowly here that you cool down too much.
- There will also be transitional sets to bring you into and out of the main set. There's usually a pulling set at the end of the warm-up to get your stroke going and a kicking set just before the cool-down because, although your arms will probably be tired by this point, you will have some strength left in your legs.
- Training devices are recommended at this phase of your fitness program to help to develop your strength.
- Follow the tips suggested in the Advanced Workouts (pages 269–71) if you swim in organized workouts or use anything other than a 25-yard pool.
- The crawl stroke will be called the freestyle. (Although in competition the term "freestyle" means any stroke that you want, virtually all swimmers choose the crawl for these events.)

- "Easy swim" means either a less strenuous stroke, such as sculling or the elementary backstroke, or any other stroke that you choose to swim slowly.
- Adjust all timed interval swims according to your own speed (see page 227).
- All warm-ups are approximately twice the length of the cool-downs. Both of these should be easy swims, and can incorporate stroke/kick drills.

SUPER LEVEL 1

Highlights: 100s with even splits (see page 234); one-arm freestyle drill (see page 125); wind-up racing dive (see page 198)

Total Distance: 1,800 yards/meters

Warm-up (400 yards/meters)

1 × 200 freestyle: alternate breathing (page 128)
4 × 50 freestyle: pull on 1:30

Main Set (1,200 yards/meters)

1 × 200 freestyle: one-arm-stroke drill; use right arm for odd laps and left arm for even laps
5 × 100 freestyle: even splits; 30 seconds rest after each 50
5 × 50 freestyle on 1:15: alternate breathing
5 × 50 kick on 2:00: freestyle

Cool-down (200 yards/meters)

4 × 50 easy swim: start each 50 with racing dive

SUPER LEVEL 2

～

Highlights: Use of hand paddles (see page 329); descending pulling set (see pages 231 and 232); freestyle kicking drill (see page 127)

Total Distance: 2,000 yards/meters

Warm-up (400 yards/meters)

3 × 100 reverse IM on 2:30
1 × 100 pull: swimmer's choice

Main Set (1,400 yards/meters)

3 × 200 freestyle; 30 seconds–1 minute rest after each 200:
    1 × 200 pull with paddles and pull-buoy
    1 × 200 pull with pull-buoy only
    1 × 200 swim with paddles only
1 × 100 swim down: easy backstroke
6 × 50 freestyle pull: descending set on 1:30; paddles optional
4 × 50 kick drill: freestyle side kick, or swimmer's choice, on 1:30
2 × 100 IM on 2:00

Cool-down (200 yards/meters)

1 × 200 easy swim

SUPER LEVEL 3

～

Highlights: Descending/ascending set (see page 231); 200-yard/meter time trial

Total Distance: 2,200 yards/meters

Warm-up (400 yards/meters)

1 × 150 freestyle: alternate breathing on odd-numbered 25s
1 × 150 freestyle: catch-up drill on odd-numbered 25s
2 × 50 freestyle pull: one-arm drill

Main Set (1,600 yards/meters)

$3 \times$ $\begin{cases} 1 \times 200 \text{ freestyle on 4:00} \\ 4 \times 50 \text{ freestyle on 1:00} \end{cases}$

Rest as needed

1×200 freestyle time trial: start from racing dive

4×50 freestyle: descending on 1:30; alternate breathing

Cool-down (200 yards/meters)

4×50 freestyle: ascending on 2:00

SUPER LEVEL 4
∼

Highlights: Flip turn (see page 213); alternate breathing; build-up set (see page 233)

Total Distance: 2,400 yards/meters

Warm-up (400 yards/meters)

1×100 freestyle: alternate breathing

4×25 freestyle build-up set on :45

4×25 kick drill on 1:00: freestyle side kick or choice

1×100 freestyle pull: one-arm drill, alternating arms every 4 strokes

Skill practice: 10 × flip turns, swimming to wall prior to turn

Main Set (1,800 yards/meters)

4×100 freestyle on 2:30; use flip turns

5 × flip turn

4×100 freestyle on 2:00; use flip turns

5 × flip turn

2×250 freestyle with alternate breathing and flip turns; alternate breathing on odd-numbered 50s

5 × flip turn

10×50 freestyle build-up set on 1:00 (use flip turns)

Cool-down (200 yards/meters)

1×200 easy IM kick

Super Level 5

~

Highlights: Glide freestyle drill (see page 125); glide backstroke drill (see page 140); catch-up backstroke drill (see page 139); backstroke flip turn (see page 217)

Total Distance: 2,500 yards/meters

Warm-up (500 yards/meters)

1 × 100 freestyle catch-up drill
4 × 25 glide freestyle drill
1 × 100 IM
4 × 25 backstroke
1 × 100 IM pull
Skill practice: 10 × backstroke flip turns

Main Set (1,800 yards/meters)

4 × 150 backstroke; 1 minute rest after each 150:
    1 × 150 backstroke
    1 × 150 backstroke; catch-up drill on odd-numbered 25s
    1 × 150 backstroke; glide backstroke on odd-numbered 25s
    1 × 150 backstroke
1 × 100 freestyle: bilateral breathing
5 × backstroke flip turn
3 × 200 mixed swim; 1 minute rest after each 200:
    1 × 200 backstroke; catch-up drill on odd-numbered 25s
    1 × 200 breaststroke
    1 × 200 backstroke; glide backstroke on odd-numbered 25s
1 × 100 freestyle: controlled breathing—choice of breathing patterns
5 × backstroke flip turn
4 × 50 backstroke kick on 2:00
4 × 50 backstroke swim on 1:30

Cool-down (200 yards/meters)

4 × 50 backstroke kick with fins

SUPER LEVEL 6
～

Highlights: Time trial of 500 yards/400 meters; build-ups (see page 233)

Total Distance: 2,500 yards/2,400 meters

Warm-up (500 yards/meters)

5 × 100 freestyle; 30 seconds rest after each 100:
    1 × 100 freestyle
    1 × 100 one-arm pull drill; alternate arms every 4 strokes
    1 × 100 catch-up freestyle; may use alternate breathing
    1 × 100 pull with hand paddles
    1 × 100 pull with controlled breathing (every 4 strokes)

Main Set (1,800 yards/1,700 meters)

5 × 50 freestyle pull build-ups on 1:20
5 × 50 freestyle swim build-ups on 1:00
1 × 100 swim-down: easy swim
Rest as needed
1 × 500-yard/400-meter time trial; racing dive, freestyle or choice
1 × 100 swim-down: easy double-arm backstroke
8 × 50 mixed swim on 2:00: butterfly alternating with breaststroke
2 × 100 IM kick; 30 seconds rest after each 100

Cool-down (200 yards/meters)

1 × 200 easy IM

SUPER LEVEL 7

～

Highlights: Grab start (see page 199); broken swims of 200 yards/meters (see page 233)

Total Distance: 2,600 yards/meters

Warm-up (500 yards/meters)

1 × 500 crescendo set: freestyle or choice; easy/hard:
 2 × 25
 2 × 50
 2 × 75
 2 × 100 pull

Main Set (1,900 yards/meters)

5 × 200 broken swim on 4:00 (on odd-numbered 200s, 10 seconds rest at the 50 and 150; on even-numbered 200s, 15 seconds rest at the 50 and 100, and 10 seconds rest at the 150)
1 × 100 swim-down: easy breaststroke
4 × 50 freestyle build-ups on 1:00
Skill practice: 6 × grab start
4 × 50 freestyle on 2:00 (use grab start for each)
1 × 400 kick: swimmer's choice or combination; alternate 1 minute easy with 1 minute hard kicking

Cool-down (200 yards/meters)

4 × 50 easy swim: alternate easy breaststroke with double-arm backstroke

SUPER LEVEL 8

➤

Highlights: Starts and turns practice (see pages 189–219); ascending/descending timed interval set (see page 227)

Total Distance: 2,800 yards/meters

Warm-up (600 yards/meters)

4 × 100 reverse IM: descending set on 2:30
4 × 50 freestyle pull: descending set on 1:15

Main Set (1,900 yards/meters)

3 × 300 mixed swim: begin each with racing dive or start; 1 minute
    rest after each 300:
      1 × 300 freestyle
      1 × 300 backstroke
      1 × 300 breaststroke
1 × 100 double-arm backstroke with dolphin kick
3 × 100 IM on 2:00
Rest as needed
10 × 50 freestyle ascending/descending time intervals (from 1:00 to
    :45, by 5-second intervals):
      1 × 50 on 1:00
      1 × 50 on :55
      1 × 50 on :50
      1 × 50 on :45
      1 × 50 easy swim; begin next 50 on following :60 mark on clock
      1 × 50 on :45
      1 × 50 on :50
      1 × 50 on :55
      1 × 50 on 1:00
      1 × 50 easy swim
1 × 100 easy IM kick

Cool-down (300 yards/meters)

4 × 50 IM; use in-the-water start for each stroke
1 × 100 easy swim

SUPER LEVEL 9

～

Highlights: Time trial with negative split (see pages 234 and 235) for 1,000 yards/meters swim

Total Distance: 2,900 yards/meters

Warm-up (600 yards/meters)

12 × 50 pull-kick-swim set, swimmer's choice; 10 seconds rest after each 50:
   4 × 50 pull
   4 × 50 kick
   4 × 50 swim

Main Set (2,000 yards/meters)

4 × 100 freestyle pull on 2:00
Rest as needed
1 × 1,000 freestyle time trial with negative split; record your time; pulse check
1 × 100 swim-down
1 × 200 IM kick
1 × 100 IM swim
1 × 200 IM kick

Cool-down (300 yards/meters)

1 × 300 easy swim: swimmer's choice

SUPER LEVEL 10

～

Highlights: Individual medley and mixed-stroke combination sets; controlled breathing swim

Total Distance: 3,000 yards/meters

Warm-up (600 yards/meters)

3 × 200 pull-kick-swim set: reverse IM
   1 × 200 reverse IM pull
   1 × 200 reverse IM kick
   1 × 200 reverse IM swim

Main Set (2,100 yards/meters)

1 × 1,800 mixed stroke set: 200s alternating with 50s
   1 × 200 IM on 4:00
   8 × 50 freestyle on 1:15
   1 × 200 IM on 4:00
   6 × 50 breaststroke on 1:15
   1 × 200 IM to 4:00
   4 × 50 backstroke on 1:15
   1 × 200 IM on 4:00
   2 × 50 butterfly on 1:15
1 × 100 easy double-arm backstroke
4 × 50 freestyle controlled breathing set: start each 50 from dive; swim
   odd-numbered 25s on one breath; even-numbered 25s easy swim

Cool-down (300 yards/meters)

1 × 100 easy supine whip kick
1 × 100 easy freestyle kick
1 × 100 easy double-arm backstroke

To Vary the Workouts
～

Vary your workout program, following these guidelines and suggestions:

> Total distance: 3,000 yards/meters
> Warm-up: 600 yards/meters
> Main set: 2,100 yards/meters
> Cool-down: 300 yards/meters

- Use Levels 1–10 as a basis for mixing and matching strokes, skills, drills, and distances
- Use the suggestions on page 264 to vary your workouts. You can also do timed intervals, time trials, broken swims, build-ups, and ascending/descending pyramids.
- See also the specialized workouts suggested in "Swimming to Win," pages 306–13.
- Mix and match the following samples of warm-ups, cool-downs, and main sets to make up a total workout.
- Use pulling equipment at beginning of main set; use kicking equipment at end of main set.
- Include the following freestyle drills in your Super workouts: fist closed pulling, dig freestyle, end head-up freestyle (see page 126)

Suggestions for 600-yard/meter Warm-ups:

1. 6 × 100 IM or reverse IM; swim continuously or on a 2:00 interval; pull on odd-numbered laps
2. 1 × 60 freestyle; on odd-numbered laps, do drills such as one-arm pull, catch-up freestyle, and glide freestyle
3. 6 × 100 freestyle, with controlled breathing; continuous or on an interval:
   1 × 25 regular rhythmic breathing
   1 × 25 alternate breathing
   1 × 25 inhaling on every fourth stroke
   1 × 25 inhaling on every fifth stroke
4. 1 × 600 freestyle pull; controlled breathing (inhale every fourth pull) on every even 25

5. 12 × 50 freestyle descending set on 1:00 (swim each 50 faster than previous one)

6. 4 × 150 pull-kick-swim freestyle or reverse IM; 30 seconds rest after each 150

7. 12 × 50 freestyle pull-kick-swim on intervals:
   4 × 50 pull on 1:15
   4 × 50 kick on 1:30
   4 × 50 swim on 1:00

8. 12 × 50 swimmer's choice:
   3 × 50 swim on 1:00
   3 × 50 pull on 1:15
   3 × 50 kick on 1:30
   3 × 50 swim on 1:00

9. 1 × 200 best-stroke pull
   1 × 200 second-best-stroke pull
   1 × 100 third-best-stroke pull
   1 × 100 worst-stroke pull

10. 1 × 600 freestyle easy/hard on alternate 50s

Sample Main Sets (total distances vary as indicated)

1. Total Distance: 2,000 yards/meters
   Ascending/descending set; swimmer's choice of stroke:
   8 × 50 on 1:00
   4 × 100 on 2:00
   2 × 200 on 4:00
   4 × 100 on 2:00
   8 × 50 on 1:00

2. Total Distance: 1,000 or 2,000 yards/meters
   4 × 250 broken swim in IM order; rest 5 seconds per lap:
   1 × 250: 1 × 25 fly (:05 rest); 1 × 50 fly, back (:10 rest); 1 × 75 fly, back, breast (:15 rest); 1 × 100 fly, back, breast, free (:20 rest)
   1 × 250: 1 × 25 back (:05 rest); 1 × 50 back, breast (:10 rest); 1 × 75 back, breast, free (:15 rest); 1 × 100 back, breast, free, fly (:20 rest)
   1 × 250: 1 × 25 breast (:05 rest); 1 × 50 breast, free (:10 rest); 1 × 75 breast, free, fly (:15 rest); 1 × 100 breast, free, fly, back (:20 rest)

1×250: 1×25 free (:05 rest); 1×50 free, fly (:10 rest); 1×75 free, fly, back (:15 rest); 1×100 free, fly, back, breast (:20 rest)

Repeat these four sets (in reverse order, if desired) to total 2,000 yards/meters.

3. Total Distance: 2,100 yards/meters

   Fins Set; 50s alternating with 400s. Use fins for entire main set.

6×50:	dolphin kick on 1:30; 8 breaths per 50
1×400:	200 butterfly; 200 freestyle
6×50:	supine flutter kick on 1:00
1×400:	200 backstroke; 200 freestyle
6×50:	flutter kick on 1:30; 8 breaths per 50
1×400:	freestyle

4. Total Distance: 1,000 yards/meters

   Individual Medley: pull-kick-swim:

   5×200: repeat the following sequence for each of 5 strokes (butterfly, backstroke, breaststroke, freestyle, swimmer's choice):

   For example:
1×50:	pull
1×50:	kick
1×100:	swim

5. Total Distance: 2,000 yards/meters

   Controlled Breathing and Stroke Work:

1×200:	1 breath per 3 strokes; every fourth 25 butterfly
3×100:	freestyle on 2:30; every third 25 butterfly
1×200:	1 breath per 4 strokes; every fourth 25 backstroke
3×100:	freestyle on 2:30; every third 25 backstroke
1×200:	1 breath per 3 strokes; every fourth 25 breaststroke
3×100:	freestyle on 2:30; every third 25 breaststroke
1×200:	freestyle or choice
3×100:	freestyle descending on 2:30

6. Total Distance: 1,000 or 2,000 yards/meters

   Individual Medley: pull-kick-swim (equipment optional throughout)

   1×600 (1×50 pull, 1×50 kick, 1×50 swim for each stroke): 30 seconds rest after each 150

        1 × 150:   butterfly
        1 × 150:   backstroke
        1 × 150:   breaststroke
        1 × 150:   freestyle
1 × 300 (1 × 25 pull, 1 × 25 kick, 1 × 25 swim for each stroke, without equipment):
        15 seconds rest after each 75
        1 × 75:   butterfly
        1 × 75:   backstroke
        1 × 75:   breaststroke
        1 × 75:   freestyle
1 × 100 Individual Medley: easy swim
Repeat workout to total 2,000 yards/meters

7. Total Distance: 2,000 yards/meters
Broken freestyle and/or your best stroke, descending:
   3 × 400:
      1 × 200; rest 20 seconds
      1 × 100; rest 15 seconds
      2 × 50; rest 10 seconds after each 50
   2 × 300:
      2 × 100; rest 15 seconds after each 100
      2 × 50 best stroke; rest 10 seconds after each 50
   1 × 200:
      1 × 100; rest 15 seconds
      2 × 50; rest 10 seconds after each 50

8. Total Distance: 2,100 yards/meters
Individual Medley and sprints:
   1 × 200 IM on 3:30
   2 × 50 best stroke on 1:00
   2 × 100 freestyle on 2:00
   1 × 200 IM on 3:30
   2 × 50 best stroke on 1:00
   2 × 100 freestyle on 1:50
   1 × 100 easy swim
   1 × 200 IM on 3:30
   2 × 50 best stroke on 1:00
   2 × 100 freestyle on 1:40
   1 × 200 IM on 3:30
   2 × 50 best stroke on 1:00
   2 × 100 freestyle on 1:30

9. Total Distance: 1,800 yards/meters
   Sprints: best stroke
   > 4 × 50 on :50
   > 3 × 100 build-ups; best stroke
   > 1 × 100 easy swim
   > 4 × 50 on :55
   > 3 × 100 build-ups; best stroke
   > 1 × 100 easy swim
   > 4 × 50 on 1:00
   > 3 × 100 build-ups; best stroke
   > 1 × 100 easy swim

10. Total Distance: 2,000 yards/meters; Estimated Time: 40 minutes
    Swim for a specific number of minutes (i.e., 5 minutes) for each stroke or do a descending/ascending length of time for each stroke:
    20-minute set:
    > 8 minutes best stroke
    > 6 minutes second-best stroke
    > 4 minutes third-best stroke
    > 2 minutes worst stroke
    > Rest as needed
    > 2 minutes worst stroke
    > 4 minutes third-best stroke
    > 6 minutes second-best stroke
    > 8 minutes best stroke

    VARIATIONS: If there is no clock, do a set distance (i.e., 250 yards/meters) for each stroke, as above. Or do the strokes in IM order, then repeat in reverse IM order.

    Repeat this set for a total of 40 minutes. This is good for a small or irregularly shaped pool (perhaps you can swim in circles around the perimeter).

Suggestions for 300-yard/meter Cool-downs:

1. 1 × 300 easy swim, any stroke
2. 3 × 100:
   > 1 × 100 glide or catch-up freestyle drill
   > 1 × 100 catch-up backstroke drill
   > 1 × 100 freestyle

3. 6×50 easy kick:
    2×50 whip kick
    2×50 supine flutter kick
    2×50 dolphin kick

4. 6×50 freestyle, or swimmer's choice, ascending on 1:00 (swim each 50 slower than previous 50)

5. 3×100 easy kick:
    1×100 dolphin side-kick drill
    1×100 flutter alternating with dolphin every 10 beats
    1×100 dolphin kick-and-roll drill

6. 3×100 pull-kick-swim, any stroke or combination

7. 3×100 easy-stroke drills:
    1×100 double-arm backstroke
    1×100 glide backstroke
    1×100 catch-up freestyle

8. 6×50 easy kick alternating with sculling on every 50

9. Easy pull-kick-swim, swimmer's choice:
    1×50 pull
    1×100 kick
    1×100 swim

10. Easy 5-minute kick-swim, swimmer's choice

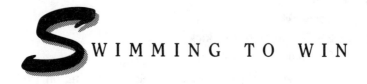 SWIMMING TO WIN

~

"SWIMMERS, TAKE YOUR MARKS!"

~

"Why am I here? What do I need this for? I thought swimming was supposed to be fun, but I feel terrible . . . I'm going to be sick. I should have gone to the bathroom . . . maybe I should go *now*. What if they start the race without me? I hope I don't make a false start; what if my goggles slip off or fog up? I just know my bathing cap is going to fall off . . . How many laps is this race? I wonder if this new suit looks okay. I should have worn my lucky one—so what if it's last year's model and falling apart. My lucky chain! Oh no, I forgot my lucky chain! That's okay, I'm going to beat that swimmer over there this time, anyway. What if the timing system goes out of whack . . . just my luck—I'll do my best time and no one will know for sure and I'll have to do it all over again, and I'll bet I won't swim as fast as the first time . . . IM? What's that . . . let's see fly, back, breast, free—or is it fly, breast, back, free . . . or . . . uh-oh . . . I'd better concentrate, the starter is raising his arm, the gun's going to go off . . . this is it! . . ." BANG!

Something like that goes through my mind every time I'm on the starting block, and if it sounds like fun to you . . . welcome to the world of competitive swimming! Only true aqua-nuts need apply; but not all aqua-nuts need compete. Advanced and Super fitness swimmers can benefit from the more intense and varied workouts and training concepts in this section, too. So I hope you'll take at least a peek and discover what goes on here.

"THE SMELL OF CHLORINE, THE ROAR OF THE CROWD," OR "WHY COMPETE?"

~

As you may have gathered, I get very, very nervous before a race. When I'm up on the starting block I usually ask myself, Why am I doing this?

Not only is no one paying me, but I'm investing my own time, money, and energy to be here! For what?

Well, part of it is the discipline, the serious training that's necessary if you're going to compete. It's been a part of my life for just about as long as I can remember. But the thing that's most interesting to me is the race against time—against the clock that measures your speed, and against the calendar that measures your age. When I started swimming in the Masters Program, in which adults nineteen and over compete against swimmers in their own age group, I was almost thirty. Since then (and now in my fifth decade), my times for the most part have steadily improved! Theoretically, as you get older, you get slower. But I'm not the only swimmer who's beaten Father Time. This is one case where the well-worn phrase "You're not getting older, you're getting better" really does apply. (Or at least if you are getting older, you're getting better at the same time.)

Time is so *objective*—there is just no arguing with it. I compete in synchronized swimming, too, where one is judged according to other people's standards and tastes, but in racing, when the clock stops, you know exactly how good you were—period. You can win a race and still not be satisfied with your own time; or you can come in last and be ecstatic at your performance.

Why *you* choose to compete, if you do, will depend on your particular circumstances and personality. But the bottom line will probably be the challenge . . . to test your abilities to the utmost . . . and then to improve on them. You'll find it an amazing "high" to swim competitively, though it's habit-forming—ask any chlorine junkie. Of course, it's an even greater high when you win. And don't say that you couldn't possibly win. *You can.* It's no pie-in-the-sky dream. Even if you don't finish first, you'll still win—in one form or another—no matter what age or shape you're in. This is especially true if you swim for fitness as part of the Masters Program, in which you're matched against swimmers in your own age bracket. But even when there are other swimmers on the starting blocks, you are really swimming against *yourself*—and against your previous best times, using the adrenaline-boosting tendency of competition to help you.

There's definitely something about performing under pressure, with family, friends, and teammates rooting for you, that brings out the best in some people. You may be able to draw on reserves that you never knew you had. Having a competitive goal to strive for may give you the incentive to drive yourself to see if you have "the right stuff"—to satisfy that curiosity that almost all people have (but won't always admit to) about just how good they really can be.

So, if you've been lap swimming for a while and are doing a mile or so during a workout, and you ask yourself, Where do I go from here? you should consider competing. If you're swimming that much, you "might as well be getting some more out of it," as one recent convert put it. You have nothing to lose and everything to win!

Why You Should Join a Swim Club
～

If you compete, you can swim either as part of a team or "unattached." I recommend that you join a swim club if at all possible. Here's why. First of all, it's a great way to make steady friends with whom you share the joys (and the woes!) of swimming. This sense of camaraderie, of belonging to a team, is one of the best things about competitive swimming. My Empire Masters Swim Team, in New York City, for instance, has over one thousand members. One is a dermatologist; another is an art dealer; there's a fashion model and a swim coach; one couple writes music in their Manhattan loft; and our club founder, Jim Forbes, is, fittingly enough, a retired U. S. Coast Guard-licensed tugboat captain. So not only do you meet many people, you have the opportunity to enjoy many types of people. You can broaden your horizons while you train your body. You also have a unique relationship with your teammates—you train together, help one another over the rough spots, and empathize with one another; but you may also be racing against some of your own club members as well as swimmers from other teams.

Clubs enable you to whip your body into magnificent shape under the watchful eye (and the barking voice) of a coach. Workouts may be scheduled daily, and may include dry-land exercises such as running, weight training, calisthenics, and drills in each competitive stroke. It's very much like the workouts you've been doing on your own, only more intense. And perhaps at an earlier hour—some clubs meet as early as 6 A.M. so that swimmers can have the pool to themselves. Some people travel for miles to work out at that insane hour. Why? As one club member says, "Because it's fun; and I need the discipline. I'd never push myself that hard. I need someone telling me what to do, that I *can* do it. To yell at me, 'Go, go, go!' or 'Shut up and swim.' "

If you want to compete, call your local Masters group, Y, recreation center, high school, college, or swim club to find a team to train with.

SPECIAL TIPS FOR COMPETITIVE SWIMMERS
～

Swimmers who want to compete should take certain factors into consideration when they train in order to make sure they're swimming their best.

Types of Events

First, you should have some idea of the event or events you'd like to participate in. Here's a sampling of a line-up for an average swim meet:

Freestyle events:
   50 yards/meters
   100 yards/meters
   200 yards/meters
   500 yards/400 meters
   1,000 yards
   1,650 yards/1,500 meters

Backstroke, breaststroke, and butterfly events:
   50 yards/meters
   100 yards/meters
   200 yards/meters

Individual Medley events:
   100 yards
   200 yards/meters
   400 yards/meters

Relay events (These events may mix various ages, sexes, distances, and strokes):
   200 yards/meters
   400 yards/meters
   800 yards/meters

Open or "freestyle" events: Usually 200 yards/meters in stroke of your choice. There are also longer distances and marathon events both poolside and in open water.

As you'll see later, the way you train will depend in part on the types of races you will swim.

A Swimmer for All Seasons

There are two main competitive swimming seasons: the indoor (short course, or 25-yard/meter pools), which usually occurs October to May, and the outdoor (long course, or 50-yard/meter pools), which occurs June through September. Both of these seasons are classically divided into three stages or parts, and each season culminates in your main meet. Which part of the season it is and which event or events you specialize in determine the kinds of workouts you do. Here is a description of each part of the swimming season, as well as suggestions for specialized workouts to be done at specific times to help you train most effectively for your event.

As you train, fine tune your skills, paying careful attention to the checklists and catalogs of common errors provided for each stroke in Part Two, "The Techniques of Swimming." Make sure you're proficient in those little extras that can make a crucial difference in your final times: flip turns; open turns for the breaststroke and butterfly; wind-up, grab, and relay starts. Chances are that the other swimmers will be using them to advantage—so why shouldn't you?

1. Early Season (approximately four to eight weeks): At this time, concentrate on general conditioning, using long, easy swims and a variety of strokes and distances up to two miles (such as those suggested in the Super Workouts). In addition, I suggest that you supplement your swimming with dry-land activities that will improve your strength, flexibility, and cardiovascular conditioning—such as aerobics, stretching and running, and exercises using stretch cords and weights. (See "Swimmers' Shape-ups," page 371.) Samples of early season workouts begin on page 306.

2. Mid-Season (six to twelve weeks): Your workouts should include a relatively consistent yardage (about 3,000 yards/meters), and you should begin to fine tune your strokes, particularly your specialty or specialties. You should do some stroke work as well as some distance and timed swims. Dry-land training should be held at maintenance level during this time. You should also pay particular attention to your resting and eating habits and your flexibility, and perhaps take vitamin and mineral supplements (go easy on the junk-palace foods!). Typical mid-season training workouts begin on page 308.

3. Taper and Peak (average two weeks before your biggest meet): This, the shortest part of the swimming season, is the time during which you prepare yourself physically and mentally for your stiffest competition. Generally the aim is to concentrate on higher-quality, lower-quantity swimming. As you get nearer and nearer the actual race, your total yardage decreases, but your times should approach racing speed. You do this by resting more between sets, doing broken swims, swimming descending sets, doing stroke drills, and practicing starts and turns to improve technique.

The average taper lasts one to two weeks, but this depends on how long and how hard you've trained during the rest of the season, and on your event and distance specialty. The longer your event, the shorter the taper. For example, a sprinter would taper about ten days, whereas a distance swimmer's taper might be only five days. Because of the taper, you bring your mind and your body to peak performance. The length of your peak may last about half as long as your taper. Suggested taper and peak workouts begin on page 312.

After your big race, you may experience a physical and mental letdown. At this time you may want to take a break from your training. Or you may want to abbreviate your workouts.

SPECIALIZED WORKOUTS—NOT FOR COMPETITIVE SWIMMERS ONLY

➤

The workouts below are really meant to be used by Super-level swimmers whether they compete or not. They're for any swimmer of any age who simply wants to swim faster and better. Many fitness swimmers (I hope) will reach the stage where they're ready to specialize, to concentrate on doing one or more strokes and/or distances really well even if they never attend a single meet.

These workouts are about 3,000 yards/meters, and so will give you plenty of ideas for varying the Super Workouts, too. The workouts are organized to coincide with the three parts of a competitive season, and include samples and training concepts for distance and marathon swims, sprints, middle-distance swims, and for peaking and tapering.

When following the workouts, make sure that you adjust all intervals to your own needs and capabilities. Don't forget to take it easy during the warm-ups and cool-downs, which are an important part of every workout.

EARLY SEASON WORKOUTS
⁓

Distance, Overdistance, and Marathon Swims

Early in the season, concentrate on distance swims to build your endurance. One good way to do this is a timed broken swim of 1,650 yards/1,500 meters; variations follow.

1. *Timed Broken 1,650 yard/1,500 meter workout*

Warm-up (800 yards/meters)

8 × 100 freestyle/swimmer's choice:
 2 × 100 easy swim
 1 × 100 with paddles
 1 × 100 with paddles and pull-buoy
 1 × 100 with pull-buoys
 1 × 100 catch-up freestyle
 2 × 100 easy swim

Main Set (2,300 yards/2,150 meters)

2 × 300 (sustain pace of first 50 for entire set):
 1 × 50; 5 seconds rest
 1 × 100; 10 seconds rest
 1 × 150; 15 seconds rest
 Repeat
 Rest as needed
1,650-yards/1,500-meter freestyle: broken
 1 × 500; 30 seconds rest
 1 × 400; 25 seconds rest
 1 × 300; 20 seconds rest
 1 × 200; 15 seconds rest
 1 × 100; 10 seconds rest
 (If you're swimming in a long-course pool, this completes your 1,500-meter broken swim.)
 Variation (slightly shorter distance): Divide swim into thirds (490 yards/450 meters) with a 30-second rest interval after each third.
 1 × 100; 5 seconds rest

1 × 50
(If you're swimming in a 25-yard pool, this completes your broken
   swim.)

Cool-down (400 yards/meters)

1 × 200 easy kick, with or without fins
1 × 200 easy swim

2. **Descending 2-mile distance swim;**   rest 1:00 between each
swim:
   1 × 1 mile
   1 × ½ mile
   1 × ¼ mile
   2 × ⅛ mile

3. **Fartlek Swim**   (Easy-hard, pyramid-fashion, continuous, 3,400-
yard/meter swim)
   2 × 50
   2 × 100
   2 × 200
   2 × 300
   2 × 400
   2 × 300
   2 × 200
   2 × 100
   2 × 50

4. **Circle Swimming**
If you are in a small or irregularly shaped pool, or a small area of open
water, swim in a circle around the perimeter; change direction after half
your swim, and perhaps change your stroke. (Count your circles, if you
like.)
To cool down, tread and/or swim easily for 5–10 minutes.

5. **Open-water Swimming**
Another way to get in your overdistance is to swim long stretches in
open water, such as a lake or the ocean. This can be most enjoyable. Here
the idea is to swim from one point to another at a steady pace. (It's also
done as a competitive event for time or distance, such as in a triathlon.)

Warm up thoroughly on land, with jumping jacks, arm circles, jogging in place, and easy stretching. Begin your swim at an easy, steady pace for the first 1,000 yards/meters, or approximately fifteen minutes. Concentrate on pulling.

As you continue into the main part of your swim, focus on the following:

- Keep a steady pace throughout the swim.
- Periodically check your time and/or distance.
- Swim in as straight a line as possible. Do bilateral breathing.
- If you get tired or bored, or if you get a "stitch," change strokes.
- Think about your stroke techniques when your mind begins to wander.

Heed the following open-water Safety and Comfort Tips:

- Prior to your open-water swim, check tides, temperature, currents, sea life, and salinity of the water.
- If you're in an open-water race, check the positioning at start. Stay clear of other swimmers (unless you like contact swimming).
- Keep an eye on your swimming course, using buoys and markers and/or other swimmers as guides.
- Use alternate breathing to change your pace, check your position, and relax your neck muscles.
- If signs of impending hypothermia, or cooling of the body's core temperature, develop (such as blue or numb fingers), don't be a martyr.

MID-SEASON WORKOUTS
～

Specialty Strokes, Distances, Individual Medley Workouts

During this part of your swim season you want to hold to a total distance of approximately 3,000 yards/meters per workout and concentrate on your specialty. The following two freestyle workouts are examples that can be adapted to other strokes.

1. Sprint Freestyle: This includes a time trial to help you achieve the "perfect 100": suppress the kick on the first 50, and accelerate it for the second 50.

Warm-up: (600 yards/meters)

6 × 50 pull on 1:00

4 × 50 catch-up freestyle drill; alternate breathing on 1:00

4 × 25 body position drill on 1:00: prone position, head up; arms extended forward underwater; scull as you flutter kick and keep shoulders as high as possible.

Main Set: (2,100 yards/meters)

4 × 200 freestyle broken swim on 4:00; rest 10 seconds at 100 and 150; pull first 100

1 × 100 easy breaststroke

5 × 100 freestyle on 2:00; pull first 50

1 × 50 easy swim

10 × 50 descending set: time interval decreases by 2 seconds; starting interval 1:00

50s	Leave on	Time interval
1	:60	1:00
2	:60	:58
3	:58	:56
4	:54	:54
5	:50	:52
6	:44	:50
7	:36	:48
8	:26	:46
9	:14	:42
10	:60	Set ends on 40

1 × 50 easy swim; rest as needed

1 × 100 timed swim: to swim the "perfect 100," try to pull the first 50, suppressing the kick, then accelerate the kick during the final 50. Record your time and make a pulse check.

Cool-down: (300 yards/meters)

6 × 50 easy kick-swim set

2. **Middle-distance Freestyle:** This workout includes a broken 200-yard/meter swim during which you should approach your best time. To get your final time, subtract your rest periods.

Warm-up: (600 yards/meters)

1 × 200 easy swim
4 × 50 catch-up one-arm pull on 1:00 (swim easily, so that you just make the interval and get very little rest)
1 × 200 easy IM

Main Set: (2,100 yards/meters)

1 × 400
1 × 200 pull
1 × 200 swim
1 × 100 pull with pull-buoy at ankles (with paddles)
1 × 100 swim
30 seconds rest
1 × 100 pull with pull-buoy above knees (with paddles)
1 × 100 swim
30 seconds rest
1 × 100 pull with paddles only
1 × 100 swim
Rest as needed
1 × 150 IM without freestyle (butterfly, backstroke, and breaststroke only)
1 × 50 easy swim
1 × 100 flutter kick with fins
1 × 50 easy swim
Rest as needed
1 × 200 broken swim
1 × 100: concentrate on pull (rest interval: 10 seconds)
1 × 50: sprint
Check pulse.

Cool-down: (300 yards/meters)

2 × 150 easy pull, kick, swim

3. *Butterfly Main Set:* Do mixed swim sets, because the butterfly is such a strenuous stroke. For example, you might break up a set of 150s this way:

4 × 150 on 4:00:

first and third 150: 1 × 50 freestyle, 1 × 50 butterfly, 1 × 50 free-style

second and fourth 150: 1 × 50 butterfly, 1 × 50 freestyle, 1 × 50 butterfly

Add some dolphin-kick drills, some butterfly pulling, and some controlled breathing drills to your workout, too.

4. *Backstroke Main Set:* You can also do descending sets and/or negative splits during a main set (this is more appropriate for freestylers and breaststrokers, than for butterfliers or IM specialists). For example:

2 × 200 backstroke on 3:30: negative split by swimming second half of each 200 faster than the first half (glance at the clock when you make the first 100)

and/or:

6 × 50 backstroke swim, descending on 1:00: swim each 50 a second or two faster than the previous one.

5. *Breaststroke Main Set:* One thing to concentrate on here is stroke drills. Since there have been so many innovations in this stroke, most swimmers' breaststroke could use some technique work. For example, you could begin the main set this way:

4 × 150 breaststroke drills (30 seconds rest between each 150):

1 × 150 pull with dolphin kick

1 × 150 pull-pull-kick drill

1 × 150 whip kick (keep hands at buttocks)

1 × 150 one-arm breaststroke drill

You could also add a descending set of 5 × 100, and some controlled breathing swims to help your underwater pull-out.

6. *Individual Medley Main Set:* Here the trick is to swim all four competitive strokes as a separate "event" in the workout, each event, or set, being introduced with an IM swim. For instance, in an IM 4 × 450 main set of 2,100 yards/meters, the butterfly set might be:

1×450 on 11:00

1×200 IM on 4:00

1×100 dolphin kick on 2:30

2×50 butterfly on 1:30 (1×50 pull, 1×50 swim)

1×50 easy swim-down on 1:30

Repeat for the backstroke, breaststroke, and freestyle, beginning each 450-yard set with a 200 IM, followed by a kick drill, a pull-swim drill, and a swim-down, as above, for each stroke. (Adjust the interval times if needed.)

For variations in your Individual Medley workouts, you can also reverse the order of the IM (i.e., freestyle, breaststroke, backstroke, butterfly). Also, in a 50-meter pool you can do 100 IMs by changing strokes at the halfway mark.

END-OF-SEASON TAPER-AND-PEAK WORKOUTS
‿

Quality Versus Quantity

A typical taper workout is about 2,000 yards/meters, with approximately one third allocated each to the warm-up, main set, and cool-down. Peak workouts are about 1,000 yards/meters, and are divided up this way: two fifths warm-up, one fifth main set, and two fifths cool-down.

1. Taper workout for middle-distance (200 yards/meters) swimmers: This might include a timed broken 200-yard/meter freestyle swim. Be sure to practice your starts and turns during the swim and add a few practice drills at the end of the cool-down.

Total Distance: 2,000 yards/meters

Warm-up (700 yards/meters):

3×200 easy pull-kick-swim, freestyle or swimmer's choice

1×100 freestyle: catch-up stroke drill

Main Set (700 yards/meters)

8×50 freestyle descending on 1:00

1×100 easy swim

Rest as needed.

Timed Swim: 1×200 broken swim 5–10 seconds rest after each 50

Check pulse.

VARIATIONS:

During the timed 200, you can break the distance into swims other than 50s; for example, 100, 50, 50; or 50, 100, 50; or 100, 50, 25, 25. (Go for 90 to 100 percent effort.)

Cool-down (600 yards/meters)

3 × 200 easy swim-kick-swim

2. *Race Pace Workout:* Approach your racing pace by expending 80 to 90 percent effort.

Total Distance: 1,000 yards/meters

Warm-up (400 yards/meters)

1 × 200 easy swim
4 × 50 build-ups on 2:00

Main Set (200 yards/meters)

- For distance swimmer: to get feel of and approach racing pace
  Timed 2 × 100: 10 seconds rest between
- For middle-distance swimmer: to get the feel of the first 50 of a 200
  3 × 50 on 2:00
  Rest as needed
  Timed 1 × 50: swim this distance as though it were the first 50 of a 200-yard race
- For sprinters: to get a fast turnover (speeding up the entire stroke cycle)
  2 × 75 on 2:00; broken at 50 with 10 seconds rest
  Rest as needed
  2 × 25 timed swim: start from racing dive
  Rest as needed

Cool-down (400 yards/meters)

1 × 100 easy swim
3 × 100 pull-kick-swim
Starts and turns

Your First Swim Meet

Get Ready . . .

To find out where and when local meets are to be held, contact your local Y, school swim team, or community center. You can also write the U. S. Masters Swimming office or use the listings in one of the periodicals listed, beginning on page 332.

Once you've decided to enter a meet, the first thing you have to do is become registered with U. S. Masters Swimming, Inc. Then get an official entry blank from the sponsoring organization. Fill it out and sent it in as instructed. There is usually a specified fee for each event you wish to enter.

Be sure to enter events that you're comfortable with. In addition to your fitness level, consider the distance, stroke, and the spacing of events. For example, for your first meet you should choose events near the beginning and end of the schedule, so that you'll have plenty of rest in between.

For your first meet, you should probably enter one to three individual events. Next time you can enter more if you feel up to it. And remember, you don't have to swim even if you've entered; you can change your mind at the last minute. But sending in your entry is a commitment, and most people who enter actually compete.

A few days before the race you'll probably experience pre-meet jitters. This is a phenomenon that affects almost everybody—young or old, new or experienced. I still get them, and I've been competing for forty plus years. So don't be surprised if you feel anything from a few butterflies in your stomach to all-out nervous diarrhea.

You may begin to feel unsure of yourself. You'll hear yourself saying, Oh, God, I feel so out of shape. I'm sick. I feel paralyzed. Why am I doing this? Here I am spending another perfectly good Saturday at the Y. All my friend and family think I'm crazy—maybe they're right.

This time your teammates come in really handy. An understanding spouse, friend, or relative can help, too. Lucky for me, I come from a swimming family—my mother, father, brother, and sisters all swim. Invite your family to the meet, whether they're swimmers or not, so that they can give you support. Nothing will give you a bigger kick than having your own rooting section.

Of course, you'll be more confident if your body has been trained, tapered, and peaked properly. But have you trained your mind? The best athletes know that mental preparation is one of the most important parts of any training program. You'd be surprised at the difference the state of your psyche can make in your performance.

To help improve performance, many swimmers use mental imagery, imagining beforehand every second of an upcoming race: the pool, the crowd, the lane markers, the starting block, the signal go, the feel of the water, their first stroke, their breathing pattern, their turn, and so on until the end of the race, where they win (or swim their best time). This mental practice can also be used during workouts (just before a sprint or a timed swim). Like a dancer or an actor, you must rehearse the race physically and mentally many times before the actual "performance," thinking through every lap, stroke by stroke and turn by turn, from start to finish, until you're sure you know every nuance of the race.

Get set . . .

On the day of the meet, it's psychologically and logistically (and sometimes ecologically) a good idea to travel with other people—especially if they're swimmers. (You'll find sympathetic company valuable.)

What to Take

In all the excitement, you might forget an item or two, so use this checklist as a reminder. I find a large water-repellent duffel bag with extra pockets ideal for carrying my paraphernalia.

- A copy of your U. S. Masters Swimming Registration Card.
- Bathing suits. Take one for warm-up and one racing suit for each event in which you'll be competing. Change into a dry suit after each event.
- Bathing cap, if you wear one (take an extra, just in case).
- Goggles. Take two pairs.
- Towels. Take at least two. (Chamois are great.)
- Toiletries and grooming aids. Don't forget your shampoo and conditioner, baby oil, soap, cotton swabs, ear, eye, or nose drops. Use plastic bottles for safety.
- Plastic bags. To tote wet things home.
- Lambswool or earplugs. If you need to keep water out of your ears.
- Sneakers, socks, warm-up suit, and T-shirts. To wear between events, over your suit; helps to keep you from getting chilled.

- Lock. For storing your valuables in a locker.
- If you're competing outdoors, take a hat, appropriate SPF suntan lotion, sunglasses, maybe an umbrella to protect you from the sun.

You might want to have team T-shirts printed up. Of course, T-shirts (and bathing caps) can be made to say anything these days; my favorites are my "excuse" T-shirts and caps, which give such tried-and-true explanations as:

- I put my earplugs in my nose
- I thought it was the backstroke
- The stopwatch didn't work
- I was saving something for the finals
- My suit fell off
- I tapered too much
- I'm allergic to chlorine
- My goggles leaked
- It was a false start

You may want to take some healthful snacks like nuts, fruit, or juices—you may find a snack bar, gratis buffet, or vending machines at the meet, but you never know.

There will be a check-in post in the lobby or at pool-side, where you pick up the entry cards that you sent in earlier or a program, or heat sheet. Your cards will now have been filled in with your *heat,* as well as your lane number. The program indicates the order or events and heats, the entrants, their age groups, and their seed times. These heats are usually set up so that you swim with people close to your seed time. Within each heat, the swimmers are arranged so that the fastest are in the center lanes and the slower swimmers are in the outer lanes.

Next, proceed to the locker room. Locate the bathroom for future reference, a locker, and change into your warm-up swim suit. If you have long hair (this goes for guys, too) secure it with an elastic band before you put on your bathing cap; if your cap shifts during the race, this will keep your hair from falling in your eyes. Remove all jewelry.

In most cases, it's best to lock your valuables in the locker and to keep out only what you need—extra suits, towels, sweatsuit, etc. Leave the essentials in your bag and take it pool-side with you.

Next, do a warm-up and check out the pool. Get in the water and loosen up with a few laps. As you do so, see how "fast" the pool is. Check the wall of the pool; some may be slippery and others may cause the water to splash up in waves as you turn. Is the pool wavy? If so, it may affect your comfort and speed. If the backstroke is one of your events, count the number of strokes it takes you to go from the overhead flags to the wall. See whether *touch pads* for electronic timing are in place against the wall, just under the starting block.

If so, be sure to touch the pad strongly when you finish, so that it stops your time. (There are usually back-up hand timers just in case.) Take a few practice dives to test the starting blocks. If you're in a relay, practice a few exchanges with your teammates. *Goggles* are optional during a race. For a longer distance, you may even want to use an in-the-water start so that you don't risk your goggles slipping off. However, if you tighten them up and keep your chin tucked on entry, they should be fine.

The pre-race warm-up should bring your pulse up the same way it does during a workout. It should get you loose, stretched, and relaxed; establish your breathing pattern; and warm up your stroke. If you're in shape and ready, a warm-up will not tire you out. On the contrary, it will help *get you going*. If you're not in your best shape, do an abbreviated, easier warm-up.

A *pre-race warm-up* should begin with a long, easy swim, followed by stroke drills, then by a set to bring your heart rate up. It should total approximately 1,000 yards/meters (or about one third of your daily yardage).

Here's a sample pre-race warm-up:

1 × 200 easy swim

1 × 200 stroke and kick drills

1 × 200 pull

1 × 300 pace set: 6 × 50 on a comfortable interval; sprinters should do faster interval, with build-up 50s

1 × 100 easy swim

Finish by practicing starts and turns. Diving starts are permitted in designated sprint lanes, swimming only in one direction.

After warming up, go back to the locker room and change into a dry racing suit. If you were a bit nervous before, warming up should have calmed you down a bit (although you may find that your suit is awfully difficult to get on!).

Go!

When it's time for you to step onto the starting block, concentrate on how you're going to swim the race. Try to be relaxed but alert. Take a few deep breaths to calm you down, but don't overdo it.

During the race, concentrate on your actual performance. Try to swim it exactly as you've planned; don't let the presence of your competitors cause you to deviate from your strategy. They may be ahead of you or behind you—but who knows how they've planned to swim the race?

Try to get someone to note your intermediate times (your splits). Usually the timer for your lane will do this if you ask, or have a friend with a stopwatch take them for you. During longer races, such as 500s or 1,650s, lap counters will tell you (visually or orally) how many laps you've completed.

After the race, whatever the results, stay in the water to cool down and to allow your pulse to return to normal. If there's a warm-up/cool-down pool nearby, do a few easy laps. If not, do some bobbing, sculling, or floating. It's much better to cool down in the water. The cool water will help disperse the extra body heat.

During the cool-down, think about your reasons for competing. You may be disappointed this time, but there's always a next time; no one can be the best or even do his best at every meet. And remember that the word "compete" comes from the Latin *competere*, meaning "to strive together." Most people assume that the idea is to strive *against* one another, to put winning above all else. But if you think of swimming as a constructive, creative activity that helps you develop as a person, that mixes seriousness with fun, you'll realize that, whatever the order of finish, you have nothing to lose.

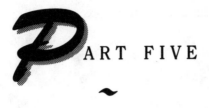

PART FIVE

~

EQUIPMENT

*A*ll you really need to swim is a pool, a suit, and perhaps a cap and goggles. When used judiciously, though, the training devices described here can help you to vary your workouts, refine your techniques, learn new skills, and accelerate and intensify the conditioning process. They can be invaluable in getting you over a hump or in surmounting a plateau. They're also fun to use—either alone or in the combinations suggested. (Don't get carried away and try to use everything at once!)

The pool where you work out may supply some training devices; if so, they may be lying around pool-side. If you don't see any, ask for them; they may simply be stored away somewhere. If your pool doesn't provide basic equipment, you can always take your own. All of the equipment discussed here can be found at a well-equipped sporting goods store, but if an item isn't available locally, contact one of the supplier manufacturers listed at the end of this chapter. Sources of information about swimming, the best books, periodicals, and films, are listed there, too.

POOLS
~

All pools are definitely not created equal. A good pool is worth looking for, paying for, and even traveling for. So carefully consider your needs, preferences, and level of ability when selecting one. When you're away from home, you may not have much of a choice; but shop around for your regular pool, keeping the following factors in mind.

Size: Pool sizes vary greatly. Let's begin at the top, with the two sizes that are the most desirable. First, there are the "long-course" pools. These

50-meter (sometimes 55-yard) pools are common on the West Coast, where they're usually outdoors. Many universities throughout the country also have indoor and outdoor long-course pools, though, and they often allow community members to use them during certain hours. In addition, private clubs with good facilities often house a 50-meter pool complex and have a team that you can train with. Long-course pools are terrific for intermediate, advanced, and competitive-level workouts. They're usually well designed and fully equipped with lane markers for lap swimming, pace clocks, and training devices such as kickboards, pull-buoys, and hand paddles. This is the only truly "Olympic size" pool; anything shorter, no matter what advertisers may claim, is not. (By the way, you should be aware that swimming in a long-course pool is a different experience from swimming in a shorter pool: it's more strenuous because you have fewer turns and therefore fewer rests.)

Next come the 25-yard, 25-meter, and 20-yard pools for competition. However, although only the 25-yard and 25-meter pools qualify as "regulation short course," all these lengths are fine for any swimmer at any level. (Beginning swimmers should make sure that there's an area that is shallow enough for practicing new skills, though.) You'll find pools in this group in many places—Ys, some health clubs, swim clubs, public recreation areas, schools, park department facilities, etc. They sometimes have lane markers, pace clocks, and various training devices. You may also find 33⅓-yard/meter pools located in the above places as well.

After these two groups, the sizing situation is a mess. The length of hotel, motel, health club, and health spa pools often depends upon how much space and money the owner has, and may be anything from 10 to 15 yards. These are fine when you're at the beginner stage; since there's a large shallow end, it's easy to swim the shorter laps or widths, and it's unlikely that there will be lap swimmers for you to dodge. As you improve, though, you'll probably outgrow this size pool fairly quickly. But don't forget swimming if that's the only kind of pool that's around: you'll still be able to swim mini-laps, do drills, practice starts and turns, do some kicking and a variety of water exercises. You can also swim around the perimeter of the pool, first counterclockwise, then clockwise.

Shape: Kidney-shaped pools are fine for beginners, for practicing certain skills, and for water exercises, but persons who want to improve their fitness by swimming longer distances won't be satisfied in anything but a standard-sized, rectangular pool.

Cleanliness: The pool and its surroundings should be spotless. However, cloudy water doesn't necessarily mean that the pool is dirty or unsafe; it could just be a temporary chemical imbalance. (Generally, if you can see the drain at the deep end, the water is clear enough for safe swimming.) Inspect the wall at water level—if the pool has a case of "ring around the collar," it may mean that maintenance isn't up to par. All pools have a filtration system for recirculating the water and balancing the chemicals; the lifeguard or pool manager can probably tell you whether there are any problems there.

Indoors or Outdoors?   If you can, by all means swim outdoors: it's much more pleasant when the sunlight is filtering through the water and you're breathing fresh air. And unless it's a thunderstorm, there's nothing wrong with swimming even in the rain (just swim underwater if you don't want to get wet!). Depending on the climate in your area, you may be able to swim outdoors all year round; if you live in a colder climate, switching from indoors during the winter to outdoors during the summer can provide a welcome change in your routine.

Traffic: While having the whole pool, or at least one lane, all to yourself is nice, it's hardly possible all the time. Observe pool courtesy by circling counterclockwise within the lane and you'll find that crowding is not a problem. Of course, if there are hundreds of persons splashing around, you might schedule your swims for less popular times. There should be at least one lane marked off for lap swimming, if that's what you plan to do.

Also, when turning, wait at the wall, if at all possible, to allow a faster swimmer to pass you. You'll know that someone is eager to pass if you felt a little toe tickle on the preceding lap.

Temperature: The ideal water temperature for comfort and safety is between 78° F and 84° F. For light workouts such as those done by beginning swimmers, or for water exercises, water at the warmer end of the scale is preferable. For heavier workouts, cooler water is better because it helps dissipate your increased body heat. The American National Red Cross recommends that the air temperature be about four degrees higher than the water temperature.

Ambience: What's your style: no-fuss, no-frills—or music, lush vegetation, chairs for lounging, and fancy mirrors and murals? You want to feel comfortable at your pool, so make sure that you like the atmosphere at your chosen watering hole before you commit yourself and your money. Remember, you'll be spending about an hour there at least three times a week. In addition to the ambience, you may also want a well-equipped gym, exercise room, and/or whirlpool and sauna facilities, under one roof.

Lifeguard: The presence of a qualified person in case of emergency is something swimmers at all levels should insist upon. Never swim alone.

SWIM SUITS

～

We've come a long way since 1909 when Annette Kellerman, the Australian national swimming heroine, was arrested for wearing a daring one-piece tank suit. Looking and feeling like a woolly body stocking, her suit would be considered a real drag (literally and figuratively) by today's standards—but it was a definite improvement over the fussy, skirted monstrosities that women were wearing at the time. (Although men's suits have always been more practical and comfortable than women's, the fellows wore suits similar to Annette's until the end of World War II.) But Ms. Kellerman definitely had the right idea about eliminating resistance. Since then, suits have become steadily lighter, sleeker, and skimpier, in an effort to increase streamlining and reduce swimming times.

The arrival of the aptly named skinsuit, worn by the East German women's team in the 1972 Olympics, generated a shock similar to that of the Kellerman suit in its day. But a more serious shock was the record-breaking times achieved by the swimmers who wore the contour-revealing suits, and now these "disgraceful" suits that fit like a second skin are commonplace on serious fitness swimmers and competitors alike. They're seen on recreational and fashion-conscious swimmers, too, in the form of the comfortable and practical Lycra.

Men's suit styles have also undergone a streamlining, from the conservative wool tank suit, to the heavy cotton boxer shorts, and finally to the Lycra "skin" bikini brief seen on serious competitive and fitness swimmers today.

Almost any suit will do when you begin your program. But eventually women should get rid of the excess fabric such as decorative bows, buckles, buttons, and skirts, and men should graduate from baggy shorts. These all create drag in the water and slow you down, making swimming harder than it need be. So pare down to the minimum with a suit that fits well without binding at the arms, legs, or waist. When buying a suit, be sure to try it on. If you can, simulate swimming movements in the dressing room to make sure it won't slip or rub; you won't want to have to interrupt your workouts to adjust your suit every lap or two. For women a one-piece tank or maillot-type suit is best. Some well-constructed dance leotards also fit the bill, and many sportswear manufacturers have designed suits that are hard to distinguish from their inspirations—real racing suits.

Fitness and racing suits are available at sporting goods stores and are a must for competitive swimmers, when an extra ounce or two can make a crucial difference in the time. Even if you don't compete (yet), consider getting a suit designed for serious swimming. Why should you be held back by a suit that's one iota heavier than it has to be? A racing suit will help you swim better. It has strategically placed straps that allow the greatest possible freedom of movement. It's sleek, taut, and practically weightless. It gives your body a streamlined feel and allows you to slip through the water more smoothly and quickly. In fact, while you're swimming you'll probably forget that you're wearing one.

Fitness and racing suits are available in seemingly endless variations. There are numerous styles that affect their shape, style, back, straps, leg height, type of fabric, thickness, design, and therefore prices will vary.

To prolong the life of any suit, avoid sitting on rough edges or surfaces. Most manufacturers suggest that you rinse your suit out in fresh water after each swim, and allow it to air-dry.

GOGGLES
⁓

Goggles may not be the most attractive thing you'll ever wear, but they're surely an improvement over "red eye." And not only do goggles protect your eyes, they help you to see better underwater. For contact lens wearers, of course, goggles are a must. Prescription goggles are available, as well.

Goggles come in various shapes, sizes, eye socket cushioning, anti-fog features, variable adjustments for nosepieces and head straps, casing and more.

Finding a comfortable pair of goggles is largely a matter of trial and error. Manufacturers naturally try to design models to fit everyone, but as this is impossible, you'll just have to buy a pair and keep your fingers crossed.

Goggles come in a variety of tints. Clear is the all-purpose color, and the blue, green, or gray ones are made to shield your eyes from bright sunlight. Yellow or rose-colored lenses, on the other hand, actually make indoor light seem brighter.

When you wear goggles, get the proper fit by adjusting both the rubber headband and the center piece over the nose. If you wear a cap, the goggles should be over it. For diving and for fast flip turns, wear your goggles a bit tighter than usual. The cushioning around the lenses keeps the water out. To help form a tighter seal, press the goggles gently against your eye sockets to help create a vacuum. The slight indentations they leave around your eyes disappear quickly, but to minimize this effect you can push the goggles up on your forehead whenever you don't really need them, such as during a rest period or while doing a kick drill.

If you have trouble with your goggles fogging up (and most swimmers do, because of the condensation formed by the difference in the air and water temperatures), you can try several remedies. The best are the special defogging products that deposit a thick oily film on the inside surface of the lenses. Made especially for this purpose, these solutions really work, swim after swim after swim. This means only a small squeeze bottle will last virtually forever, so you can share one with a fellow swimmer.

However, before you rush out and buy such a specialized item, you might experiment with one or more alternatives. The handiest and cheapest, and most popular, is good old saliva—something swimmers have been relying on for years.

BATHING CAPS
➤

Remember the days of flower-petal bathing caps, or wiglike caps? Well, today, caps are just as streamlined as suits are and come in a variety of colors, shapes, thicknesses, and materials (e.g., latex, Lycra, and silicone). Some pools require a cap for long-haired swimmers of either sex, but even persons with relatively short hair will find that, although no cap can keep your hair perfectly dry, it will keep your hair out of your eyes and will spare it the brunt of chemical abuse. If you have long hair, you can gather it into an elastic band before slipping on a bathing cap. A sweatband helps to keep out water by acting as an absorptive barrier. A Lycra cap may be worn under a rubber one; wearing it also makes donning the rubber one easier and more comfortable. (This is especially helpful when you're swimming for long periods.)

After each swim, let your bathing cap air-dry. Then dust it lightly with corn starch or talcum powder; this keeps it from sticking to itself and so makes it easier to put on next time.

KICKBOARDS

If you're going to use any "extra" piece of equipment, let it be a kickboard. Few things can compare to this simple device—a rectangular slab of compressed plastic—for versatility and usefulness. And that applies for all swimmers, be they beginners, fitness seekers, or competitors.

A kickboard can support the upper part of your body, allowing you to breathe normally as you practice your kicks (hence the term "kickboard"). Thus you can learn a new kick or improve a familiar one; you can strengthen your legs for a trimmer look and stronger, faster kicks; and you can vary your workouts.

One method of using a kickboard in the prone position is to hold it comfortably with your arms straight along the top, fingertips curled around the upper (rounded) edge. Or you can hold the board farther away from you, so that you have room to put your face in the water to practice your rhythmic breathing. Excessive prone kicking with a kickboard may cause discomfort in your lower back. Switch to back flutter kick for variation.

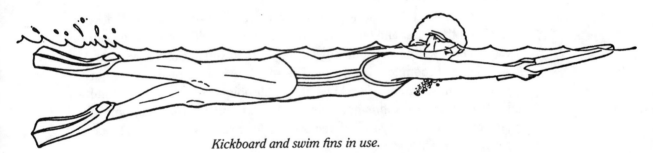

Kickboard and swim fins in use.

SWIM FINS

Fins are more than a child's plaything or a scuba diver's must-have; they're a useful training device for the fitness and competitive swimmer alike. In the first place, they add variety to your workouts. Second, they help you develop muscles in your thighs, calves, and abdomen. Third, the overload placed on these large muscle groups helps to improve your cardiovascular capacity as well. Fourth, they help make your feet and ankles more flexible. They also make you go faster. There are a variety of styles, shapes, sizes, contours, and colors to fit most every need, including a "monofin"!

According to one theory, once your body is attuned to faster action, it continues to respond quickly, whether the fins are on or not. The added propulsion also causes your body to ride higher in the water *(to hydroplane)*, which is important for most strokes, especially the butterfly; combined with the fins' tendency to accentuate the undulating body motion, this means that your arms can recover higher and smoother, resulting in a more fluid stroke. In the backstroke, fins counteract "low legs," a common problem in that stroke. They also give you a feel for the efficient whipping action that your feet should develop while swimming every stroke. (Unfortunately, fins aren't good for practicing the breaststroke or the sidestroke because of the nature of the kick.) Thus, wearing fins makes your kick more effective and efficient by forcing you to do it "the right way"; theoretically, this efficiency becomes a habit that stays with you even when you take the fins off.

Swim fins come in several sizes, shapes, colors, weights, designs, function and foot attachments. The shoe type are more comfortable and stable, for some people, than the strap-backed. To put them on, bend the heel back inside out, insert your foot, and flip the back up in place. If you develop soreness or blisters when wearing fins, slip on a pair of thin cotton socks to protect your feet.

Observe safety precautions when you wear fins—always walk backwards, in the water and out. Be aware, too, that the added propulsion can cause a pool wall to sneak up on you sooner than you'd think: leave yourself plenty of room for your turns. The added resistance really works out your leg muscles and your knee and ankle joints, so start slowly, and increase your use of fins gradually. And watch out for the phantom fin phenomenon—when you first remove the fins, you'll feel as though you have no feet left!

PULL-BUOYS

～

Pull-buoys are made of Styrofoam or similar material. They come in several sizes, shapes, colors, designs, and methods of adjustment.

A pull-buoy is like a kickboard for your lower body: it supports your legs so that you can work on your arm strokes. Thus, you can do pulling drills to learn a new stroke, to improve technique, to build proper upper-body strength, and to vary your workouts.

To use a pull-buoy, place it with the center or straps between your thighs, so that when you assume a horizontal position one cylinder will

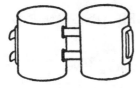

Pull-buoys

be on top of your legs and one will be under them. Press your thighs together to hold it in place and to contribute to stability and streamlining. It can also be used as a kickboard and as an upper-body support during supine kicking drills.

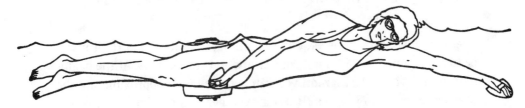

Pull-buoy and hand paddles in use.

HAND PADDLES

⮜

Hand paddles fit on your palms and act the way fins do for your feet— using them strengthens your shoulder, chest, arm, and back muscles by increasing the water's resistance. Hand paddles come in several shapes, sizes, and colors, resistance designs, hand attachments, and materials (e.g., gloves, mitts). Most are one half inch to two inches larger than your hand all around, but there are also half-sized paddles as well as forearm paddles.

Paddles also help you to improve your form, first by telling you whether you're lifting your elbow high enough during overwater recovery: if your elbow is too low, the paddle dips into the water and the added drag throws off your stroke noticeably. The paddles' larger surface area also insures that your hand enters the water at the proper angle; if not, the slap, splash, and added resistance will be obvious. Some paddles also have a lip at the wrist end that tells you whether you're ending your pull too flat or too early. Hand paddles are often used in conjunction with a pull-buoy.

Like fins, hand paddles put an extra strain on your muscles and joints. So use them sparingly at first and gradually increase their use during your workouts.

OTHER RESISTANCE DEVICES
～

Swimmers—especially competitive swimmers—sometimes wear resistance devices during workouts in order to create more "drag" and so to improve their conditioning. Such devices include small rubber "donuts" that are twisted around the ankles in a figure 8, pull-buoys worn between the ankles, and two or three swim suits worn one over the other.

CLOCKS AND OTHER TIMING DEVICES
～

The more involved you become in swimming, the more important it will be to have some way of timing your swims and rest periods. At the beginning of the workout program, you can get away with approximating the time by counting to yourself. But once you get to the point where you're doing timed swims, paced swims, intervals, repeats, sprints, and timed distance swims, you need a more accurate way of telling time.

A *pace clock*, which is standard equipment at many pools, is the best instrument for this. Pace clocks have only a minute and a second hand, and are usually large enough to be seen one pool length away.

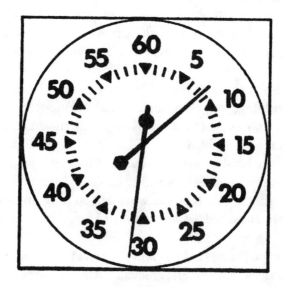

A pace clock.

Other timing devices that you can use are:

- Pool facility digital timing equipment
- Digital lap counters
- A wall clock with an easily visible second hand
- A waterproof wristwatch
- A stopwatch

SUPPLIER/MANUFACTURERS

~

Arena, N.A.
109 Inverness Drive East
Englewood, CO 80112
(303) 799-1856

Competitive Aquatic Supply
15131 Triton Lane
Suite 110
Huntington Beach, CA 92649
(714) 898-2655

The Finals
1466 Broadway
New York, NY 10036
(212) 302-1308
1-800-431-9111

Hind Corporate
3765 South Higuera
San Luis Obispo, CA 93401
1-800-235-4150
1-800-544-8555 in California

Jantzen, Inc.
P. O. Box 3001
Portland, OR 97208
1-800-626-0215

Kast-A-Way Swimwear
9356 Cincinnati/Columbus Road
Route 42
Cincinnati, OH 45241
1-800-543-2763

Metro Swim Shop
1221 Valley Road
Stirling, NJ 07980
(908) 647-8121
1-800-258-0272

Ocean Pool Company, Inc.
45 Mall Drive
Commack, NY 11725
(516) 543-1110
1-800-645-5316

Rothhammer-Sprint International,
   Inc.
P. O. Box 5579
Santa Maria, CA 93456
1-800-235-2156

Speedo® America
7911 Haskell Avenue
Van Nuys, CA 91410
(818) 376-0300

TYR Sport
P. O. Box 1930
Huntington Beach, CA 92649
(714) 897-0799

The Victor
2725 W. 81st Street
Hialeah, FL 33016
1-800-356-5132

World Wide Aquatics
10500 University Center Drive
Suite 250
Tampa, FL 33612
1-800-726-1530

SWIMMING MAGAZINES
～

Aquatics International Magazine
6151 Powers Ferry Road N.W.
Atlanta, GA 30339-2941
(404) 955-2500

Fitness Swimmer Magazine
12 East 26th Street
New York, NY 10010
(212) 683-3701
1-800-998-0735

Masters Sports
1633 Broadway
New York, NY 10019
(212) 767-5036

Swim Magazine
P. O. Box 91870
Pasadena, CA 91109-1870
(818) 304-7755

Swimming Technique
P. O. Box 91870
Pasadena, CA 91109
(818) 304-7755

The Swimming Times
P. O. Box 1132
Lowell, MA 01853
1-800-821-4776

Swimming World/Sports
   Publications
P. O. Box 91870
Pasadena, CA 91109
(818) 304-7755
1-800-538-9787

World Aquatic News and Travel
P. O. Box 70366
Pasadena, CA 91117
(818) 793-2582

ORGANIZATIONS

~

AAHPERD
American Alliance for Health,
    Physical Education, Recreation
    and Dance
1900 Association Drive
Reston, VA 22091,
(703) 476-3400

Amateur Athletic Union of the U.S.
3400 West 86th Street
Indianapolis, IN 46268
(317) 872-2900

American National Red Cross
    Health and Safety
431 18th Street N.W.
Washington, DC 20006
(202) 639-3542

American Swimming Coaches
    Association
c/o 1 Hall of Fame Drive
Fort Lauderdale, FL 33316
(305) 462-6536

Council for National Cooperation
    in Aquatics (CNCA)
P. O. Box 351743
Toledo, OH 43635
(419) 867-3326

F.I.N.A.
Fédération Internationale de
    Natation Amateur
425 Walnut Street
Suite 1610
Cincinnati, OH 45202
(513) 381-2793

International Swimming Hall of
    Fame World Headquarters
1 Hall of Fame Drive
Fort Lauderdale, FL 33316
(305) 462-6536

National Collegiate Athletic
    Association
6201 College Blvd.
Overland Park, KS 66211
(913) 339-1906

National Recreation and Park
    Association
Aquatics Section
650 West Higgins Road
Hoffman Estates, IL 60195
1-800-677-2236

National Safety Council, Aquatics
1121 Spring Lake Drive
Itusca, IL 60143
1-800-621-6244

National Spa and Pool Institute
2111 Eisenhower Avenue
Alexandria, VA 22314
(703) 838-0083

President's Council on Physical
    Fitness and Sports
701 Pennsylvania Avenue
Suite 250
Washington, DC 20004
(202) 272-3421

Special Olympics International—
  Aquatics
1350 New York Avenue N.W.
Suite 500
Washington, DC 20005
(202) 628-3630

Underwater Society of America
Fin Swimming
P. O. Box 628
Daly City, CA 94017
(415) 583-8492

U. S. Masters Swimming, Inc.
2 Peters Avenue
Rutland, MA 01549
(508) 886-6631

United States Swimming, Inc.
1750 Boulder Street
Colorado Springs, CO 80909
(719) 578-4578

United States Synchronized
  Swimming, Inc.
Pan Am Plaza
Suite 510
201 South Capitol Street
Indianapolis, IN 46225
(317) 237-5700

United States Water Polo, Inc.
Pan Am Plaza
Suite 520
201 South Capitol Street
Indianapolis, IN 46225
(317) 237-5599

YMCA of the U.S.A.
101 N. Wacker Drive
Chicago, IL 60606
(312) 977-0031
1-800-USA-YMCA

Young Women's Christian
  Association of the U.S.A.
726 Broadway
New York, NY 10003
(212) 614-2700

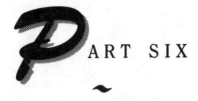

PART SIX

DR. J's Q's & A's

CHLORINE, SKIN, AND HAIR[1]

❧

Q: Why do they put those chemicals in the pool water?

A: In the first place, to keep the water clean, safe, and swimmable. Chlorine (slightly different from the kind found in laundry bleach) is one of the most effective chemicals found so far to sanitize water. It helps to kill the bacteria and algae, and may be introduced as a gas, liquid, or powder. Chlorine also "consumes" substances that would otherwise cloud the water: perspiration (did you realize that you sweat when you swim?), suntan and other lotions, deodorants, and so on. So it keeps the water clear, too.

Chemicals also serve to balance the pH level. If the water becomes either too alkaline or too acidic, it may cause eye, ear, and skin irritation, and it promotes the growth of bacteria. Sodium bicarbonate (soda ash) is added to raise pH level. Muriatic acid is used to lower pH.

Q: Isn't there some other way to keep the water clean and swimmable?

A: There are several nonchemical purification systems that substantially reduce the need for chemicals. One uses short-wave ultraviolet en-

---

[1]Consultants for this section:

- Stephen B. Kurtin, M.D., Assistant Clinical Professor of Dermatology, Mount Sinai School of Medicine (and Masters swimmer).
- Milton A. Gabrielson, Ph.D., editor of *Swimming Pools, A Guide to Their Planning, Design and Operation,* Council for National Cooperation in Aquatics Publication; Special Assistant to the President, Nova University, Fort Lauderdale, Florida.

ergy, which causes microorganisms literally to explode, and thus kills algae, bacteria, viruses, and other uninvited "swimmers." Another is ionization, in which ion-producing electrical currents kill bacteria and algae in the water return line; filters then remove the dead organisms. A third technique uses chlorine/chlorozone generators to manufacture chlorine in a form that doesn't alter the water texture and does away with the need for adding salts, acids, or chlorine. Finally, there are ozone generators that sterilize water by breaking down organic matter into carbon dioxide and water—at a rate about sixty times faster than chemical purification! These methods are currently being tried in hot tubs, spas, and pools; let's hope they catch on.

Q: Does chlorine penetrate the skin?

A: No, but you should at least rinse, and preferably wash it off with soap, after each swim.

Q: Why is it important to get rid of all the chlorine on my skin?

A: Because chlorine and salt water remove the oils that keep your natural moisture in. Paradoxically, prolonged immersion in water of any kind can actually dry your skin. So use a moisturizing soap when you shower off after a swim. Then, while your skin is still slightly damp, apply a moisturizing lotion; those containing urea or lactic acid are best. People with dry or "delicate" skin or eczema must be extra careful, because chlorine will worsen their condition, so it's especially important to apply a moisturizer if you fall into this category.

Q: Does that mean that chlorine will help people with oily skin?

A: Yes; chlorine will help clear up oily skin by removing excess oil. People with acne will tend to see an improvement, too. And swimmers are generally immune from "athlete's acne," caused when excess body heat and sweat increase oil production and clog the pores.

Q: Sometimes my skin gets itchy between swims. Why?

A: That's probably "swimmer's itch," which occurs especially in open water. It's an allergic reaction to a parasite (one of the schistosomes) that superficially penetrates the skin. Repeated exposure eventually results in an itching rash that lasts about three days. The best treatment is calamine lotion and antihistamines.

You may also experience temporary itchiness after a really strenuous swim. This frequently happens after hard exercise of any kind, and has nothing to do with swimming, chlorine, or water per se. When you're exercising, the blood vessels dilate from the extra blood flow, and when you stop, they constrict, sometimes causing "the blotchies."

Q: Are swimmers especially prone to athlete's foot or jock itch?

A: These are both fungus infections that are actually much less common among swimmers than other athletes. Funguses prefer warmth and moisture to grow. Since swimmers don't generate as much heat or perspire as much as dry-land athletes, infections of this type aren't much of a problem. Unless, of course, you don't dry off your feet and groin properly after your shower. Ears, too, can become infected with a fungus. Apply a small amount of rubbing alcohol to the affected areas with a cotton swab to hasten evaporation of excess water. It's also a good idea to sprinkle a little powder on the feet. Walking around the locker room and shower areas with shower clogs does absolutely no good, because funguses are all around you, all the time, just waiting for a chance to grow. (There is a one out of three chance that you have funguses between your toes right now.)

If you do develop either athlete's foot or jock itch, the over-the-counter preparations may get rid of them, but if you don't get quick results, see a doctor for some stronger medication to keep the fungus from spreading.

Q: Can I still get sunburned when I'm in the water?

A: Yes; few people realize that the sun's rays penetrate water. So if you're swimming outdoors, use a sunscreen or sunblock. For best results, apply it at least one hour before going outdoors, and reapply after you've come out of the water. Use an appropriate SPF. The higher the number, the greater the protection.

Q: Are there any special steps I should take to protect my hair?

A: Water, especially if it's chlorinated or salty, dries out hair just as it dries out your skin. After a swim, at least rinse out your hair to remove as much of the chlorine and other chemicals (or salt) as possible. Better still, wash it with a mild shampoo for dry or damaged hair. Lather only once; then apply creme rinse or conditioner to replenish the oils and to help untangle the hair. If you find your hair feeling dry, sticky, or dull, consider changing shampoos. Some are able to remove certain chemical deposits that others don't. There are specially formulated shampoos and conditioners for those who swim in chlorinated water.

To minimize the exposure to chemicals in the first place, and to keep hair from tangling more than it has to, wear a bathing cap—even if you have short hair. Though none are completely leakproof, caps do offer some protection. If you don't wear a cap, your hair is completely exposed to the pool chemicals, and it is whipped around in the water the way your clothes are in a washing machine. I've discovered that it's also a good idea to wear a Lycra cap under a latex or silicone one. The Lycra isn't waterproof, but it's a smooth, absorbent lining that acts as a buffer between my hair and my outer cap, which sometimes pulls and tangles the hair.

Q: Does my tinted (or permanented) hair require special care?

A: Chlorine enters the hair shaft, causing hair to swell and stretch more than normal. Hair that's already been chemically treated is more porous and delicate than "virgin" hair, so you may be more prone to breakage, split ends, and even discoloration. Make an extra effort to keep your hair dry (there are Velcro bathing caps available), and treat it very gently when wet—comb out tangles with a wide-toothed comb, starting at the ends and working your way up toward the scalp.

Q: Should I cut my hair if I'm swimming often?

A: Short hair does make sense for swimming. And since you'll be in the pool, and therefore shampooing, at least three times a week, choose a style—whether long or short or medium length—that doesn't need fussing to look good. Styles that you can just wash and let dry naturally are ideal. Keep blow-drying and electric curlers to a minimum, since they're time-consuming, space-consuming, and damaging to the hair. To cut down on shampooing and drying, try to schedule your swims on the days you'd normally wash your hair anyway (or vice versa).

EYES, EARS, NOSE, AND THROAT[2]

━

Q: My eyes get really bloodshot and my throat gets scratchy when I swim. Am I allergic to the chlorine?

A: It's very rare to be "allergic" to chlorine in the usual sense, but after repeated exposures, many people experience an "irritant reaction" which looks and feels like an allergic reaction with swelling, itching and sneezing, sniffling, and red eyes.

Sometimes a scratchy throat and coughing are caused by free chlorine particles in the air, especially in poorly ventilated indoor pools.

Q: Why do I see halos around lights after I've been swimming?

A: When your eyes are exposed to chemically treated and/or hypotonic water (containing less salt than the cornea), the cornea may swell up. This edema causes the light rays to bend as they pass through, which results in the halos around lights that sometimes plague swimmers. The eyes may also turn red, tear, and become overly sensitive to light and cigarette smoke. A nap, rinsing the eyes, and time, will alleviate this condition; goggles will prevent it.

Q: What causes the sensation of having something in my eye after I've been swimming?

A: That's another, but related, story. Exposure to chlorine can cause superficial punctate keratitis—the outer cells of the cornea actually fall off, leaving a nerve exposed and giving you the feeling that you have something in your eye. It takes a day or two for this condition to heal—that's how long it takes your body to replace the lost cells. Again, wearing goggles is the best way to prevent this condition.

---

[2]Consultants for this section:

- David H. Abramson, M.D., Attending Surgeon at Manhattan Eye and Ear Hospital (former international competitive swimmer).
- Milton Costello, B.M.E., Licensed Professional Engineer, Wantagh, New York.
- Bruce M. Hyman, M.D., Director of Adult Out-Patient Eye Clinic, Roosevelt Hospital, New York.
- John S. Rodman, M.D., Attending Physician at Lenox Hill Hospital in New York (and Masters swimmer).

Q: Can I get an eye infection from swimming?

A: Not if you're swimming in a pool that's adequately chlorinated. The current standard of at least 2.0 parts per million of free available chlorine is sufficient to kill all bacteria and most viruses.

Fresh-water swimming holes such as quarries and lakes, as well as underchlorinated pools, can harbor harmful bacteria and viruses, however. You can protect yourself from them by wearing goggles—but not someone else's goggles, since the infection may spread this way. Consult a physician if you have any eye condition that persists.

Q: Can I wear my contact lenses when I swim?

A: Yes, but most recent experiments by the Centers for Disease Control show soft contact lens wearers face certain risks. Although contact lenses can protect your eyes from chlorine, wearing soft lenses while swimming is associated with eye infections; in addition, you run a 4–15 percent chance of losing the lenses. Other studies recommend you use goggles whether or not you wear contact lenses to protect your eyes from microorganisms and bacteria normally found in pools and natural bodies of water. And if you do wear contacts during swimming, you should remove them and disinfect them after twenty to thirty minutes to minimize the risk of problems.

If you wear contacts, you might want to discuss with your optometrist the possibility of having prescription goggles made. You can also purchase goggles "ready made" in a variety of diopter powers.

Q: I seem to get a lot of water in my ears. Is this harmful? What's "swimmer's ear"?

A: Getting water in your ears is annoying and can lead to "swimmer's ear." When you swim, water sometimes travels up the Eustachian tube, the connecting tube that stretches from behind the nose to behind the eardrum. If you have an infection in your nasal passages, therefore, the water can transfer the inflammation to your middle ear; this is known as "swimmer's ear." This problem is pretty unusual, though, and it may occur in scuba divers because of the changes in pressure that they're subjected to. And it's more common in children than in adults, because adults have a little kink in the Eustachian tube that tends to catch the water. If you do develop a persistent pain in your ear, see a doctor; you may have developed a middle-ear infection that requires professional attention.

Q: How can I prevent water from getting in my ears? Once it's in, how can I get it out?

A: Wearing earplugs made of rubber, plastic, or wax may protect your ears. The main concern with these is that, if water does get trapped behind the plug, it could be worse than having water flowing in and out of your outer ear. A bathing cap pulled over your ears may be sufficient protection. Another method is to use lamb's wool.

Wrap a small wad of lamb's wool (sold in foot-care departments) around your index finger; coat it with a little petroleum jelly and insert it into the ear canal. This takes a bit of practice, so experiment a few times until you find just the right amount and depth. I apply it every time I swim and haven't had "swimmer's ear" since I have used it. It helps to keep water out and forms just enough of a soft, absorbent barrier to make sure that ear problems stay away.

To get water out of your ears, dry them with a hair dryer or *gently* use cotton swabs. Also, there are fast-drying, antibacterial eardrops available, made especially to prevent "swimmer's ear."

Q: Do swimmers get more colds than other people?

A: Swimming, of itself, doesn't increase your chances of upper respiratory infections. Not dressing sensibly, however, can cause problems. In cold weather, it's just not smart to walk outside without a hat or scarf after swimming, since 30 to 40 percent of your body heat escapes from your head.

Q: Sometimes I feel as though I can't catch my breath. What's happening?

A: It may be a result of breathing too fast too deeply. This is called hyperventilating, or perhaps you're not giving yourself enough rest.

Q: Can I swim with a cold?

A: Time-honored tradition takes swimmers out of the water when they have colds. But I've never heard any really convincing argument as to why people should avoid swimming when they have a mild upper respiratory infection. It's true that vigorous exercise does cut down your body's ability to fight infection, and that chlorine does irritate respiratory passages a little. But a mild cold, the tail end of one, or a chronic runny nose (which can happen in winter even when no infection is present) doesn't mean you have to stay out of the water. It depends on how you feel.

However, it's a different story if you have a fever, in which case you should absolutely stay away from the pool. If you have a bad cough you shouldn't swim either—not only for your own sake, but to avoid spreading disease. And don't fool around with bad respiratory problems; see a doctor if you're really sick.

Q: I have a sinus condition—should I wear nose clips?

A: In case of a full-blown sinusitis, when there's pain below the eyes, especially when you press on the area, tremendous pressure in the sinus cavity, and a foul taste in the mouth, you shouldn't go in the water; consult a physician.

However, nose clips are a matter of personal preference. Some people are never bothered by water getting up their noses, while others seem to get an inordinate amount of it. If you're one of those people, it's reasonable to consider using nose clips. But even then they shouldn't be used routinely—they can be annoying and uncomfortable in themselves, and they become one more thing that you have to concern yourself with. In any event, there are several styles, shapes, and sizes available to fit most noses. But nose clips should still be worn only by those who are prone to sinus infection.

Q: Why does it burn when water gets up my nose?

A: The stinging is caused when the chlorinated water penetrates the sinus cavities, irritating the delicate membranes that enclose them.

ACHES AND PAINS[3]

~

Q: What kinds of injuries do swimmers have to watch out for?

A: Very few; swimming is a relatively safe sport, perhaps the safest of all. (In fact, sports medicine specialists often recommend swimming or some other form of hydrotherapy to their patients who have injured themselves during some other activity.) The water's buoyancy makes swimming easy on the joints and muscles, unlike dry-land sports such as running and even bike riding. Injuries are usually a matter of overuse—subjecting the body to something for which it is not adequately prepared, either because the warm-up was inadequate or because the body isn't strong or limber enough to do as much as it's being asked to. In addition to simple muscle soreness, overzealous swimmers may sometimes suffer from "swimmer's shoulder," which is caused by too much freestyle, backstroke, or butterfly; knee problems, which can affect the breaststroker; and low back pain from doing too much butterfly, or kicking too much with a kickboard.

Q: Why do I sometimes feel stiff and sore after swimming?

A: A little bit of muscle soreness is a way of life for those of us who exercise in order to improve our level of fitness. Theoretically, someone who's on a carefully designed *maintenance* program shouldn't get sore. But for most of us, slight soreness is actually desirable, because it means you've been working hard enough to cause a change in your body, which, eventually, means an improved physical condition. Although it's really difficult to cause a sprain or strain while swimming, you should always *listen to your body*. If it hurts while you're swimming, don't push yourself. Simple muscle soreness is caused when waste products such as lactic acid build up in the muscles, and is usually evident the next day.

---

[3]Consultants for this section:

- Burton Berson, M.D., Chief of the Sports Medicine Clinic, New York; Assistant Clinical Professor of Orthopedic Surgery at Mount Sinai Hospital, New York.
- Willibald Nagler, M.D., F.A.C.P., Psychiatrist-in-Chief, Department of Rehabilitation Medicine at New York Hospital–Cornell Medical Center.
- Max M. Novick, M.D., Clinical Professor of Surgery, Director of Sports Medicine CMDNJ–New Jersey Medical School, Perth Amboy, New Jersey.
- Patrick O'Leary, M.D., Attending Orthopedic Surgeon, Lenox Hill Hospital, New York.
- John L. Xethalis, M.D., Attending Orthopedic Surgeon, Lenox Hill Hospital, New York.
- Lenore R. Zohman, M.D., Director of Montefiore Hospital Exercise Laboratory and Cardiology Program, The Bronx, New York.

Q: What can I do to prevent or ease achy muscles?

A: To reduce simple muscle soreness, begin your exercise program slowly and progress gradually. Try not to be that weekend athlete who exercises furiously on Saturday and Sunday, then limps to work on Monday. Exercise regularly so that your muscles stay in shape. For best results, swim every other day so your body has a chance to recover. Remember to warm up and cool down to ease your muscles from a state of rest to one of activity, then back to relative inactivity. There is no medical treatment for muscle soreness; liniments containing oil of wintergreen may ease the pain but do not promote healing. Relaxed, easy swimming is the ideal therapy for mild soreness. If the pain is severe, apply ice for the first day, then switch to heat. If discomfort persists, see a doctor; the problem may be a real injury that requires professional help.

Q: Will taking a sauna or steambath help soreness?

A: These dilate the blood vessels so that more blood flows to the muscles, which helps to carry away the excess lactic acid. Whirlpools, saunas, and steambaths therefore can be helpful. But they're not the real answer—stretching and a proper warm-up and cool-down are. (Saunas, etc., are not recommended instead of a warm-up just before you go into the water because of the extreme change in temperature.)

Q: Will a massage help my aching muscles?

A: Yes. A good massage will not only ease already sore muscles but will help prevent soreness from occurring. Massage can release muscle tension and help to remove the accumulated toxins that cause muscle fatigue. Massage also improves your circulation in general and so helps to calm your nerves, aid digestion, and leave you with a feeling of well-being.

Q: What about pains in my joints?

A: These are very few and far between among swimmers, and usually occur only when you are swimming great distances, as competitive swimmers do. But they can affect any one of us when overenthusiasm induces us to do "too much too soon." Even those who know better occasionally overdo it, as one intermediate swimmer can testify: "There I was, on my first winter vacation since I'd taken up swimming for fitness. I had access to a beautiful 50-meter outdoor pool, and, boy, did I take advantage of that. I saw it as a golden opportunity to increase my distance—and I did: from 500 meters to 2,500 meters in four days! I was in pretty good shape generally, from calisthenics, dancing, and jogging, so my muscles didn't hurt much; they just felt nice and tight. But after my fourth day, my left shoulder began to hurt. I figured it was just a sore deltoid—I'd switched breathing sides and my left arm was getting more than its accustomed workout. But the next day, I heard a clicking sound when I did the freestyle and figured something more serious was up."

She was right. She had the beginnings of tendinitis—an inflammation of the connective tissue. The constant repetition of the arm motions was just too much for her shoulder to bear at this point in her development.

Q: How do I prevent or treat tendinitis?

A: To prevent tendinitis, increase your workload gradually by following my step-by-step programs. Not only will that keep you from overdoing it, it will make sure that your technique is correct—another possible cause of injury and discomfort. And always warm up thoroughly before every workout, and cool down properly afterward. Between workouts, do some resistance exercises to build up muscle strength. If you're a "weekend athlete," don't overestimate your ability; you may regret it on Monday morning.

If you do develop joint problems, avoid the motion that caused it until the problem clears up (usually less than a week): Avoid resistive devices or kickboard use if your knees or shoulders are sore. Try other strokes such as sculling, the breaststroke, maybe the backstroke, or treading. If your knees or ankles are sore, do more arm-stroke drills.

Once the tendinitis is under control, you should modify your stroke (i.e., don't swing your arms quite so high, or do a modified whip kick) to prevent a recurrence. If possible, have your stroke techniques critiqued to identify movements that may be causing the condition.

Try alternate breathing during the crawl, too; the arm opposite your breathing side sometimes pulls deeper and harder than the other, so tendinitis usually occurs, if at all, there. Alternate breathing not only helps to balance your stroke, it creates an even load on both arms.

Unless the pain is severe, usually a little sensible attention, some heat, and perhaps an anti-inflammatory drug such as aspirin are the best treatment—try them before you consult an orthopedist.

Q: Why is water so good for therapy?

A: For many reasons:

- It reduces the effects of gravity, so that there's less strain on the joints. The water's buoyancy supports and cushions the entire body.
- At the same time, the water's resistance helps build muscle strength and tone—but gently, because the same resistance precludes fast, jerky movements that could lead to injury.
- The water also relaxes muscles, especially if it's 80 degrees F. or above. (Muscles aren't tense while they're working.) This also extends your range of motion, thereby helping to keep your body limber.
- Water stimulates the circulation, increasing the flow of oxygen and energy to the muscles.

So it's no wonder that therapists prescribe gentle swimming and special hydrotherapy exercises for patients who have been injured or who suffer from chronic joint problems (such as post-fracture patients and victims of arthritis).

Q: Can water exercise help my back problem?

A: Yes, except in the case of severe neck injuries. In particular, the elementary backstroke is easy on your back.

Q: Can water exercise help my shoulder and knee pain?

A: Do gentle water exercises that will increase the range of motion of these joints; progressive exercise to build up the surrounding muscles gradually will help take the strain off the joints. A gentle breaststroke (for shoulder problems) and crawl stroke (for knee problems) will help loosen up the affected areas.

Q: The common cramp—what is it, what causes it, how do I deal with it?

A: A cramp, an abrupt, powerful contraction of the muscle fibers, may be caused by fatigue, overexertion, cold, or lack of warm-up. Most commonly, it occurs in the leg, particularly in the calf muscle.

Treatment of the cramp is aimed at releasing the contraction. This is often best accomplished by alternately flexing and extending the affected area, and by kneading with the thumbs.

ESPECIALLY FOR WOMEN[4]

◆

Q: Can I swim while I'm menstruating?

A: It's up to you. But thanks to the tampon, you can swim at any time of the month.

Most of the available research indicates that menstruation itself is no reason to stop swimming (or any other exercise). During your period, mild exercise is usually at least as effective (and healthier overall) as crawling into bed with a hot water bottle and a snifter of brandy.

Some women do say that their performance is affected while they're menstruating. In several surveys, about half of the women said they didn't notice any difference; of the rest, about half said they performed worse—but the other half said they performed better! Some of this may be psychological, some may be due to very real fluctuations in the blood pressure and resting pulse rate. And if you take medication for your discomfort, that may affect your performance, too.

Q: Will exercise affect my periods?

A: Yes—for the better. In general, women who exercise regularly suffer fewer of the discomforts associated with menstruation: fewer headaches, less tension, and fewer and less severe cramps and lower back pains. And studies have shown that exercising five days prior to the onset of your period can even curb premenstrual tension and depression by letting you sweat away extra water and sodium. And since swimming is a natural diuretic, it helps to combat the common problem of water retention, which in turn helps banish "bloat" and the myriad of discomforts it's responsible for.

Occasionally, competitive athletes experience dysmenorrhea (painful periods) or amenorrhea (cessation of periods). No one is quite sure why this happens, but it may be that their lowered percentage of body fat

---

[4]Consultants for this section:

- Donald M. Pearlman, M.D., Associate Professor of Surgery, Albert Einstein College of Medicine.
- Patricia Berland and Cindy Kurtin, who swam through their pregnancies.

affects the production of hormones. In any event, this effect does not last once the training regimen is lightened. And lest you think that this is the perfect form of birth control—this phenomenon is evident only among the highest level of competitive athletes.

Q: Can I swim if I'm pregnant?

A: Unless there are special circumstances, there's absolutely nothing wrong with swimming while you're pregnant. As a matter of fact, exercise assists the circulation, which helps the growth of the fetus, and it tones the muscles, which helps the mother during labor and delivery.

During the middle and later stages of a pregnancy, dry-land exercises may prove uncomfortable and even dangerous. Even if you're been exercising all along, you might fall and/or jar the internal organs. But water's buoyancy, along with its natural cushioning properties (remember, nature chose water to surround and protect the developing baby), makes swimming the safest and most comfortable exercise for those who are exercising "for two." In fact, you may feel even better in the water than on land because of water's gravity-defying properties. All these reasons are why obstetricians often recommend that you swim your way through pregnancy.

Many pregnant women who were fitness swimmers have swum through their pregnancies. They have mentioned that, even though they might feel tired when they begin, they finish their swim with a sense of well-being and relaxation. However, they've pointed out that they usually depend more on their arm strength than on their legs, so as not to put any unnecessary strain on the uterus. Swimming also helped them to keep their weight in check and eased their deliveries.

Q: But surely I shouldn't be doing fifty yards of the butterfly in my eighth month?

A: True, the nature of your workouts will change as your body does; when you're pregnant, you should never swim so hard or so long that you feel uncomfortable. (Be sure to check with your obstetrician before beginning any exercise program.) In general, you should gradually begin to swim more slowly as your pregnancy progresses. Do fewer and/or longer intervals if your workouts usually include them. Concentrate on long, slow, easy swims. Your stroke mechanics will change slightly because you'll become more buoyant, but chances are that your crawl, backstroke, and breaststroke will remain relatively intact. The butterfly, flip turns, and dives, on the other hand, may have to be eliminated. Do more and more water exercises during a workout, too. Swim as late into the pregnancy as your doctor will allow, and resume swimming afterward to regain your figure.

Q: Can I swim if I have a vaginal or bladder infection?

A: Mild cases of vaginitis or cystitis are no reason to stop swimming. The water won't enter the urethra; and the small amount that may enter the vagina is negligible. However, if your condition is serious enough to warrant medical attention, follow your doctor's advice. In the case of a yeast infection, which is affected by excess moisture, your physician will probably recommend that you stay out of the pool.

Q: How can I prevent yeast infections?

A: Wear a dry suit whenever possible (e.g., in between events at swim meets). When changing, be certain to dry yourself thoroughly with a fresh towel, paper towels, or a blow dryer. Also, your diet plays an important part in preventing these infections.

NUTRITION, DIET, WEIGHT LOSS
☙

Q: Do I have to follow a special diet to be on a fitness program?

A: Not really, except that it is extra important that you get the right amounts of all the nutrients your body needs. It's a myth that athletes need more protein than sedentary people; the average 150-pound person, whatever his or her level of activity, needs about 50 grams a day, and some authorities maintain that even that's an overestimate. Although muscles are composed of protein, extra protein alone doesn't increase your muscle mass.

Q: So what's a balanced diet?

A: That's still a pretty controversial subject as far as vitamins and minerals go. However, it is clear that, in terms of protein, carbohydrates, and fats, a balanced diet is definitely not the typical American fare, which is far too high in refined carbohydrates, fat, and salt, and often unnecessarily high in protein. According to the United States Senate Nutrition

Committee's report, "Dietary Goals for the United States," the typical American should adopt a diet that, compared to his present one, is:

- lower in calories
- lower in salt
- lower in refined carbohydrates (ideally, approximately 15 percent of total calories)
- lower in fats of all kinds (no more than 30 percent of all calories and some authorities recommend even less fat)
- higher in complex carbohydrates such as fresh fruits and vegetables and whole grains (ideally 55–60 percent of total calories)

It's best to eat a wide variety of wholesome foods, including plenty of fresh fruits and vegetables; lots of whole grains and beans; and some low-fat dairy and meat products such as skim milk, fish, poultry, and beef (if you eat meat). The more active you become, the more calories you'll need to maintain your weight and supply your body with nutrients and energy. There's a bonus to this kind of eating pattern, too; studies suggest that low-fat, high-fiber diets help keep you healthier by reducing the risk of many diseases, including heart disease, diabetes, and cancer.

Q: Do active people need more vitamins and minerals than other people? Should I take supplements?

A: The evidence is not completely clear on this controversial subject; however, some studies indicate physical exertion does require higher levels of certain nutrients, and that certain nutrients can improve your physical performance. In addition, many published reports show that, even in affluent and presumably well-fed societies such as ours, some people are highly deficient in certain nutrients. For example, one of the most common deficiencies in Americans is that of iron—particularly in women of childbearing age. The fact that a woman loses two to four ounces of blood every month means that many women don't have enough iron in their systems to produce hemoglobin, which is what carries oxygen to the body's muscles. Since women store less iron in their bodies than men do, and have a lower hemoglobin count to begin with, they may have a problem with utilizing oxygen properly. Because a muscle needs adequate oxygen to perform, an active woman may need to supplement her iron intake.

A lack of potassium has been indicated as a cause of muscle cramps—

something that an avid exerciser should watch out for. Since strenuous exercise causes you to excrete potassium to help your body dissipate the additional heat generated, it's wise to replace this mineral by eating fruits and vegetables. Magnesium is another mineral the level of which plummets during heavy exercise; good sources are dark bread, nuts, and vegetables. So, as insurance, many athletes and active people take vitamin and mineral supplements. But remember, these are supplements to—not substitutes for—healthful foods.

Q: What's a good reducing diet?

A: Swimming (or any other strenuous, regular exercise) will help cure "spoon-in-mouth disease," even if you maintain your present caloric intake. If you swam enough to burn up about 500 calories every day, you'd lose one pound per week. However, since most fitness swimmers don't swim that long or that hard, they also need to modify their diet in order to lose weight at a reasonable rate.

Diet plans come and go, but crash diets and fad diets simply won't work over the long haul. You can't stay on them forever because they are either too boring, too extreme, or too impractical. Diet plans that help you take off weight and keep it off are ones that are designed to change your eating habits for a lifetime. They'll also reduce the risk of vitamin and mineral deficiencies. According to nutritionist Shari Lieberman in *The Real Vitamin and Mineral Book* (Avery Publishing Group, Inc., 1990), researchers found that none of the eleven best-selling diet books supplied a full 100 percent of the Recommended Dietary Allowances (RDAs) for thirteen vitamins and minerals.

There are many appropriate and healthful weight-reducing options now available. Since weight-reducing requirements, goals, and motivation vary among individuals, you might find it helpful to get an overview of the various weight-loss programs. Two books that might aid you are *Diets That Work* by D. Scanlon, R.D. (Contemporary Books, 1992), and *Straight Talk About Weight Control* (Consumers Union, Mount Vernon, New York, 1991).

But whatever your diet, be sure that it's properly balanced. If you cut down too much on protein, for example, your body actually begins to consume the protein of which your muscles are made. And active people actually need plenty of complex carbohydrates, for energy and for the B vitamins that your body needs to convert food into energy. Fats and junk foods you can do away with—your body requires only one to two ounces of fat per day, and you'll probably get at least that much from other foods.

Q: How can swimming help me to lose (or keep from gaining) weight?

A: In many ways. That's why I say to people: "You like to eat? You'd better swim!" I love to eat. Most babies' first words are something like "Mama" or "Dada"; mine was "cheesecake!"

If you think lying around all day drinking diet sodas and nibbling on plain lettuce sprinkled with lemon juice will do the trick . . . think again. Exercise is the magic ingredient in the recipe for successful dieting.

- It's physically impossible to eat while swimming (I know—I've tried!). So nip a potential binge in the bud: slip on a swim suit and get thee to a pool.

- Strenuous exercise actually helps to curb your appetite. Experiments have shown that, although *moderate* exercise may increase your desire for food, *vigorous* activities such as running, jumping rope, or swimming (which also burn the most calories) have just the opposite effect. In other words, the last thing you'll feel like doing after a two-mile swim is stuffing yourself.

- Exercise raises your metabolism (the rate at which you burn calories), not only during the activity itself, but for long afterward. So hours after you're out of the pool, you're still reaping the rewards.

- It seems a paradox, but exercise actually gives you more energy, so you may not feel as tempted to gobble a candy bar as a "pick-me-up." By the same token, once you've reached a certain level of fitness, you'll notice that empty-calorie junk foods clog up your finely tuned system.

- Exercise relaxes you, and so cuts down on the compulsive eating that results from nervous tension. Next time you "need" a slice of pie, take a brisk swim instead.

So do what I do—leave those pounds in the pool.

Q: How many calories will I burn if I exercise in the water?

A: Although the oxygen consumption level of the muscles most accurately determines the calorie burn, your heart rate is more easily used as a reference for your workout intensity. Recent research has been done with water exercise which indicates that the number of calories burned during water walking increases with the depth of the water. Walking 3 miles per hour can burn up to 500 calories in thigh-high water. A half hour of deep-water running burns about 300 calories, compared with about 200 to 250 for running, 150 for playing tennis, and 150 to 200 for aerobics. For a 150-pound person, swimming at his target heart rate (THR) burns approximately 10–15 calories a minute; this is approximately 600 calories per hour.

There is some evidence that swimming is not as effective as dry-land exercise for losing *body fat,* if you're already fat. This may be because swimming is basically an arm exercise; you need to use big muscles in the legs and buttocks to burn fat. And if you are doing water aerobics, the body weighs much less in water than on land, so the leg muscles don't have to work as hard as on dry land. In addition, exercising in water also helps keep muscles cool. The more the muscles heat up, the harder the heart beats to pump blood through the body to carry the heat away; if the water already is doing this job, the heart rate doesn't need to rise as much.

The bottom line is: are Olympic swimmers fat? No! Not in my book!

SWIMMING FASTER AND FARTHER[5]

～

Q: What are the key elements of my workout?

A: To get the most out of your workout, whether you swim for fitness or competition, you should focus on the following:

- *Safety Considerations*
  Including how you feel throughout your workout.

- *Environmental Considerations*
  An awareness of other swimmers, as well as potential dangers including equipment usage.

- *Pacing Your Workout*
  Recognizing your energy output and speed as you progress through your workout.

- *Stroke Technique*
  Awareness of your body position, your arm and leg motions when swimming, as well as when practicing drills.

---

[5]Consultants for this section:
- Paul Katz, La Salle swim coach and former All-American butterfly champion from Yale University, New Haven, Connecticut.
- Herbert Erlanger, M.D., Associate Clinical Professor of Anesthesiology, Cornell Medical Center, New York Hospital, New York.

- *Keeping Track of Your Workout*
  With respect to number of repetitions and/or laps.

- And above all—remember to *breathe* rhythmically and continuously.

- And enjoy your workout!

Q: What should I do when I feel discouraged about my swimming progress?

A: You need a pep talk—what coaches usually hand out to raise their teams' spirits and to help them over the rough spots. Everyone—fitness and competitive swimmer alike—needs a little boost now and then. Remember that your swimming is a long-range project. It requires dedication and self-discipline; depending on how far you want to go with it, you may find it taking up considerable chunks of your time and energy. Stick with it during the plateaus, when you seemingly are making little progress. Remember, good swimmers aren't born; they're made. Hang in there!

Q: Why do men generally outperform women in sports?

A: In head-to-head competition, the best man in a particular sport will virtually always beat the best woman. Generally, men are stronger than women are. They have larger bones and muscles; their hearts and lungs are 10 percent larger, and they have higher levels of oxygen-bearing hemoglobin. This seems to be brought about by the male hormone testosterone since, until puberty, male and female capacities don't differ that much. But strength isn't the final word in athletic endeavors—skill and endurance account for a lot—especially in swimming.

Consider this: the differences between men's and women's times in all sports are rapidly shrinking. Women today are breaking records set by men during the 1960s, and many male Olympic champs of only a few games ago wouldn't even qualify for women's Olympic teams these days. The difference in swimming (and track) times is diminishing so fast that one scientist, K. F. Dyer, an Australian, has gone so far as to say that they will vanish completely, at least in the long-distance events, quite soon. The theoretical explanation of why women give men a run for their money in longer-distance swimming is twofold. For one thing, women are more buoyant than men; for another, women's bodies have more energy reserves (in the form of fat), which they are able to tap more efficiently. And although women's narrower shoulders sacrifice some upper body strength, they make up for it by allowing a more resistance-free passage through the water.

Some older people recognize that women weren't given the chance to train and compete the way men were. Title IX of the Education Amendments, passed in 1972, which provides that "no person in the United States shall, on the basis of sex, be excluded from participation . . . in any education program or activity receiving Federal financial assistance," began to turn things around. But as anyone familiar with either the civil rights movement or the women's movement must be aware, it's a long hard battle toward equal opportunity.

Q: Why are some people better at sprinting and others at swimming long distances?

A: Partly because of training, and partly because of heredity. Every muscle is made up of two types of fibers. Red fibers, also known as slow-twitch fibers, give you endurance. White, or fast-twitch, fibers are for speed and strength. Everyone has a different ratio of red to white fibers, which is fixed at birth. You can, however, develop whatever you have. That's why it's best for persons with a higher percentage of red fibers to swim long distances; and for persons with more white fibers to train for short distances. (Unfortunately, the only way you can tell to which group you belong, short of a muscle biopsy, is trial and error.)

Q: How can I develop my white fibers so that I swim faster?

A: First of all, you should swim against the clock. Interval training makes you aware of how long it takes you to swim a specific distance. (It also gives you an incentive to swim faster, since the quicker you go the more rest you get.) Once you've developed this internal clock, you have to train harder and/or develop a more efficient technique in order to reduce your times. Ultimately, your body will figure out its own little tricks (in addition to the tips in this book) to speed you through the water. You will reach a point where your mind and body will work together to find the best way for *you* to swim.

A coach or a more advanced swimmer can accelerate this process by conveying to the developing swimmer those little nuances that improve performance. This is truer of swimming than of many other sports in which, if you don't "have it" naturally, there's very little that you can do about it. In swimming, there's plenty of room for those who aren't "naturals" to apply techniques as effectively as those who are considered natural talents. As with anything else, it takes time to learn these subtleties, and many swimmers go through a long period of trial and error. Hopefully, this book will reduce that time as much as possible.

Q: What causes the muscles to feel tight after a hard swim?

A: This tight feeling is caused by lactic acid, a by-product of the chemical reaction that occurs in the muscles. The muscle cells are converting food fuel into energy, using oxygen. Lactic acid builds up when the cells don't get enough oxygen. As you swim regularly over time, your body learns to use oxygen more efficiently. So, the better condition you're in and the longer it takes you to go into oxygen debt, the longer you can function in that state and the faster you'll recover from it. Also, learning how to pace yourself evenly can help reduce the buildup of lactic acid in the beginning of your swim.

Q: Why do my legs get tight and tired quickly when I'm swimming fast?

A: During a workout, a timed swim, or a race, many swimmers have a tendency to overkick. When this happens, the large muscles in your legs, particularly the quadriceps along the front of the thigh, use up tremendous amounts of oxygen even though they push more water up and down than backward, they don't add that much to your forward propulsion. As a result, you tire quickly. Since kicking also works your abdominal and chest muscles, and your diaphragm, overkicking may also throw off your rhythmic breathing pattern. To avoid oxygen debt during sprints or fast swims, try to establish a kicking pattern that's proportionate to the rest of the stroke. Once you've worn yourself out by overkicking, it's difficult to resume comfortable breathing and get a second wind, because you have to "repay" your oxygen debt. (See page 117 for the relative power of the pull and the kick in the various strokes.)

Q: My arms, shoulders, and the muscles along my upper body get sore after a long swim. What should I do?

A: Distance swimmers especially rely on their upper bodies to supply most of the forward propulsion. So during a long swim, such as 1,500 meters (metric mile), or a 2-mile "marathon," the muscles you mention get a tremendous workout. The best way to prevent them from tightening up, especially after a race, is to take a slow, easy cool-down swim (or "swim down"). Then stretch the upper body for a few minutes (see "Swimmers' Shape-ups," page 371); repeat the stretch several times during the first half hour afterward, if possible.

Q: Where and when did the competitive swimming begin?

A: Although swimming wasn't part of the ancient Olympics, it was enjoyed by the Greeks and other early civilizations. Young men swam in ancient Greece and Rome as part of their military training. The first recorded swimming competitions were held in Japan in 36 B.C.

Modern competitive swimming began in the mid-nineteenth century. Shortly thereafter, what later came to be known as the Amateur Swimming Association was formed and established rules for competition. In 1908, FINA (Fédération Internationale de Natation Amateur), the world governing body for swimming and other aquatic competition, was founded. When the first modern Olympiad was held in Greece in 1896, there were three men's freestyle events, which were swum in the ocean. It wasn't until the games held in Stockholm in 1912 that swimming events for women were included. Now, swimming is a major part of the summer games.

Q: Does shaving down (shaving the arms, legs, and chest) before a race actually increase a swimmer's speed?

A: This can help—psychologically as well as physically. Shaving, which you usually save for your biggest meet of the season, can be an important part of the psych-up that you do for the big event. It makes your body feel lighter, more slippery; you feel as though you're getting more out of your kick, riding higher in the water, and slicing through it cleanly and smoothly.

Q: What and when should I eat before a competition?

A: It's best to eat a relatively light, easily digestible meal about three to four hours before the event. Some favorites are tuna sandwiches, lean meat or poultry, milk, or fruit. Foods high in fat should be avoided because they take a long time to digest and may therefore cause discomfort. Highly refined carbohydrates, such as candy bars, should be avoided, since they stimulate the production of insulin, which eventually lowers your blood sugar and results in a let-you-down instead of a pick-me-up.

Q: What's carbohydrate loading?

A: Muscles get their energy from glycose, which the body manufactures from carbohydrates. However, since the body has a limited capacity to store this sugar, athletes often load up on carbohydrates—especially pasta, potatoes, and bread—before an event in order to make sure that their glycogen stores are filled to capacity. However, for swimming a workout or even a meet (unless it's a marathon swim), carbohydrate loading is not really needed, since, in this case, the demand on your glycose reserves is not that severe.

Q: What is Masters swimming?

A: Masters swimming is a nationwide competitive swimming program. It began when Dr. Ransom Arthur, of the Navy Medical Neuropsychiatric Research Unit in San Diego, became inspired by the Amateur Athletic Union's Masters track and field program and joined forces with John Spannuth, then president of the American Swimming Coaches Association. The Navy supported the idea of establishing a regular swimming program for adults, and the first Masters swim meet was held in May 1970. From that humble beginning (there were only fifty participants), the program grew: as of this writing, there are approximately thirty thousand Masters swimmers, and their ranks are ever expanding, due in part to the continuing interest and sponsorship for promoting adult fitness Masters activities by the U. S. Masters Swimming, Inc.

Q: What are the goals of the Masters Swimming Program? What benefits will I derive if I join?

A: The program's primary purpose is to promote physical fitness via training and competitive swimming. The competition is relatively low-key and is held in five-year age groups (from twenty-five to twenty-nine, to ninety and over) so that you're competing against swimmers who are approximately the same age you are. By setting goals toward which older participants can work, the program provides motivation for continuing a training regimen despite inconveniences and time pressures. Competition is a useful way of measuring your progress, and it's exciting. A fringe benefit is to foster fellowship and camaraderie among the participants. If there are no Masters clubs near you, help to start one. (I did.)

Q: Where can I find more information about Masters swimming?

A: Ask for information from either your local Masters swimming club or contact U. S. Masters Swimming, Inc.

U. S. Masters Swimming, Inc.
2 Peters Avenue
Rutland, MA 01549
Tel: (508) 886-6631
FAX: (508) 886-6265

Q: What are the Senior Olympics?

A: In addition to Masters swimming, there are also competitions locally, regionally, nationally, and internationally that encompass senior age groups, including the United States Senior Sports Classic. There are competitions for men and women aged fifty-five and over in a variety of individual and team sports including swimming. For further information, write to:

U.S.N.S.O. (United States National Senior Olympics)
14323 South Outer Forty Road
Suite N300
Chesterfield, MO 63017

Q: What about swim camps?

A: Aside from attending regular organized workouts, you can go to camp. There are many swim camps around the country, open to swimmers of all ages and abilities, where you can spend five to seven hours a day in the water, learning from coaches, trainers, and other swimmers. Activities include videotapes of your technique, with various films and lectures, to learn about conditioning, stretching, dry-land exercises, and nutrition for swimmers. Length of camp, cost, and amenities will vary. Novice fitness swimmers and Masters swimmers can benefit greatly from attending a swim camp.

To find swim camps, browse through the swim magazines listed on page 332. Check them also for the local swim clinics that are held near you throughout the country.

ODDS AND ENDS

～

Q: I'm a runner who is considering beginning a swimming program; how does swimming compare with running?

A: Both are excellent aerobic exercises. If you compared a champion runner with a champion swimmer, the runner would go one mile in about four minutes; the swimmer would cover a mile in about four times as long, or sixteen minutes. The training effect follows the same ratio: the benefits of swimming a half mile are comparable to those of running two miles. (Of course, skill is a mitigating factor—if you're a good runner but an inefficient swimmer, for instance, swimming a half mile may be harder for you than running even four miles.)

If you've been running for fitness and switch over to swimming, you'll notice that there are fewer injuries and pains—no shin splints, no foot problems such as blisters, and a far lower incidence of joint problems— because there's no pounding the pavement. When you swim, there's less danger of overheating while you exercise, too, since the water acts as a natural coolant for your body.

Since swimming uses the arms and upper body more than the legs, you may want to balance your program with some dry-land exercises. I think jogging, walking briskly, jumping rope, bicycle riding, skating, skiing, and dancing are all good adjuncts to your swimming regimen. You may want to do them especially on the days when you don't swim.

Q: How can I swim if the pool is crowded?

A: The first thing to do is to try to swim in a counterclockwise direction within your lane, staying to the right side much as if you were driving along a two-way road. Try to find a lane with swimmers that go about the same speed as you. (Some pools label their lanes according to speed.) If this isn't possible, you can pass on the left if you're faster (assuming that no one is coming in the opposite direction); or let others pass you if you're slower. Another possibility is to swim one fast lap, then get out and walk back to your starting side and do another lap. (These are "windsprints.") If worse comes to worst, do some stationary kicking, bobbing, treading, or other water exercises until the traffic clears up. Swimming isn't supposed to be a contact sport; nor should you have to wait around for your own lane—depending on the length of the pool, up to twelve swimmers can use one lane if they observe principles of pool courtesy.

Q: I'm discouraged that I can't seem to make much progress in my swimming. What can I do?

A: At any stage of the game, swimmers can reach a plateau. Usually the support and advice of another swimmer is the key:

- Swim with a buddy if you haven't been already. Having another person there can make all the difference in the world.
- Join a swim class to obtain some general pointers.
- Take private lessons from an instructor who makes you feel at ease.

Q: What's the difference between a "lap" and a "length" in a pool?

A: In the United States, at least, they're usually the same thing. Although a few people prefer to count a lap as one round trip, the term generally means one length of the pool.

Q: Why do I have the urge to urinate while I'm swimming?

A: Although there's no physiological explanation for this widely observed phenomenon, various medical experts have speculated that it may be caused in part by the difference between the air and water temperatures and by the increased activity.

Q: Why do I get so thirsty during and after a swim?

A: Even though you may not realize it, you perspire when you swim. You also exhale water vapor, and you produce more urine, as discussed above. Finally, the alum added to the pool water tends to make your mouth feel dry.

Q: Should I learn all those different strokes?

A: Although it's no crime to do the doggie paddle, the strokes described in this book are much more efficient—and therefore, once you get the hang of them, actually easier. Learning and improving the different strokes also makes swimming more fun, more interesting, more challenging, and a better all-round exercise.

Q: How can I keep track of my laps when I'm swimming a long distance?

A: It's easy to lose count, but the more you swim, the easier it becomes. Here are a few tricks to help you remember. The first is to divide the swim, mentally, into smaller ones. Let's say you're swimming 1,650 yards or 1,500 meters (almost one mile) straight. In a 25-yard pool, you can divide the swim into four 400-yard swims (and subdivide that if needed), plus two laps. For shorter swims, you can divide the distance into 100s; just count "1" for every 100 yards. To help you mark the end of each segment, do a different turn: alternate closed and flip turns after every 100 yards, for instance.

You can also keep track by varying your breathing pattern. Breathe rhythmically (on the same side) during every odd-numbered 100; breathe alternately (every three arm strokes for the crawl) during the even 100s. You could base a whole workout on a pyramid-type breathing pattern: breathe every other stroke, then every third stroke, every fourth stroke, every fifth stroke, and back down again.

An alternate approach is to swim "by the clock." If you know that you cover 50 yards (two laps in a 25-yard pool) in one minute, for example, swimming for a straight 10 minutes means that you will cover approximately 500 yards, or twenty laps.

An amusing alternative is to sing to yourself, as Diana Nyad does during her marathon open-water swims. (Her version of "Row, Row, Row Your Boat" takes seventy-five choruses to make a mile; another of her favorites is "Frère Jacques" in three languages.) Anyone know the words to "Ebb Tide"?

Q: What is a "swimmer's high"?

A: This is a state, comparable to "jogger's high," in which you get the feeling of simultaneous exhilaration and calmness. It usually occurs once you've gotten into the main set of your workout. Your mind has drifted away from your daily concerns; your breathing is not labored; your muscles are loose. It's a mental as well as a physical high that leaves you feeling better, with more energy and direction than you had before. (Or maybe you're just hooked on chlorine!)

Q: Sometimes I forget the combination to my lock; any tips on how to remember it?

A: You can write the combination on the inside of your goggles strap or bathing cap, or on your bathing suit tag. You might want to use indelible ink, but I find that most ballpoint pen inks last and last.

Q: *Why is it best to swim three times a week?*

A: According to recent studies, your body needs aerobic exercise approximately every sixty hours in order to maintain a level of fitness. That's about every two and a half days, which works out to approximately every other day, or three times a week.

Q: *Is it possible to swim too much?*

A: Yes. If you feel overtired, run down, achy or listless, or that you're working hard without seeing any improvement, you may be swimming too much. Even in your training, you can go overboard and become "stale," especially if you don't peak and taper for a meet (see page 304). Fitness and competitive swimmers alike should remember that there's more to life than swimming; no matter how dedicated you are, leave some time and energy for other interests.

Q: *My spouse (child, friend) swims so much that I never see him or her anymore. What should I do?*

A: Perhaps you should consider getting in the swim, too. Not only is it more enjoyable if both of you swim, but you'll both be healthier, and you'll have an interest to share. And if you become a swimming family, chances are that you'll become more active, change your eating habits for the better, and meet new friends.

Q: *Why do some people call swimming the "Fountain of Youth"?*

A: Dr. Paul Hutinger, a Masters swim champion in his mid-sixties and a research specialist in the physiology of exercise at Western Illinois University, has called swimming the "Fountain of Youth." You can slow down and even help reverse the aging process if you follow a regular, year-round fitness program. But this exercise must continue throughout life if it is to have an extended effect. Swimming is the ideal sport to enjoy your whole life long, because it causes very little wear and tear on your joints. Aging is also affected by heredity and pathology, and the benefits of a fitness program depend to a certain degree on your age at its inception. So, although swimming may not be the "Fountain of Youth" for everyone, it may at least prove to be the "Fountain of Middle Age." And if that doesn't impress you twenty-year-olds—wait till you're seventy!

Q: Where can I swim when abroad?

A: Purchase a copy of the F.I.N.A. handbook. It will tell you how to contact the people who can advise you about suitable pools in various countries. Also contact U. S. Masters Swimming and Masters Swimming International.

Q: Sometimes my muscles begin to feel a little tight when I swim. What should I do?

A: Do these in-between loosening-up exercises.

- Bob in place for a minute or two.
- Swim a few very slow laps, exaggerating your stroke roll and recovery of arms.
- Shrug your shoulders, rotate your head and arms, stretch your legs and back, and do water exercises. Then resume swimming.

Q: Will smoking affect my swimming ability?

A: Definitely. Cigarette smoking speeds up your heartbeat, increases your blood pressure, and lowers the supply of oxygen in your blood. Over a period of time, smoking causes inflammation of the bronchial tubes, an increase in the secretion of mucus, changes in the epithelial cells, and a destruction of the lungs' elasticity.

Of the hundreds of chemical substances in cigarette smoke, nicotine, "tar," and carbon monoxide are the most dangerous. Nicotine constricts your blood vessels, cutting down the flow of blood and oxygen and making your heart pump harder. "Tar," which contains chemicals that have caused cancer in laboratory animals, forms a brown sticky coating over your lungs. Carbon monoxide inhibits the red blood cells' ability to carry oxygen throughout the body—and stays in your system for as long as six hours after your last cigarette. All of these effects cut down on your "wind" and so prevent you from becoming the swimmer you might be. I strongly urge you to give up smoking as part of your fitness program. Swimming can help you here, by reducing tension, and by giving you a glimpse of what healthy lungs, filled with clean air, feel like.

Q: What's synchronized swimming? Where can I find out more about it?

A: Synchronized swimming is the competitive form of water ballet, which you may have seen in Esther Williams films. It's like figure skating in the water. Here, stroke variations with "figures" similar to gymnastic stunts are combined to form a graceful routine to musical accompaniment. It's beautiful to watch and fun to try. I've included a few water exercises (page 377) that are also synchronized swimming workout skills; these are excellent for developing upper body strength.

If you're interested, you can subscribe to a bimonthly publication that will tell you what's happening in this exciting sport:

Synchro
c/o Dawn Bean
11902 Red Hill Avenue
Santa Ana, CA 92705

Your local Y, swim club, or recreation center can advise you on synchronized swimming activity in your area.

Q: *Does caffeine affect my swimming?*

A: It may—but exactly how depends on your own body chemistry. It may raise your heart rate, make you jittery, short of breath, even light-headed. On the other hand, you might be the type (like me) who does well with caffeine coursing through your veins.

Why? In an article in the June 1978 *RunnersWorld,* Dr. David Costill, an exercise physiologist at Ball State University, recommended two cups of coffee taken about one hour before exercise, because research found that this caused a 19 percent increase in the length of time needed to reach exhaustion. In another study, caffeine taken two hours before exercise increased the amount of work performed by 7 percent. The reason is apparently that caffeine increases the amount of fat burned for energy (40 percent as opposed to 22 percent without caffeine), which lessens the amount of glycogen used by the muscle cells, which, in turn, forestalls exhaustion.

Q: *Will swimming give me bulky muscles?*

A: No. Swimming is an exercise that results in smooth, firm, elongated muscles. If you want more bulk and "definition" you need to do more dry-land exercises such as running, calisthenics, and particularly weight lifting.

368 ~ *Swimming for Total Fitness*

Q: Am I too old, obese, or uncoordinated to swim?

A: No! Everyone, whatever his or her age, weight, or level of ability (or sex, color, creed, national origin, or political persuasion), can enjoy the lifetime benefits of swimming!

JUST FOR FUN
❧

Throw these fascinating facts around at the next pool party.

Q: Where did the idea of swimming pools come from?

A: For centuries, natural bodies of water were the only swimming facilities available. The eighteenth century, however, added a new wrinkle in fresh- and salt-water dipping: "floating swimming baths." Popular in England, France, and the United States, these were floating docks in natural water. Eventually they gave way to stationary ones that stayed put on the beach floor. Landlocked pools finally arrived in this country, Germany, and England in the middle of the last century.

Q: What are some of the more unusual pools that have been built?

A: There was William Randolph Hearst's 18-karat gold-lined indoor pool at San Simeon. And Wilt Chamberlain's moatlike pool that allowed visitors the option of either using the front door or swimming right into a small pool in his living room. Then there were the Hollywood models: Jayne Mansfield's heart-shaped hole in the ground, and Liberace's grand-piano look-alike.

Q: Where is the world's largest swimming pool?

A: According to the *Guinness Book of World Records,* it's the Orthleib pool in Casablanca, Morocco: 1,547 feet long and 246 feet wide. This salt-water pool is especially recommended for lap swimmers who have trouble keeping count.

Q: How fast are the fastest swimmers?

A: The fastest human swimmers move through the water at 5 to 6 miles an hour. Contrast that with dolphins, which swim up to 24 miles an hour, and whales, which swim up to 35 miles an hour. (But, as a look at the records will show, we're getting faster all the time.)

Q: Where can I see a 12-ton sculpture entitled Swimmer *and a 3,200-tile mosaic depicting King Neptune?*

A: At the International Swimming Hall of Fame in Fort Lauderdale, Florida. This huge swimming complex devoted to the glory of the sport contains a pool and diving complex, an auditorium, a film library, the world's largest bookstore devoted exclusively to aquatics, and a gift and souvenir shop where you can buy all sorts of swimming memorabilia— bumper stickers, T-shirts, post cards, bathing suits, and novelties.

Over forty thousand people visit the Hall of Fame every year—many to view the major swimming and diving competitions held there, and to browse through the Hall of Fame's exhibits devoted to its honorees (such as Johnny Weissmuller, Buster Crabbe, Gertrude Ederle, and Esther Williams), to gaze at its treasure trove of memorabilia including Lloyd Bridges's *Sea Hunt* wetsuit, and an elegant 800 B.C. Greek bas-relief of swimmers.

Q: Who was the first person to swim across the English Channel?

A: Captain Matthew Webb, in 1875. Since then, hundreds of other hardy souls have followed in his wake. Gertrude Ederle was the first woman to cross it, in 1926. The first double crossing was achieved by Antonio Abertondo, an Argentinian, in 1961; it took him 43 hours and 10 minutes. The fastest single crossing to date was made by Penny Dean, on July 29, 1978; her time was 7 hours, 40 minutes. The youngest was Marcus Hooper, age twelve, who made the swim August 5–6, 1979; his time was 14 hours, 37 minutes.

Q: Who is the greatest swimmer that ever lived?

A: Most people would agree that that title should go to Johnny Weissmuller, even though his world records were all topped long ago. Over the course of his career, he won five Olympic gold medals, fifty-one National Championships—and never lost a single race during his ten-year career! The record he set in 1927 for the 100-yard freestyle (51 seconds) stood for seventeen years. (Today records rarely hold for more than seventeen months.)

Q: What about some other remarkable swim personalities?

A: Of course, there's Mark Spitz, who became an international celebrity by winning an unprecedented seven gold medals in the 1972 Olympics in Munich. And one of the world's most impressive marathon swimmers is Diana Nyad, who has swum around Manhattan Island (28 miles), crossed Lake Ontario (32 miles), swum from Capri to Naples (22 miles), and from the Great Barrier Reef to the Australian Coast (50 miles). In 1979 she was the first person to defy the Gulf Stream by swimming from the Bahamas to Florida (80 miles).

Duke Kahanamoku, both a freestyle sprinter and a water polo player, and Juno Stover Irwin, tower and platform diver, were the only competitors in history to make the U. S. Olympic swimming and diving teams for four separate Olympics. (Juno also has another unique record—she mothered a child between each of her Olympic diving stints!)

Coach George Haines holds the distinction of being on the U. S. Olympic swim coaching staff since 1960, and is recognized as one of America's top coaches of the sport. One of Coach Haines's teams, in fact, the one that competed in 1976 in Montreal, won every event except one (the 200-meter breaststroke) in an unprecedented Olympic sweep.

APPENDIXES

APPENDIX A:

SWIMMERS' SHAPE-UPS

*T*he best way to improve your swimming is to swim. But there are literally hundreds of exercises, activities, and pieces of equipment that can help you to improve your strength, endurance, and flexibility as well as to add variety to your fitness program. So, if you enjoy doing sit-ups, jumping jacks, push-ups, yoga, bicycle riding, jogging, and so on, by all means continue to do so.

But remember the principle of "specificity of training": certain exercises are especially useful for swimmers because they concentrate on developing those skills and those areas of the body most important for swimming. Some of these are done on dry land, others can be done in the water (water exercises), and some use equipment such as weights and resistance devices.

371

Whether you elect to do your own favorite general conditioning exercises or the swimming-specific exercises described below, or a combination of both, remember that they're an adjunct to, not a replacement for, swimming. You might incorporate a few of them into the warm-up or cool-down of a swimming workout. Or, on a nonswimming day, you could do a relatively long dry-land workout (though many of the shape-ups may also be done in the water, where buoyancy and water resistance add a new dimension).

The following exercises are mostly light strength-building calisthenics (ideal for warm-ups) and stretches. Many of the stretches may be done either as short, easy movements to get the creaks out before a swim or held as a single, longer position to get a full stretch. The latest research shows that most people are better off reserving such full stretching for a dry-land cool-down after the rest of the workout, when stretching will elongate the fibers of your muscles and counteract their tendency to tighten up. Stretching after a workout serves two purposes: it helps prevent stiffness and soreness the next day, and it increases your overall flexibility, since at this time your body is warm and oxygenated and so most accommodating. The best full stretch is a long, slow, static one (that is, held steady with no bouncing), for thirty seconds for each of two phases. The first phase is an easy stretch, during which you totally relax while the tension should actually diminish. During the second, or developmental, phase, you stretch farther, but never so that it's painful. Stretching, both in and out of the water, can be an important asset to your swimming and to your total health. Be careful not to overdo it, though. Stretching should never be painful. If it is, either stop or stretch more gently.

LAND EXERCISES
～

Tug-of-war (stretches forearms, chest, shoulders, latissimus dorsi, or "lats"; benefits all strokes):   Bend one arm up behind your head and the other arm down behind your waist. Slide your hands between your shoulder blades, until the fingers touch. If you can, grasp one hand with the other and pull gently as in a tug-of-war. Change arm positions. (Use a handkerchief to extend your reach if you can't touch hands at first.)

Shoulder Hang (stretches arms, shoulders, and back; benefits all strokes):   Grasp a bar or other sturdy object, with hands shoulder width apart. Relax and just hang as long as is comfortable.

Trunk Press (stretches chest, shoulders, hamstrings, and back; benefits all strokes):   Bend forward at the hips with a straight back, resting your hands on the back of a chair. Keep your legs straight as you arch your back and shoulders up and down like a cat.

Trunk Twisters (good for body roll used in crawl and backstroke): Stand with hands on your waist; twist your right elbow and trunk to the left; return to center, then twist to right.

Torso Turn (good for developing body roll, particularly if one side is not as flexible as the other; helps stretch the shoulders and upper arms): Face a fixed object such as a diving board ladder or a lifeguard stand, and grasp it with your left hand at shoulder level. Twist your torso to look over your right shoulder, feeling the stretch in the front of your shoulders. Reverse, and repeat.

Knee Bends (strengthens legs for push-offs during dives, starts, and turns):   Stand with hands on your waist (or one hand on chair back for balance). Bend your knees and go down as far as possible, keeping your heels planted on the floor.

The Sky Is High "Plyometrics" (strengthens the legs and increases their explosive power, which is good for starts and turns): Rub some chalk on the index finger of one hand. Stand next to a wall, facing it. Bend your knees slightly, then, raising both arms in the air, jump as high as you can, touching the chalked finger to the wall to mark your height. Leave the mark for future comparison.

Forward Lunge (stretches and strengthens legs for all kicks, especially the whip kick):   Lunge forward like a fencer, with one foot well in front of the other. Facing in the direction of the forward foot, press your hips forward and down toward the floor. Change legs.

Kneeling Arch (stretches toes, feet, and ankles for all kicks; stretches thighs for the whip kick):   Kneel with legs hip width apart. Lean back, resting your weight on your hands, and gradually continue backward toward the floor, until your weight is resting on your elbows. Eventually ease your back onto the floor between your legs, keeping your knees on the floor.

Bridge (stretches and strengthens back, shoulders, chest, and front of thighs; good for all strokes, especially the butterfly and the backstroke): Lying on your back, bend your knees and place your feet on the floor under your buttocks. Push your hips off the floor to rest your weight on your shoulders, rolling up through the pelvis and lower back. If you can, place your hands palms down under your shoulders and press yourself all the way up into a full arch, resting your weight on your hands and feet. Roll down slowly.

Lower Back Arch (stretches lower back for dolphin kick):   Lying face down, bend your elbows and place your hands palms down under your shoulders. Push up, arching your back and looking up, keeping the pelvis down. Roll down slowly.

Toe Touching (stretches back and hamstrings; benefits all strokes): Sitting on the floor, legs together in front of you, bend forward at the waist to touch your toes. Eventually try to straighten your back and touch your chest to your thighs.

Ankle Circles (good for all kicks; encourages whipping action):   In a sitting position, rotate your feet from the ankle, aiming for full motion. Do one ankle at a time, first clockwise, then counterclockwise. Switch ankles.

Ankle Rocking (for additional ankle flexibility; good for all kicks): Kneel on the floor, legs together, with the tops of your feet against the floor. Sit down on heels; rest your hands on your knees, stretching the toes and ankles by rocking forward and backward gently.

Resistance Devices for Swimmers

The dominance of the East German swimmers in the 1972 Olympics began to focus the spotlight on the benefits of weight training. Though we aren't all Kornelia Ender, weight training, when used properly, can result in the added strength needed for increased speed and endurance for all strokes and distances.

In weight training, you pit your strength against gravity, in the form of a *free weight,* such as dumbbells or barbells; modern stationary *weight machines,* such as Universal and Nautilus; *pulley devices or stretch cords;* or *swim benches and mini-gyms.* By gradually increasing the resistance of such devices and the number of times you move them, you build muscle strength. Again, apply the principle of specificity of training, and concentrate on exercises that will most help your swimming. For swimming, it's best to use relatively light resistance and relatively high numbers of repetitions (eight to twelve) within each set. Gradually increase the number of sets to three, with a thirty-second rest between.

Pulleys and Stretch Cords: Pulleys, which are often available at gyms and health clubs, are cords attached to movable weights that slide up and down along a channel. Stretch cords, one length of elastic cord with a handle on either end, are an outgrowth of pulleys, and are inexpensive and easy to make. (To make your own, buy a length of surgical tubing approximately twice as long as you are tall. Make a loop handle at each end simply by doubling it back on itself and tying a knot. When you're ready to use it, slip it through or around a stationary object such as an eyescrew, doorknob, pole, railing, or pool-side fence.)

You can use pulleys and stretch cords in a similar way. Grasp one handle in each hand. Then, for example, you can bend over at the waist and simulate all of the swimming arm motions, keeping elbows high and concentrating on the accelerated phase 2 of each stroke. As you pull through your stroke using stretch cords, the tension increases; for more tension and a more difficult arm pull, stand farther away from where it is fixed. A good rule of thumb is to still be able to feel some resistance during the part of the stroke cycle when your hands are all the way forward. Here, more repetitions can be done—approximately twenty per set, three sets per stroke, at a faster pace than you would swim.

The Exer-Genie is a device consisting of a cylinder through which a rope passes, like a portable pulley. The adjustable tension, which is created by friction on the rope, is especially good for practicing your arm stroke pulls.

Mini-Gym and Isokinetic Swim Bench: This whole line of resistance equipment, designed especially for swimmers, lets you move your arms through a full range of swimming motions. The resistance automatically adjusts to the force applied by your muscles (an *isokinetic* exercise), so that, as your arms tire and your pull weakens, the resistance also decreases, thereby lessening the chance of injury. The Vasa-Trainer and the Isokinetic Swim Bench, outgrowths of the Mini-Gym concept, have digital gauges that measure the force of your pull.

Free Weights and Universal and Nautilus Machines: The principle behind all three of these systems is similar, each one having certain advantages. Individuals can easily buy or even make their own *free weights*—barbells and dumbbells. This equipment is also common at Ys, health clubs, gyms, and fitness centers. Swimmers should do tricep extensions, bench presses, bicep curls, seated presses, straight-arm pull-overs, knee bends (if your knees permit), leg presses, rowing exercises, wrist curls, and other exercises that strengthen the muscles used in swimming. Use of free weights provides certain advantages not found in all other weight-training systems. Their use requires balance, develops neurological coordination, permits free acceleration and deceleration during exercise movement, and allows for a full range of motion and an almost infinite variety of movements.

The *Universal Gym* and other similar systems are large, multi-exercise systems of stationary weight-lifting apparatus. Their advantages over free weights are the easily adjustable resistance, the large number of exercises that can be done on one piece of equipment, and the reduced danger of falling weights. Although you can't accomplish a full range of swimming motions, you can use Universal to strengthen important swimming muscle groups.

Nautilus, now one of the standards in weight training, is another alternative. Although you still can't perform swimming motions, Nautilus does allow you to isolate and strengthen individual muscle groups. It's also unique in that it utilizes a cam device that enables the resistance to vary with the degree of muscle contraction. Thus, it provides resistance throughout the movement—at the beginning, middle, and end. An added plus is that the apparatus allows you to move through a full range of motion.

There are over twelve hundred fitness centers in America that feature Nautilus equipment, including many health clubs. The Nautilus hip and back, pull-over, and tricep-extension machines are the best for swimmers. The chest press, leg press, shoulder press, arm curl, wrist curl, leg extension, leg curl, and pull down are also good.

WATER AEROBICS
～

Sometimes conditions just aren't ideal for a swimming workout. The pool may be too crowded to swim laps comfortably. You may be away from home and have only a mini-pool available. Maybe you have a cold and don't want to put your head in the water. You could have an injury that restricts the use of your arms and legs. Or perhaps you're just ready for a change of pace, or a way to vary your warm-ups or cool-downs.

That's the perfect time to try a new approach to body conditioning: water exercises. These special exercises are designed to take advantage of the water's buoyancy and resistance. Unlike swimming, they keep you relatively in one place. And water exercises can be done by virtually anyone, at any level: by nonswimmers, beginning swimmers, and advanced swimmers, by super athletes and by those who are just at the beginning of a fitness program. Some of these are more difficult than others, and many are based on exercises I do to practice synchronized swimming. Others are slow, easy stretches ideal for relaxing, or as the perfect finale to a fitness swim. Many can be done in chest-deep water, and should be repeated for between thirty seconds and two minutes each. If done as a stretch, the water exercise should be done in the same way as a dry-land stretch: in two phases, first an easy one, followed by the more demanding developmental stretch.

Wall Kicking (tones the lower body; strengthens arms and chest; aerobic benefits if you do it long enough):   This exercise, described earlier in the book, consists of holding on to the pool wall and practicing the flutter kick, scissors kick, whip kick, or dolphin kick in either prone or supine position.

Stationary Pulling (tones arms and shoulders; tightens buttocks; practices arm motions of the various strokes):   In a prone position, hook your feet over pool gutter. Practice the arm motions of the various strokes, using rhythmic breathing, alternate breathing, and controlled breathing.

Stationary Swimming: There are tethered swim devices available that harness your body to a line that prevents you from moving through the water, and so allows you to swim in place. If you're handy, you can make your own stationary swim harness and affix it to a pool ladder.

Bobbing (good all-round strengthener and toner for the lower body— and possibly the upper body, depending on the variation used; aerobic benefits if you add a jumping action and do it long enough):   Bobbing has many variations—your head can stay above the water or can submerge with each bob; you can raise and lower arms as you bob; or you might add jumping action—either in place or moving forward, to side, or backward. All bobbing is based on the simple knee bend: bend your knees as you go down, and straighten them as you come up. This is the basis of "plyometrics."

- Alternate your legs front and back in a wide lunging position, front leg bent and back leg straight.
- Bob on one leg, keeping the other bent close to chest; reverse legs.
- Bob with both knees facing out to the side and away from each other (like a plié).

Treading (all-over toning; aerobic benefits if done long and vigorously enough):   This is a kind of vertical swimming; do it in water that's deep enough so that your toes don't hit bottom. As with bobbing, there are many variations:

- Regular treading (see page 68) is a wide, horizontal scull for the arms combined with a bicycle leg motion.
- Tread with a frog or scissors kick instead of the bicycle leg motion.
- Tread using dolphin kick.
- Tread, turning your feet inward toward the center of your body ("the egg beater").
- Using any kick, lift alternate arms vertically out of the water; then lift both simultaneously. When you need to rest, do so in the prone position with limbs relaxed; then continue.
- Tug-of-war: starting with your back to pool wall for support, practice sculling with your palms facing up—this "support sculling" will cause your body to move downward. Then move away from wall and add the "egg-beater" kick, which will tend to push you upward and counteract the downward "tug" of the support sculling.

Sculling (tones arms, chest muscles and abdomen, buttocks, back, thighs and/or calves, depending on the variations used; aerobic benefits if done long enough):   This is a small figure-8 motion done with the hands near the hips, usually while in a stationary supine position (see page 81). Keep legs straight and your toes pointed to prevent your body from "sitting" in the water.

- Place both feet on the edge of the deck, legs straight, with your body in a supine position. Scull while you lift each leg alternately, so that it forms a right angle with the water and with your body (the other leg remains straight, your foot resting on the deck to help support you). Eventually, try to do this exercise without the wall for support.

- Repeat the above exercise, lifting both legs at the same time.

Leg Sweep (stretches and tones the whole leg, the buttocks, and the lower back):   Stand with one side to the pool wall, holding on to it with the nearer arm. Lift one leg forward and up. Straighten and extend the leg. Bring the leg straight down, through the standing position, then as far in back of you as possible, keeping your legs straight. Return the leg to a standing position. Repeat with the other leg.

Leg Circle (tones and stretches thighs and buttocks; stretches lower back):   Face the pool wall, holding on with both hands. Bring one leg out to side, knee straight. Bend your knee and twist the leg around behind you, trying to touch your toes to the wall on your other side. Repeat an equal number of times with each leg.

Lower Leg Press (stretches calves and lower legs):   Stand in chest-deep water, facing the pool wall, with your arms extended in front of you and your hands grasping the gutter. Bend one leg and place your foot flat on the bottom in front of you, keeping the other leg straight behind you. Slowly move your body forward until you feel a stretch in the calf of your straight leg. Reverse legs.

Wall Push-ups (strengthens arms, shoulders, and back; this is also a good way to exit the pool):   Face the wall and rest your palms on the deck edge, your hands shoulder width apart and your elbows bent. Bend your knees and jump up, straightening your arms and lifting your body so that your thighs rest on the deck edge. Contract your body and hold for five seconds. Variation: do the exercise with your back to the wall.

Sit-ups (tones abdominal and leg muscles):   With your back to the wall, grasp the edge or gutter as though you were doing a supine flutter-kick drill. Bend and lift both legs together, tucking your knees to your chest. (You can also do this in a supine position, holding a kickboard over your abdomen.) Repeat continuously.

Side-winders (strengthens the abdominals, legs, inner and outer thighs):   Standing with your back to wall, grasp the gutter edge. Lift your legs in front of you, keeping them straight and together, until they are level with the water surface. Then sweep your right leg to the right, trying to touch the wall. Sweep your left leg to the right to meet it. Repeat on the other side.

Push-away (tones and stretches legs, buttocks, entire back, arms, shoulders):   Face the wall, grasping the gutter with both hands. Bend your knees and place both feet flat against the wall just below the water level (backstroke-start position). Try to straighten your legs; hold for fifteen to thirty seconds.

Leg Stretch (stretches the hamstrings):   Repeat the above exercise, working the legs individually by placing one on the pool bottom as far back behind you as possible, as you straighten the other one.

Side Stretch (tones and stretches inner thigh, sides, shoulders):   Stand with one side to the wall. Raise the near leg in front of you and hook the foot over the gutter. Keeping both legs straight, bend at the waist and stretch and try to touch the raised foot with the opposite hand. Repeat on opposite side.

Loop-the-Loop (back stretch; helps backstroke start; improves breath control):   Face the wall, grasping the edge with both hands. Bend your knees toward your chest and place your feet flat on the wall at water level (backstroke start position). Spring away from the wall by straightening your legs; extend your arms overhead and arch your back. Enter the water in a back dive; then continue in a smooth, circular motion until your hands touch bottom. Maintaining an arched, streamlined body position, push off the bottom with your hands and complete the circle as you emerge from the water. (This should be done in water at least six feet deep, for safety's sake.)

Arm Circles (tones upper arms and shoulders):   Crouch in the water so that your arms and shoulders are submerged. Make tiny circles with both arms, first forward, then backward. (Use hand paddles for more resistance.)

Arch and Stretch (stretches arms, shoulders, and back):   In chin-deep water, stand with your back to the wall, your heels close to it. Reach behind you and grasp the gutter. Then lean forward, look up, and arch your chest, pushing your hips forward. Ease into this position, then hold it for fifteen to thirty seconds. When this part is easy for you, try to "walk" your feet up the wall, keeping your legs straight for more stretch.

Arm Arcs (tones arms and shoulders; stretches chest and shoulders): Stand or crouch so that your arms and shoulders are submerged. Extend your arms in front of you, palms down. Press them down and back in a semicircular motion, until the hands reach the surface behind you. Then rotate your arms so that the hands are palms down again, and arc the arms forward to the starting position. (Using hand paddles increases the effect of the water's resistance.)

Finale Stretches (for arms, shoulders, back, and chest; these feel especially good after a workout):   In a prone or supine position, interlace your fingers, palms turned away from you, and stretch overhead—first to one side, then to the other, then straight overhead. Another variation is to stand in chest-deep water; interlace your fingers behind your back, palms facing toward you. Keeping your arms straight, bring them up as high as they'll go.

There are also many new types of resistance equipment to be used in the water. You may want to experiment with them to vary your workouts.

For information on water exercises, you can read *The W.E.T. Workout*® —Water Exercise Techniques (Facts on File, 1985), by Dr. Jane Katz.

DEEP-WATER EXERCISES
～

Deep-water vertical exercise attracts marathoners, triathletes, cross-trainers, and runners for rehabilitation because deep-water aerobics provides them with the opportunity to maintain their physical conditioning and specificity of training while preventing overuse injury.

Flotation devices are generally used with deep-water exercise in order to provide a "neutral buoyancy" position to keep your chin out of the water. This enables you to jog in deep water, and concentrate on running form, regardless of your swimming ability. Most notable among these devices are the rubber flotation belts, like the "AquaJogger" and the "Wet Vest," a lightweight, snug-fitting vest made of neophrene, which keeps you upright as well as buoyant. A tether rope can also be attached to a poolside anchor and can allow you to jog in a small shallow or deep area, and to simulate sprint running in the water.

Samples of deep water exercises include:

Deep-water Running

Keep your elbows close to your body, moving your arms in opposition to your legs. Maintain your body posture, and practice your running form.

Hurdles

Simulate running a hurdle course. Begin with your knees together under your body. Then your front leg extends straight forward, and your rear leg is bent behind you. Return to the bent-knee position under your body, and repeat with opposite leg forward.

Cross-country Skiing

Simulate cross-country skiing with arms and legs in opposition. Aim for increased range of motion, forward and back; keep your range of motion as extended and equidistant as possible.

Training Tips: With a pace clock or wristwatch, count the number of strides you take in a given time period (cadence check). Rest, repeat, and try to increase the number each time. You can also Interval train by simulating a running workout with sets of fast and slow runs (fartlek method).

In addition to conventional pools, compact pools with artificial currents, as well as one-lane lap pools (both shallow and deep), extend possibilities for water aerobics, and are a consideration for homeowners.

APPENDIX B:

SAFE SWIMMING

*E*very swimming pool, beach, or watering hole is unique. Become familiar with your surroundings every time you're in a new situation. Realize that, even if there is a lifeguard, *you* are an extra pair of eyes. The first and best rule to remember is to use common sense, and try not to panic in case of emergency. For more information on water safety, contact your local American National Red Cross chapter on the U. S. Coast Guard. The Red Cross and the Ys also teach lifesaving courses. Here are some water safety tips:

- Never swim alone—there should be at least one other person around at all times. Half the people who drown were swimming alone.
- Avoid alcoholic beverages when swimming (or boating)—nearly half of the people who drown have alcohol in the bloodstream.
- In open water, check with the lifeguard or beach patrol for information about tides, currents, depths, and so on. Don't guess.
- If you're a shallow-water swimmer, observe the water-depth markers.

- Obey posted rules and regulations; swim or dive only in designated areas.

- Make sure there are no swimmers nearby before you jump or dive into the water. Only one person should use a diving platform at a time. Always be aware of other swimmers around you to avoid collisions.

- Swim after dark only if the area is properly lit and if a buddy or lifeguard is present.

- Avoid eating a heavy meal before swimming strenuously.

- Don't jump into cool water if you're overheated, since this may cause cramps. Cool off first.

- If you do get a cramp, stretch the muscle and knead the area with your thumb, alternating direct pressure and release until the cramp goes away.

- Only trained lifesavers should attempt a swimming rescue. However, you can help with nonswimming rescues in the following way: extend a pole, branch, leg, arm, oar, towel, or article of clothing to the victim. As you pull him or her to safety, stay low, keeping your weight back to prevent being pulled into the water yourself. If the swimmer is farther away, toss a life preserver (or anything that floats) to support him or her as you call for help. Even nonswimmers can save a life this way. The last thing even qualified rescuers do is jump into the water; and just because you may know some components of rescue-life skills, such as the scissors kick, it doesn't mean that you are qualified to attempt a rescue.

- Leave the water as soon as you feel chilly. Numb or blue fingers and toes mean you've been in too long, and can signal the approach of hypothermia.

- SCUBA diving (Self-Contained Underwater Breathing Apparatus) is not the same as swimming. So before you venture out into Jacques Cousteau territory, take a course of instruction. (Skin diving—the use of fins, mask, and snorkel—can be learned relatively quickly.)

- Get training in basic first aid and cardiopulmonary resuscitation (the ABC's of CPR).

APPENDIX C:

~

FOR THE RECORD

SPECIAL SWIMS

~

Once you're swimming regularly, you may want to keep track of your progress and set some long-term goals for yourself. Competitive swimming is one way to do this. Here are several alternatives.

The American National Red Cross 50-Mile Swim and Stay Fit Program: As the Red Cross says, it's "not a marathon, not a race, not competitive, not an endurance contest"; this is simply a very satisfying way the Red Cross has designed to encourage regular swimming. You simply keep a running total of the number of miles you've swum to date, by filling in each swim on a chart posted at your pool. This self-administered program is run on the honor system, although there may be a "pool monitor." Usually, the fifty miles are accomplished quite gradually; if you do it in 440-yard (quarter-mile) segments, it would amount to 200 swims, or about 70 weeks. The Red Cross awards wallet-sized certificates in 10-mile units; at the end of the 50 miles, you get a larger certificate. For a small fee, you can also obtain a pin and a patch to commemorate your feat. Many swimmers complete the distance, then enroll again to try to finish in less time.

28-Mile Manhattan Island and 300-Mile Three-Island Swims: Manhattan is a nice place to visit, you say, but you wouldn't want to swim around it. This cumulative swim converts your own pool mileage into an imagined trip around Manhattan Island. A longer version, the 300-mile

"Three-Island Swim" (around Manhattan, Staten Island, and Long Island), works the same way. Both of these swims are sponsored by the Greater New York American Red Cross Chapter. An accompanying map (on page 388) notes various attractions for the "Three-Island Swim." Try it, you'll like it!

Your Personalized Swim and Stay Fit Program: You can make up your own program of whatever distance you like. Swim to your sister's house on the other side of town, around your state, down the Mississippi, or to Rome—all on paper. For her famous swim, Dr. Joyce Brothers decided to "swim" to her daughter's college.

Swim-a-thons for raising cash: In addition to neighborhood cake sales, swim for dollars to raise money for your favorite charity. Participating swimmers (of all ages and levels) can go out and hustle up financial support in the form of pledges from sponsors.

The International Swimming Hall of Fame (address on page 333) will help you sponsor a swim-a-thon in your community.

Distance and Timed Swims: (Half-hour and One-hour Postal Swims): This event, the object of which is to see who can swim the greatest distance in an hour, gives you the opportunity to compete without the expense and inconvenience of traveling to a meet. After your swim, in any 25-yard or 50-meter pool, you simply mail in the results on an official entry blank for tabulation (hence the term "postal swim"). You can swim either as an individual or as part of a team. Meet results and awards will be mailed to you. These Masters postal swims are held annually, and others are cropping up.

Swim and Stay Fit Program
Health and Safety Services

✚ American Red Cross

SPONSORED BY:

NAME OF CHAPTER

and

NAME OF COOPERATING FACILITY

NAME OF SWIMMER	TOTAL MILES COMPLETED (50-mile segments)	DATE STARTED (New 50 miles)	M I L E S
1			
2			
3			
4			
5			
6			
7			
8			
9			
10			
11			
12			
13			
14			
15			
16			
17			
18			
19			
20			

American Red Cross Form 5348 (Rev. 1-84)

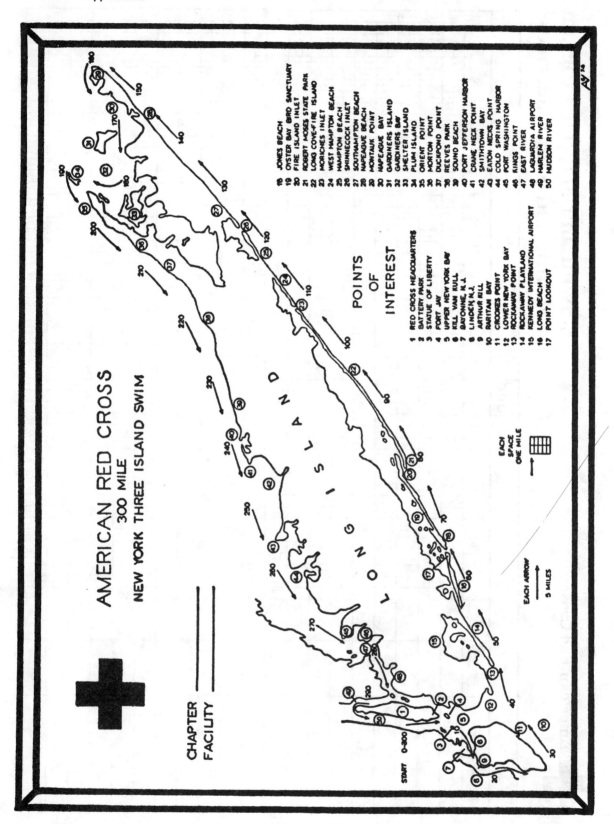

AMERICAN RED CROSS
300 MILE
NEW YORK THREE ISLAND SWIM

CHAPTER
FACILITY

POINTS
OF
INTEREST

1 RED CROSS HEADQUARTERS
2 BATTERY PARK
3 STATUE OF LIBERTY
4 FORT JAY
5 UPPER NEW YORK BAY
6 KILL VAN KULL
7 BAYONNE, N.J.
8 LINDEN, N.J.
9 ARTHUR KILL
10 RARITAN BAY
11 CROOKES POINT
12 LOWER NEW YORK BAY
13 ROCKAWAY POINT
14 ROCKAWAY PLAYLAND
15 KENNEDY INTERNATIONAL AIRPORT
16 LONG BEACH
17 POINT LOOKOUT

18 JONES BEACH
19 OYSTER BAY BIRD SANCTUARY
20 FIRE ISLAND INLET
21 ROBERT MOSES STATE PARK
22 LONG COVE-FIRE ISLAND
23 MORICHES INLET
24 WEST HAMPTON BEACH
25 HAMPTON BEACH
26 SHINNECOCK INLET
27 SOUTHAMPTON BEACH
28 NAPEAGUE BEACH
29 MONTAUK POINT
30 NAPEAGUE BAY
31 GARDINERS ISLAND
32 GARDINERS BAY
33 SHELTER ISLAND
34 PLUM ISLAND
35 ORIENT POINT
36 MORTON POINT
37 DUCKPOND POINT
38 REEVES PARK
39 SOUND BEACH
40 PORT JEFFERSON HARBOR
41 CRANE NECK POINT
42 SMITHTOWN BAY
43 EATON NECKS POINT
44 COLD SPRING HARBOR
45 PORT WASHINGTON
46 KINGS POINT
47 EAST RIVER
48 LAGUARDIA AIRPORT
49 HARLEM RIVER
50 HUDSON RIVER

EACH
SPACE
ONE MILE

EACH ARROW
5 MILES

LONG ISLAND

START 0-300

Converting Meters to Yards

~

A meter is approximately 10 percent longer than a yard; thus:

The Basics

1 meter	=	39.37 inches
1 yard	=	.9144 meters
3 meters	=	10 feet
50 meters	=	55 yards
100 meters	=	110 yards
400 meters	=	440 yards (¼ mile)
800 meters	=	880 yards (½ mile)
1,500 meters	=	1,650 yards
1,600 meters	=	1,760 yards (1 mile)

In a 20-yard pool:

¼ mile is 22 laps   (440 yards)
½ mile is 44 laps   (880 yards)
1 mile is 88 laps   (1,760 yards)

In a 25-yard pool:

¼ mile is 18 laps   (450 yards)
½ mile is 36 laps   (900 yards)
1 mile is 70 laps   (1,750 yards)

In a 25-meter pool:

¼ mile is 16 laps   (400 meters)
½ mile is 32 laps   (800 meters)
1 mile is 64 laps   (1,600 meters)

In a 33⅓-yard pool:

¼ mile is 13 laps   (433 yards)
½ mile is 26 laps   (866 yards)
1 mile is 52 laps   (1,732 yards)

In a 50-meter/55-yard pool:

¼ mile is 8 laps   (400 meters)
½ mile is 16 laps   (800 meters)
1 mile is 32 laps   (1,600 meters)

APPENDIX D:

FOR *YOUR* RECORD

FUNDAMENTALS OF SWIMMING CHECKLIST

Check off each skill as you feel you've mastered it.

NEW SKILL	SKILL CHECK	DATE/COMMENTS
LESSON ONE		
Breathing		
Bobbing		
Flutter Kicking on Wall		
Bobbing and Breathing		
Exiting the Pool		
LESSON TWO		
Controlled Breathing		
Prone Flutter Kicking with Controlled Breathing		
Prone Float and Recovery to a Stand		
Prone Glide and Flutter Kicking with Assistance		

NEW SKILL	SKILL CHECK	DATE/COMMENTS
Prone Glide and Flutter Kicking with Kickboard		
LESSON THREE		
Prone Glide to Wall with Flutter Kicking (Unassisted)		
Crawl-stroke Arm Motion (Assisted) (Unassisted)		
LESSON FOUR		
Crawl-stroke Arm Motion and Flutter Kicking		
Flutter Kicking and Rhythmic Breathing		
Crawl-stroke Arm Motion and Rhythmic Breathing		
Crawl Stroke, Flutter Kicking, and Rhythmic Breathing		
LESSON FIVE		
Buoyancy Check		
Deep-water Tour		
Treading (Chin-deep Water)		
LESSON SIX		
Supine Float and Recovery		
Supine Float and Flutter Kicking		
Deep-water Treading		

NEW SKILL	SKILL CHECK	DATE/COMMENTS
LESSON SEVEN		
Supine Sculling with Flutter Kicking		
Shallow Surface Dive		
LESSON EIGHT		
Elementary Backstroke with Flutter Kick		
Sitting Dive		
LESSON NINE		
Whip Kick		
Supine Float and Whip Kick		
Elementary Backstroke with Whip Kick		
LESSON TEN		
Windmill-backstroke Arm Motion		
Windmill Backstroke with Flutter Kick		
Changing Direction and Turning Over		

SWIMMERS' SHAPE-UP LOG
(Calisthenics, Water Exercises, Resistance Training)

EXERCISE/ EQUIPMENT	DATE	REPETITIONS PER SET	SETS	WEIGHTS	COMMENTS

WORKOUT LOG

DATE	POOL LOCATION AND LENGTH	WARM-UP	MAIN SET	COOL-DOWN	TOTAL DISTANCE OF WORK-OUT	COMMENTS

GOALS AND BEST TIMES

STROKE	DISTANCE	GOAL	BEST TIME	DATE	LOCATION	COMMENTS
Free-style	50 yds./m.	:	:			
	100 yds./m.	:	:			
	200 yds./m.	:	:			
	500 yds./ 400 m.	:	:			
	1000 yds./ 800 m.	:	:			
	1650 yds./ 1500 m.	:	:			
Back-stroke	50 yds./m.	:	:			
	100 yds./m.	:	:			
	200 yds./m.	:	:			
Breast-stroke	50 yds./m.	:	:			
	100 yds./m.	:	:			
	200 yds./m.	:	:			
Butter-fly	50 yds./m.	:	:			
	100 yds./m.	:	:			
	200 yds./m.	:	:			
I.M.	100 yds./m.	:	:			
	200 yds./m.	:	:			
	400 yds./m.	:	:			

Remember: A worthwhile goal is one that's reasonably attainable, but hard enough to be worthy of the effort.

TIMED SWIM LOG

DATE	POOL LOCATION AND LENGTH	DISTANCE AND STROKE	TIME	PULSE CHECK	COMMENTS
			..		
			..		
			..		
			..		
			..		
			..		
			..		
			..		
			..		
			..		
			..		

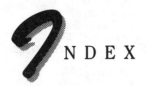

INDEX